D1453422

CLARENDON LIBRARY OF LOGIC AND PHILOSOPHY

General Editor: L. Jonathan Cohen

THE LOGIC
OF
NATURAL LANGUAGE

THE LOGIC
OF
NATURAL LANGUAGE

═══

FRED SOMMERS

CLARENDON PRESS · OXFORD
1982

Oxford University Press, Walton Street, Oxford OX2 6DP

London Glasgow New York Toronto
Delhi Bombay Calcutta Madras Karachi
Kuala Lumpur Singapore Hong Kong Tokyo
Nairobi Dar es Salaam Cape Town
Melbourne Auckland

and associate companies in
Beirut Berlin Ibadan Mexico City

Published in the United States by
Oxford University Press, New York

© Fred Sommers 1982

All rights reserved. No part of this publication may be reproduced,
stored in a retrieval system, or transmitted, in any form or by any means,
electronic, mechanical, photocopying, recording, or otherwise, without
the prior permission of Oxford University Press

British Library Cataloguing in Publication Data

Sommers, Fred
　The logic of natural language.—(Clarendon
library of logic and philosophy)
　1. Language and logic
　I. Title
　149'946　　BC57

　ISBN 0–19–824425–8

Library of Congress Cataloging in Publication Data

Sommers, Frederic Tamler, 1923–
　The logic of natural language.

　(Clarendon library of logic and philosophy)
　Bibliography: p.
　Includes index.
　1. Logic.　I. Title.　II. Series.
　BC71.S715　　160　　　　81–14199
　ISBN 0–19–824425–8 (U.S.)　　AACR2

BC
71
.S715
1982

Set by the Macmillan India Ltd.
Printed in the United States of America

For Tamler
And For The Memory Of My Parents

וְזָרַח הַשֶּׁמֶשׁ, וּבָא הַשֶּׁמֶשׁ.

Preface

The essay before you is the fruit of some fifteen years of investigation into the logical syntax of natural language. In the summer of 1965 I read a paper to the Congress on Logic and Scientific Method at Bedford College, London, that presented an algorithm for the algebraic treatment of syllogistic arguments in which categorical propositions were transcribed as fractions and reciprocals.[1] I spent the next two years looking for a more general algorithm with greater expressive power, one that could transcribe relational, multi-general propositions as well as simple categoricals. The new algorithm—presented here in chapter 9—came to me as I was sitting with a note pad in a Tel Aviv shelter during an alert on the Monday morning of the Six Day Arab-Israeli War. This shows that logic, as well as philosophy in general, has its uses in times of stress.

The first article on the more general calculus was published in *Mind*, January 1970, as *The Calculus of Terms*. Unfortunately its message had little effect although I followed it by a series of articles that exploited the new notation and exposed some important consequences for the philosophy of language. It became clear that the current Fregean logic had fully replaced the more traditional logic of terms and that articles could not do justice to the neo-classical alternative that I was advocating.

I had for some years been planning to write a book on the logic of categories but the lack of response to my more recent interests, the logic of terms and its relation to natural syntax, strongly suggested that I must first do book-length justice to these latter topics. I began writing this essay in 1975 and, after several long interruptions and two revisions, completed it in the summer of 1980. I still hope to write the book on category

---

[1] 'On a Fregean Dogma'. Apparently I was not alone in representing categorical propositions as fractions. Charles Merchant, a mathematician at the University of Arizona, subsequently wrote me of his independent work on this algorithm.

theory. In the present work (chapter 13) I do little more than indicate how traditional logic's way with contrariety leads to the conception of categories that is at the basis of Ryle's seminal work in the forties and my own more formal treatment of categories in the early sixties. Indeed it was my recognition of the need for a notion of contrariety that would allow for saying, for example, that Saturday is neither fed nor unfed (which renders both 'Saturday is fed' and 'Saturday is unfed' 'category mistakes') that prompted me to re-examine traditional Aristotelian logic with its characteristic distinction between contrary terms or predicates and contradictory propositions. This distinction is absent in modern logic which uses the forms 'Px' and '−Px' to represent contrary predicates thereby conflating the two oppositions of contrariety and contradiction so fundamental to the classical term-theoretic standpoint.[2]

The current use of propositional negation as the sole form of opposition 'precludes the kind of internal term and predicate structure that makes it possible to treat negation as a means of changing around concepts inside the meanings of terms and predicates'. The quoted words are Jerrold Katz's but they are typical of the sort of reaction one gets from linguists who find the restricted grammar of 'standard' logical languages to be at odds with their intuitions into the logical grammar of empirical languages.

More generally the theory of logical form that has its source in the formation rules for standard languages poses severe problems for the linguist. The older subject—predicate logic with its classical binary noun-phrase verb-phrase analysis of sentences has been discredited and while some linguists appear prepared to abandon the classical analysis in favour of analyses that conform more closely to the syntax of modern predicate logic others may welcome a rehabilitated classical logic of 'categorical' sentences that leaves the fundamental binary structure in place. Motivations for philosophers to welcome a return to a more classical organon also exist but these are more

---

[2] Early treatments of the distinction between negating a sentence and denying a predicate may be found in my 'Predicability' (1963) and 'Truth Functional Counterfactuals' (1964). In the present essay see especially Chapters 13, 14 and Appendix B.

complex and I shall not attempt a summary characterization of them in these prefatory remarks. They will, I think, be clear to one who reads the book itself.

The book's title was suggested to me by Michael Lockwood. Lockwood's views on the philosophy of language are generally congenial to mine and especially on the question of the propriety of predicating proper names and other definite singular terms. Lockwood holds, as I do, that these can be treated syntactically on a footing with general terms.

My former colleague Clifton MacIntosh discussed with me the problems of a semantics for the algebraic version of traditional formal logic presented in chapter 9. I have included (as Appendix F) MacIntosh's work on this problem in which he gives proof and model theory for a good chunk of the term logic. Aris Noah's observations on the relations of functor logic to my algebraic version of term logic are included as Appendix E. My student Christopher Karp offered criticisms which cost me many hours of revision. I am indebted to him for his persistence and clarity.

A number of philosophers who have been interested in my earlier work on categories as well as my more recent work on term logic have made helpful suggestions both in print and in conversation. Foremost among these is George Englebretsen in a series of papers. Ashok Gangadean's applications of category theory to the problem of relating widely variant ontological systems have rekindled my own sense of the importance of the logic of categories for general philosophy. In a similar way the recent work of Frank Keil applying category theory to conceptual development has shown how philosophical logic may help in the solution of problems in cognitive psychology. David Massie's paper on the tree theory of categories and his dissertation on the logic of terms have complemented many stimulating discussions. I am grateful to the authors of many articles that deal with my views on category structures. Some of these are included in the selective bibliography. The comments of John Bacon on early versions of the algebra of terms were very useful to me. Bacon was first to notice that the distributed terms of the older logic had negative valence in the new algebra—an observation that leads one to look favourably on the scholastic doctrine of distribution of terms whose most recent detractor is the redoubtable Peter Geach.

The success of Frege's revolution in logic is in large part due to the work of a group of exciting and clear-headed philosophers who developed and criticized his ideas and gave them currency in the larger philosophical community. After Russell, one must mention Tarski, Carnap and Quine. Gilbert Ryle applied Russell's idea of a type mistake to statements in the natural languages, introducing thereby a new and distinctive style of philosophical argumentation. My interest in Ryle's 'category mistakes' turned me away from the study of Whitehead's metaphysical writings (on which I had written a doctoral thesis at Columbia University) to the study of problems that could be arranged for possible solution. In particular I was prompted to find out how the terms of category correct sentences of a natural language are related and structured. Ryle liked and published my results in this area. I owe a great deal to him intellectually but even more for the encouragement of his steady and gentle presence during the fifteen or so years that I knew him. I am not alone in being thus indebted to Ryle.

Strawson's book on logical theory was another influence in the fifties that set me to thinking about problems that arise when one tries to be clear about the relations of logical structures to structures in the natural languages, this time in the area of logical syntax. In that book Strawson criticized the attempt by logicians to impose their theory of logical form on sentences of the natural languages. It is, I think, unfortunate that Strawson did not pursue this line of criticism by developing an alternative which would circumvent the problems raised by the bad fit of formal logic to actual inference in the natural language. But this may be unfair. The fifties were the days when philosophers could talk of 'informal logic'—a term that made it appear right to think of the syntax and semantics of natural languages as somehow incapable of rigorous treatment and which suggests that the search for a logical syntax of the natural languages could not possibly succeed. But primarily the failure of Strawson and other 'ordinary language philosophers' to provide a formal alternative to the current Fregean organon was due to the immense influence of Frege himself and to his powerful disciples among whom Quine is foremost today.

Quine's influence is inescapable. I am grateful to him for insisting that logic must be confined to the consideration of a limited number of particles such as 'some' 'not' and 'and'. This is admirable and right; one who attends to it will not waste his time on promiscuous 'logics' of this that and the other thing. This point concerns the logical particles. But Quine's Occamist zeal has also led him to remove proper names as an essential category of extra-logical expressions. This move had already been made by the scholastics who construed 'Socrates is P' as 'every Socrates is P' and it is just what the doctor ordered for an ailing term logic. Two other points of contact with Quine are his choice of conjunction, negation, and the existential quantifier as the primitive elements for logic, and his recent development of a predicate functor logic. The first point accords with my view that the basic logical particles consist of a commutative connective ('some is', or 'and') and a sign of negative quality (for qualifying sentences and terms). The second point accords with my view that logical syntax analyses sentences into terms and functors. Quine's functor syntax is unabashedly artificial. We shall favour a logical syntax of (nested) binary "categorical" forms that is classical, natural and universal.

No one defending an unpopular doctrine can do better than to have had Imre Lakatos for a friend. Lakatos understood and could articulate how ideas come to power and he encouraged me to look and fight for the older 'research program' which Frege has eclipsed.

My gratitude to some is more personal. To Marcia Zakai and to Anne Meixsell who did so much to make things neat and felicitous and to all my close friends who at times seemed even more impatient than I to see this in print, I express deep thanks. Finally there are Tamler and Leyele who showed me that there is as much truth in beauty as there is beauty in truth.

F.T.S.
Brandeis 1981

Contents

xiv   CONTENTS

A Short Glossary of Abbreviations and Symbols

MPL	Modern Predicate Logic
TFL	Traditional Formal Logic
†	The dagger. This sign represents the functor 'some is' when flanked by two terms. It represents 'and' when flanked by two statements.
$+, +$	The pair of pluses function like the dagger sign. For example '$+S+P$' transcribes 'some S is P' and '$+p+q$' transcribes 'p and q'.
$-, +$	Transcribes 'every is' and 'if then' as in '$-S+P$' (every S is P) and in '$-p+q$' (if p then q).
$\llcorner S \lrcorner$	A purely symbolic way of representing 'Some S'.
[S]	A purely symbolic way of representing 'every S'.
(P)	The symbolic way of representing 'is P'. For example '[Boy] (loves $\llcorner$Girl$\lrcorner$)' represents 'every boy loves some girl'.
SNF	The subject-predicate normal form. A sentence is in SNF when each of its subject-expressions has its own predicate. For example '[Boy] ($\llcorner$Girl$\lrcorner$ (loves))' 'every boy (some girl (loves))' is the SNF of 'every boy loves some girl'.
R^{21}	The converse of the relational expression R^{12}. For example if L^{12}_{ab} = 'a loves b', 'L^{21}_{ba}' represents 'b is loved by a'.

$+\alpha+P$	Where α is a definite singular term, '$+\alpha+P$' represents '(some) α is P', or simply 'α is P'. Because 'α' has unique denotation '$+\alpha+P$' entails '$-\alpha+P$' ('every α is P').
$*\alpha+P$	Represents '$+\alpha+P$' and indicates that '$+\alpha+P$' entails '$-\alpha+P$'.
$\pm\alpha+P$	Another variant for 'α is P'. The double sign in the subject serves to indicate that 'some α is P' entails 'every α is P'.
U-term	A term whose denotation is contextually restricted. The terms of pronominal subjects are U-terms.
G-term	General term. G-terms are not contextually restricted.
Some S_j	The subject of an antecedent sentence to which a pronoun has subsequent reference. For example: 'Some S_j is P and *J is Q' is the pronominal sequence 'Some S is P and it is Q'. The term 'J' is called the 'proterm'.
Ex	The *sentence* 'something exists'.
Ex & Px	Something exists and it is P. The intersentential form of '$(\exists x)(Px)$'.
$+[+Tx+E]$ $+[\pm X+P]$	The algebraic form of 'something exists and it is P'.
A-type pronoun	A pronoun whose antecedent has reference to a particular thing under consideration in some epistemic context. Example 'Some man is on the roof! ... It isn't a man'. Here 'It' refers to what was taken to be a man by the first speaker.
D-type pronoun	A pronoun that refers descriptively to the thing under consideration as in 'Some man is on the roof. He (the man in question) is a burglar!'
B-type pronoun	A pronoun whose antecedent does not refer epistemically. B-type pronouns are translatable as bound variables in MPL.

E-type pronouns   A type of pronoun discriminated by Gareth Evans. Its antecedent is non-epistemic but it cannot be given a bound variable translation.

Introduction

The thesis I will be arguing for belongs to the premodern—which is to say, pre-Fregean—tradition of logical theory whose major figures from Aristotle to Leibniz never doubted that the sentences of a natural language like Greek or English that entered into deductive reasoning could, for logical purposes, be parsed in ways familiar to the grammarian. Implicit in the program of traditional formal logic is the idea of a logical syntax of natural language in which the grammarians' noun-phrase/verb-phrase analysis is the fundamental pattern. If the logical syntax of a sentence like 'everyone reads a newspaper' corresponds to its natural grammatical structure it will not be incorrect to say that the noun-phrase 'everyone' is its logical subject and the verb-phrase 'reads a newspaper' its logical predicate. Of course even the traditional logician often regimented sentences for logical reckoning. He might for example find it necessary to rephrase the above sentence as 'every person is a reader of some newspaper' before using it as a premiss in some argument. Such regimentation puts sentences into logically useful patterns by isolating the terms of the sentence. If the terms from other premisses that enter into the logical reckoning are 'person', 'a reader of a newspaper' and 'a newspaper,' a regimentation into the pattern 'Every X is an R to a Y' will make these terms available. It did not, however, seriously occur to the traditional logician that logical reckoning called for more than this sort of paraphrasing. The regimented forms may be stilted but they do not significantly depart from the syntax of the sentence being regimented and in many cases they preserve its syntax intact.

The idea of a logical syntax of natural language stands opposed to what the Fregean believes about logical form. Frege himself held that an adequate account of inferences expressed in natural language requires translation into a new idiom, the idiom of a language expressly constructed for use by logicians.

This new logical language is no mere convenience: Frege believed that the syntax of natural language was logically useless, misleading, and incoherent. Being convinced of this, Frege did not criticize the grammarian for misconstruing natural language. On the contrary, from Frege's standpoint the grammarian could well be right in his description of the syntax of natural language. If so the inadequacy is not in the grammarian but in his subject-matter. Michael Dummett aptly sums up Frege's reaction to the phenomenon that the natural languages lack a perspicuous logical grammar with the words 'so much the worse for natural language'.

We may borrow from the late Yehoshua Bar Hillel the terms 'constructionist' and 'naturalist' to characterize the respective positions of Frege and his predecessors on logical syntax. The constructionist believes with Frege that a truly logical syntax is the syntax of an artificial language constructed for the purpose of formalizing deductive reasoning. The naturalist believes with Aristotle and Leibniz that logical syntax is implicit in the grammar of natural language and that the structure attributed by grammarians to sentences of natural language is in close correspondence to their logical form. If the constructionist is right a mere regimentation of 'Everyone reads a newspaper' will not reveal its logical form; for that something more radical is needed. Logicians aptly call the sentence 'for anything x if x is a person then there is a thing y such that y is a newspaper and x reads y' a *translation* of the original sentence 'Everyone reads a newspaper'. Translation versus regimentation; these alternatives divide the constructionist and naturalist positions on how to get at logical form. Translation introduces new syntax not found in the vernacular sentence, the pronominal letters, 'x' and 'y', the compound constructions 'if . . . then', and '. . . and . . .'; according to the constructionists these are needed to make perspicuous the logical form and to facilitate logical reckoning.

With Russell's elaboration and popularization of Frege's logical theories the constructionist position achieved dominance in this century. It owed not a little to the researches of Tarski who argued that the natural languages were semantically deficient and urged the use of formal languages for the avoidance of semantic inconsistency. More recently however the work of Chomsky and his followers have contributed to a naturalist climate which does not favour a dismissive attitude to the natural languages. Implicit in the linguists' belief in the coherence of his own subject-matter is a challenge to the constructionist scepticism concerning the possibility of logical syntax of natural language. This is not to say that a challenge of this kind is without its hazards. For if natural language can lay claim to a syntax that is adequate for logical purposes then this can be taken to mean that the syntax currently attributed to it by most grammarians is faulty and superficial. Where Frege himself was content to dismiss the grammarian, the contemporary Fregean makes bold to correct him. We find Geach chastising Chomsky for classifying 'some man' along with 'Socrates' as noun phrases in sentences like 'Socrates is wise' and 'some man is wise'. According to Geach it is a logical and, therefore, grammatical howler to consider 'Socrates' and 'some man' as members of the same substitution class. Geach argues thus because the formation rules for the logical languages treat 'individual symbols' like 'Socrates' and phrases like 'some man' as belonging to different grammatical categories. So we have the phenomenon that the language of modern formal logic originally devised in distrust of natural language is being deployed as a constraint on linguistic theory. And not a few working linguists are looking to the syntax of modern quantificational logic as a model for the constituent analysis of the sentences of the natural languages.

Frege condemned 'psychologism' and the idea that logic might be viewed as that part of cognitive psychology which characterizes how we think when we think correctly is foreign to the Fregean standpoint. It is not hard to see that the issues dividing the constructionist and the naturalist are relevant to the question whether logic could be said to give insight into the laws of thought in the sense of describing what is mentally happening as one moves from the premisses to the conclusion of a deductive argument. A logic whose basic syntax is that of the actual language in which inferences are made can lay claim to a psychological veracity that Frege has abjured. But here too the hands-off-psychology attitude that currently prevails among logicians could 'dialectically' turn into its meddlesome opposite. In the absence of a comprehensive naturalist alternative to modern predicate logic and in the conviction that modern logic is the only genuine logic we may soon see Geach-like objections to any empirical theory that does not model the cognitive deductive process along the familiar lines of justification of inferences in modern quantificational logic. It is on the other hand even more likely that the lack of an adequate naturalistic logic would simply make impossible the development of a plausible account of the cognitive processes involved in deductive reasoning.

A naturalist program must show itself capable of overcoming the logistic advantage enjoyed by Fregean systems of logic. In chapter 9 I indicate how this may be done. The removal of prejudice to traditional formal logic and the attempt to develop it as an alternative instrument comparable in power to modern predicate logic may be viewed by some Fregeans as an attack on the latter type of systems. That is not my purpose. I believe and hope to show that traditional formal logic is especially suited to the task of making perspicuous the logical form of sentences in the natural languages that are actually used in deductive reasoning and that, in virtue of this, traditional logic provides models for the study of what actually happens when we reckon the premises and arrive at conclusions. But Frege himself has rightly taught us that logic *need* not be concerned with either of these matters, not with the actual language and not with deductive thinking as a cognitive process. Too often the claim of greatness for Frege's theory of quantifiers and for his logistic system generally is made to rest on the claim that traditional formal logic is essentially incapable of achieving a formalization of inference comparable to Frege's logic. That this should turn out to be false does not in the least detract from the power and scope of quantification theory. Of course there are those who identify logic with modern logic (seeing in advance all adequate alternatives to it as mere notational variants). That an identification of this kind is false (and fatuously so) is one of the themes of this book.

For the contemporary philosopher the availability of an alternative to Frege is of interest because of its implications for the philosophy of language, metaphysics and epistemology. The logical subjects and predicates of the basic propositions in a non-Fregean organon differ radically from the individual

constants or variables and predicates of the atomic propositions of a standard logical language. One consequence of
this is that the existence of atomic propositions is denied by the
neo-Aristotelian and the vehicle of reference is shifted away
from individual definite subjects like 'Socrates' or 'this' to
subjects of form 'some S'. Indeed we find that the new
naturalist organon treats most definite subjects (proper names,
demonstratives, definite descriptions) as anaphoric expressions
that have back reference to propositions of form 'some S is P'.
A theory which holds that reference begins with 'some S', and
which makes reference by definite subjects pronominally
dependent on primary indefinite reference, bears on many
issues in the theory of knowledge that could not be explored in
the body of the book.

In chapters 13 and 14 I explore some of the consequences of
adopting a non-Fregean view of the logical predicate. In the
traditional organon, the relation of contrariety that two terms
like 'wise' and 'unwise' have to one another is primitive and not
definable by sentential negation. In Frege all negativity is
sentential or definable by sentential negation. Thus 'Socrates is
unwise' means nothing else than 'it is not the case that Socrates
is wise'. I have long been interested in logical systems that
distinguish between negating a proposition that affirms a
predicate of a subject and asserting a proposition that affirms
the contrary of the predicate of the same subject. This
distinction is a feature of traditional formal logic and its
philosophical implications are discussed in the later chapters of
the book.

Some terminological remarks may be helpful. In writings on
logical theory or on topics in the philosophy of language terms
like 'statement', 'proposition', and 'term' are commonly used
with systematic ambiguity, referring sometimes to a type of
expression and sometimes to a type of thing expressed or
denoted. I did not think it important to disambiguate these
different uses; it would have been tedious to do so for the
majority of contexts where there is little chance of confusion. I
have also followed a common, though not universal practice,
of using 'statement' and 'proposition' interchangeably. The
proposition expressed by a sentence is the statement made by
its use; it is what is said. (To say something is to specify a

determinate state of affairs whose presence or absence determines the truth of what is said.) I do however distinguish between the meaning of a sentence and the proposition it expresses or the statement it is used to make. If I utter any of the sentences 'I am hungry', 'Ich habe Hunger', 'J'ai faim', I will not have said anything different than I would have said by the utterence of either of the others. We say that these sentences have the same meaning. And generally a set of sentences have the same meaning if and only if for a given speaker in a given situation the use of any one of the sentences determines the same truth conditions as the use of any other sentence in the set. Having the same meaning is however neither necessary nor sufficient for being used to say the same thing. Two sentences S1 and S2 may differ in meaning and be used to say the same thing: consider 'I am hungry' said by me and 'he is hungry' said by someone referring to me. On the other hand two sentences that mean the same thing may be used to specify different states of affairs: consider 'I am hungry' and 'ich habe Hunger' uttered respectively by Russell and Wittgenstein. A sentence assumed to be in use will be referred to as a statement or proposition. In practice, two sentences are referred to as the same proposition or statement or are said to express the same proposition or to make the same statement if and only if they have the same meaning and it is being assumed that they are being used to say the same thing.

The simplest sentence consists of a subject and a predicate, each containing a term. For example, the subject 'a student' of 'a student is waiting' refers to a student; the term 'student' denotes every individual student. Terms denote individuals. The sentence itself denotes (or 'specifies') a state of affairs, namely that state of affairs which must obtain for the sentence, as it is used in an illocutionary act of assertion, to be true. A sentence in assertive use is said to express a proposition. This may be taken to say that, qua assertion, the sentence *is* a proposition. Strictly speaking only sentences in actual assertive use are propositions. But strict speaking would deprive us of the welcome convenience of using 'sentence', 'proposition', and 'statement' interchangeably. The logician analyses the logical syntax of a sentence in abstraction from its illocutionary use. The relaxed policy of referring to an assertable sentence as a proposition or statement is harmless, even though, in all strictness, an unasserted sentence is neither true nor false and so only potentially a statement or proposition. For the logician concerned to characterize the kind of sentences that enter into argument this fact that a sentence denotes a state of affairs and has the requisite indicative form for assertive use suffices for the purpose at hand.

[The policy of referring to sentences as propositions has the more serious purpose of allowing one to avoid thinking of propositions as meanings of sentences, 'expressed by sentences' and distinct from them. Propositions in that sense can be explained away at the price of 'countenancing' states of affairs. For we may understand 'Jones said that p' ('Jones expressed the proposition that p', 'Jones made the statement that p' and the like) to mean that a sentence denoting the state of affairs in which p was used in an illocutionary act of assertion. There are philosophers who are no more willing to countenance states, situations, or circumstances, than they are willing to countenance propositions. But I know of none who would explicitly deny that a sentence in assertive use is associated with certain conditions of its truth. And the existence of the state of affairs in which p is precisely the condition for the truth of 'p'. It therefore seems to me that excluding states of affairs from one's ontology transgresses the decencies of a healthy 'ontic' snobbery.

In one sense, then, a proposition is a sentence or, more precisely, an assertion. In another more suspect sense a proposition is a kind of entity that is distinct from the sentence that expresses it. The question whether non-sentential propositions can be eliminated is far from settled. Ontological propositions are the prima facie referents of sentences of form 'that p is Q', for example of 'that p is shocking (true, goes without saying, etc.)'. That a sentence of this general form does not refer to a sentence (let alone mention one) is arguable from the category deviance of 'that p is Q but (un)grammatical' and from the fact that what is shocking about William Calley's having shot unarmed villagers is something more and different from any assertion to that effect. In the majority of cases however we can plausibly construe 'that p is Q' to be referring to the state of affairs in which p. Thus we can understand that 'p is shocking' to mean that the state of affairs in which p is shocking and 'that p is true' to mean that the state of affairs in which p obtains. The reference to propositions in a sentence like 'that p goes without saying' seems more resistant to an analysis in terms of states of affairs. But if one understands 'Jones says that p' to mean 'Jones asserts a sentence denoting the state of affairs in which p' then one can construe 'that p goes without saying' to say that one need not bother to assert any sentence denoting the state in which p. I tend to the view that we may speak of propositions in two unexceptionable senses. In one sense, propositions$_1$, it simply means 'sentence' (qua assertion or statement). Sentences of form ' "p" is true' refer to propositions$_1$. Propositions$_1$ are true or false depending on the existence or non-existence of the states of affairs they denote.

The second sense of proposition is ontological: a proposition$_2$ is a state of affairs *in its role of having been denoted by an assertion* (or proposition$_1$). A state of affairs cannot be said to be true or false. Nevertheless sentences of form 'that p is true (false)' should be construed as referring to states of affairs. Thus 'that p is true (false)' is understood to say that the state of affairs in which p exists (doesn't exist). Although propositions$_2$ are 'out there', they are tied to sentences as their denotata. 'Proposition$_2$' is like the word 'denotatum'. The latter means 'individual denoted by a term', the former 'state of affairs denoted by a sentence'. Hospitality to states of affairs, situations (even counterfactual ones) and the like is a fair price to pay for exorcizing the mediating meanings that some philosophers interpose between sentences and their truth conditions.]

Only a fragment of the sentences of a natural language can enter as premisses or conclusions in arguments. The logician is in no position to characterize the syntax of *all* of the sentences of this fragment. It is, instead, his job to characterize a fragment of this fragment, a canonical set of sentences that satisfies the following conditions:

1. The syntax of the canonical set is easily specifiable (in a recursive manner).
2. The syntactic structure of the sentences reveal their logical relations to one another.
3. Every non-canonical sentence in the logically relevant fragment has a canonical paraphrase.

An example of a non-canonical sentence is

(1) If you've smelled one violet you've smelled them all.
The canonical paraphrase of (1) in the language of traditional formal logic is

(1N) Every smeller of some violet is a smeller of every violet.

The canonical translation of (1) in a standard language of modern predicate logic is something like

> (1C) Anyone is such that if there is a thing such that that thing is a violet and he or she smells it then anything is such that if it is a violet then he or she smells it.

In choosing a canonical logical language the Fregeans and their predecessors had a different fourth requirement in mind. The Fregeans required of a canonical language that its sentences be semantically explicit in the sense that each sentence must express the condition that must obtain for that sentence to be true. Thus the Fregean will not take as canonical 'some Spaniards are proud' preferring instead to take 'there exists a person such that that person is a Spaniard and that person is proud'. The traditional logician emphasized syntactic simplicity, requiring of a canonical sentence that it have a straightforward noun-phrase verb-phrase structure (or be a compound of such 'categorical' sentences).

Using sentence in the narrow logician's sense of assertion or 'statement-sentence' it was a central thesis of pre-Fregean logic that any sentence not compounded of other sentences (any *elementary* sentence) is (or is paraphrasable as) a sentence of form

$$\textit{some/every x is/isn't y}$$

in which x and y are interchangeable terms that may be *negative*, as in 'some non-citizens are farmers', or *compound*, as in 'some farmer is a gentleman and a scholar', or relational, as in 'every owner of a cow is a farmer', or *singular* as in '(some) Socrates is a Greek'.

The canonical sentences of traditional logic are distinguished by having noun phrases of form 'some/every x'. And all have the characteristic binary NP/VP structure.[1]

---

[1] Contrast the traditional doctrine of logical syntax which analyses each elementary sentence as having one dominant noun-phrase subject (of the form 'some/every x') and one dominant verb-phrase predicate with the contemporary doctrine as summarized in this respresentative passage:

Subjects must be singular and definite, excluding phrases that begin with 'a', 'some', 'no' and the like (Quine MofL p. 211 and Massey p. 225 call them 'singular terms',

In adhering to the binary form for relational sentences like

(2) Some boy was admiring every girl

the pre-Fregean faced logistical problems of how to deal with
terms containing noun-phrase objects of relational expressions
(transitive verbs). Here the desideratum of adhering to the
NP/VP constituent analysis appeared to be in conflict with the
requirement that a syntactic analysis must be logically perspicuous for every canonical sentence. In the traditional syntax
for logic all predicates, including those whose terms are
relational, are 'monadic'. Thus the predicate or verb phrase of
(2) is 'was admiring every girl' and the predicate term could
itself be given a binary analysis very much in the manner of an
embedded sentence:

This accords with the classical linguistic constituent analysis
but it gave rise to problems that have appeared insurmountable
in the judgement of contemporary logicians. Construed in the
traditional manner it was not clear how one could make out
that 'Every girl was being admired by some boy' followed from
(2). Nor, for similar reasons, was it clear that one could ever
account for the validity of an inference like 'Since every horse is
an animal, every tail of a horse is a tail of an animal'.

The accepted view that the classical constituent analysis was
hopelessly defective as a doctrine of logical form has tempted
some linguists whose semantic persuasions are stronger than
their syntactic intuitions away from a binary analysis of
relational propositions toward a ternary constituent analysis

---

others 'referring expressions'). Grammatical objects can be subjects in this logical
sense, as in 'Everyone loves Mary'. *Predicates* are what is left over when one or more
subjects are removed from a sentence, and they are called one-place (unary,
monadic), two-place (binary, dyadic) etc. according to the number of subjects, the
same or different, needed to restore them into sentences. (Christopher Kirwan, *Logic
and Argument*, Gerald Duckworth (London, 1978), p. 4.)

In standard logical language a sentence may have two or more non-dominant subjects
(John loves Mary, Tully is Cicero) and/or two or more non-dominant predicates (as in
'John loves a girl' which 'translates' as (∃x) (x is a girl and John loves x).

that conforms to the modern doctrine which treats 'admiring' (in the context of (2)) as a two-place predicate. Although, as I shall be arguing, the move to a ternary analysis is not forced; it is a good illustration of how doctrines of logical form operate (quite properly) as constraints on acceptable theories of grammar.

The negative verdict on the prospects for a viable traditional logic has had the effect of deflecting twentieth-century logic from its traditional task of characterizing the canonical fragment of natural language to the quite different task of constructing powerful but artificial logical languages. The contemporary logician has virtually lost sight of the fact that natural language is the actual medium of deductive reasoning and that logic is, in an important sense, a part of cognitive psychology.

To revive the prospects for getting on with the neglected enterprises one must be able to show that a logical language whose canonical sentences are classically categorical has the requisite inference power. In effect this means resuscitating and modernizing the older logic of terms and showing how it is systematically related to modern predicate logic. The reader will find, I trust, that the classical high road to logical syntax and the laws of thought is not blocked at all and that it offers a fine and clear prospect of the surrounding terrain.

1

Are there Atomic Propositions?

1. In the introduction to Michael Dummett's study of Frege we read the following:

He (Frege) was the initiator of the modern period in the study of Logic . . . The understanding of the fundamental structure of language and therefore of thought, depend upon possessing, in a correct form, that explanation of the construction of and inter-relationship between sentences which it is the business of logic to give. Modern logic stands in contrast to all the great logical systems of the past—of classical antiquity, of medieval Europe, and of India—in being able to give an account which depends on the mechanism of quantifiers and bound variables; for all the subtlety of the earlier systems, the analysis of the structure of the sentences of human language which is afforded by modern logic is, by its capacity to handle multiple generality, shown to be far deeper than they were able to attain. The discovery of the mechanism which enabled this analysis to be given and the realization of its significance, are due to Frege; if he had accomplished only this, he would have rendered a profound service to human knowledge.[1]

The historical judgement of the significance of Frege's contribution to logic is standard. It is generally agreed that a logical account of a sentence like 'everybody envies somebody' 'depends upon the mechanism of quantifiers and bound variables'. Frege was the first logician to give a logically useful representation of such 'multiply general sentences' and his discovery of the quantifier variable notation is seen as 'resolving an age old problem the failure to solve which had blocked the progress of logic for centuries'. Specifically, scholastic logic had failed to give an adequate logical account of inferences involving multiply general sentences. An example

[1] Michael Dummett, *Frege: Philosophy of Language*, (Harper and Row, 1973), p. xiii, hereafter referred to as *Frege*.

of a valid inference of this kind is 'Since there is somebody who is envied by everybody it follows that everybody envies somebody'. According to the modern commentators, the scholastics were unable to explain this kind of inference because they did not understand the way signs of generality ('everybody', 'somebody') and sentences containing proper names ('Peter envies John') were related. Discussing Frege's way of analysing 'everybody envies somebody',Dummett says:

Frege's insight consisted in considering the sentences as being constructed in stages, corresponding to the different signs of generality occurring in it. A sentence may be formed by combining a sign of generality with a one-place predicate. The one-place predicate is itself to be thought of as having been formed from a sentence by removing one or more occurrences of some one singular term (proper names). Thus we begin with a sentence such as 'Peter envies John'. From this we form a one-place predicate 'Peter envies y' by removing the proper name 'John'—the letter 'y' here serving merely to indicate where the gap occurs that is left by the removal of the proper name. This predicate can then be combined with a sign of generality 'somebody' to yield the sentence 'Peter envies somebody'. The resulting sentence may now be subjected to the same process: by removing the proper name 'Peter' we obtain the predicate 'x envies somebody' and this may then be combined with the sign of generality 'everybody' to yield the sentence 'everybody envies somebody'.[2]

The steps that are here outlined show how a doubly general sentence is constructed out of singular beginnings:

(1) Begin with a singular sentence with two proper name subjects and remove one proper name. This yields a predicate.
(2) Combine the predicate with a sign of generality. This yields a sentence.
(3) Begin again by removing from the sentence another proper name. This yields another predicate.
(4) Combine this new predicate with another sign of generality. This yields a multiply general sentence.

The constructional history of the sentence determines its meaning. For example, 'everybody envies somebody' is sometimes considered ambiguous. It might be taken to mean that

[2] Dummett, *Frege*, p. 10.

there is some one person whom everybody envies. More plausibly it is interpreted to say that everybody envies some-body or other (not necessarily the same person). A construc-tional history of the sentence that will yield the first interpre-tation could be:

(1) Peter envies John   (an atomic singular sentence)
(2) x envies John   (a one-place predicate)
(3) (x) (x envies John)   (a singly general sentence)
(4) (x) (x envies y)   (a one-place predicate)
(5) (∃y) (x) (x envies y)   (a multiply general sentence)

The more plausible interpretation has a different construc-tional history:

(1) Peter envies John   (an atomic singular sentence)
(2) Peter envies y   (a one-place predicate)
(3) (∃y (Peter envies y)   (a singly general sentence)
(4) (∃ y) (x envies y)   (a one-place predicate)
(5) (x) (∃y) (x envies y)   (a multiply general sentence)

Dummett's account of 'everybody envies somebody' assigns the second interpretation to it. Dummett attributes the plaus-ibility of the second interpretation to 'the *ad hoc* convention we tacitly employ that the order of construction corresponds to the inverse order of the signs of generality in the sentence;when "everybody" precedes "somebody" it is taken as having been introduced later in the step by step construction.'

The idea that we interpret 'everybody envies somebody' by inverting the surface order of its signs in tacitly analysing it is an example of the kind of claim made for Fregean analysis by some of his followers. For many linguists as well as for many philosophers Frege's analytical logic is viewed as a source of insights into structures below the surface structures of sen-tences in the vernacular and Frege's logical grammar is seen by these linguists and philosophers as belonging to the grammar of the natural languages at the level of 'deep structure'. Frege himself did not think of his logical language as contributing to empirical linguistics; it seems at times that he had too great a contempt for the natural languages to credit them with a logical syntax.

More to the present purpose, Frege's solution to the problem of accounting for inference with multiply general sentences required him to devise a logical grammar that postulates a distinction of level between singular sentences like 'Socrates is mortal' or 'Peter envies John' and general sentences like 'every human is mortal' or 'everybody envies somebody'. In this logical grammar, the former kind of sentences are elements or atoms in the construction of the latter kind of sentences.

2. Although Dummett and others stress the revolutionary importance of the solution to the problem of multiple generality, Frege's revolution in logic is perhaps better located in his doctrine of the atomicity of singular sentences. The basic sentences of Frege's logical grammar are atomic in the sense of being devoid of logical words such as 'everybody', 'not', and 'or'. Before Frege the sentence 'Socrates is mortal' was often parsed as having the form 'every Socrates is mortal' with 'Socrates' or 'Socratizer' as a term whose application is restricted to a single thing.[3] This traditional doctrine treats singular sentences as if they were universal and it implicitly denies the Fregean thesis that singular sentences are syntactically more primitive than general sentences. Instead, the difference between 'Socrates is mortal' and 'every man is mortal' is semantically accounted for by the difference between 'Socrates' and 'man'; i.e., by the difference between a term expressly designed to apply to no more than one thing, and one that is not restricted to unique application. Leibniz has an interesting variant of the traditional doctrine that singular terms are syntactically general. According to Leibniz, 'Socrates is mortal' is a particular proposition whose proper form is 'Some Socrates is mortal'. But 'Some Socrates is mortal' entails 'Every Socrates is mortal' so we are free to choose either way of representing the sentence. Leibniz thus views the singular proposition as equivalent to a particular proposition that entails a universal one. In effect, 'Socrates is mortal' has wild or indifferent quantity ('some-or-every Socrates is mortal'). That 'Socrates is mortal' has particular quantity is justified by the

---

[3] Speaking of 'logicians in past centuries' Quine says: 'they commonly treated a name such as "Socrates" rather on a par logically with "mortal" and "man" and as differing from these latter just in being true of fewer objects, viz. one'.
Willard Van Orman Quine, *Word and Object* (Cambridge, M.I.T. press, 1960), p. 181. Hereafter referred to as *WO*.

consideration that its subject purports to refer to someone. But 'Socrates' as we use it in '(some) Socrates is mortal' is a term that applies to no more than one individual and the fact that it applies uniquely allows us to infer 'every Socrates is mortal' from 'some Socrates is mortal'. Since 'Socrates is mortal' entails its universal generalization, it is understandable that neither quantity is actually specified. However, in justfying inferences we must sometimes be explicit in assigning a given quantity to a singular proposition. For example, we find in Aristotle a variant of the following valid syllogism with two singular premises: 'Pittacus is a good man and Pittacus is a wise man so some wise man is a good man'. To justify this we note that 'Pittacus is P' entails 'every Pittacus is P' which enables us to assign opposing quantities to the two premises giving—in one case—the formally valid syllogism: 'every Pittacus is a good man and some Pittacus is a wise man so some wise man is a good man' and—in the other case—the formally valid syllogism: 'some Pittacus is a good man and every Pittacus is a wise man so some wise man is a good man'. An assignment of particular quantities to both premises would not do.

Leibniz's doctrine of wild or indifferent quantity for singular propositions is an important rival to Frege's doctrine that singular propositions are logically atomic. Leibniz's theory is within the tradition of scholastic logic which treats all categorical propositions—singular as well as general—as assertions or denials of expressions of form 'some/every S is/isn't P'. According to this traditional theory, a genuine logical subject is an expression of form 'some S' or 'every S', and the subjects of singular propositions are no exception. Unless otherwise noted, we shall contrast Frege's doctrine of the atomicity of singular propositions with the scholastic doctrine in its specifically Leibnizian version. Although Leibniz's doctrine of wild quantity is a significant innovation it is important to place it within the tradition that denies to singular propositions the special syntactical position that Frege later accorded to them.

I shall refer to the doctrine that singular propositions are atomic as Frege's atomicity thesis. According to Frege, there is a class of propositions whose subjects are simple names or other singular expressions devoid of any sign of quantity. Names and other expressions of this kind are the only genuine logical subjects. Frege's atomicity thesis stands in contrast to the traditional doctrine of a logical subject as a syntactically complex expression containing a sign of quantity, 'some' or 'every', followed by a term. The traditional doctrine assimilates singular propositions to the class of general propositions. More correctly, it recognizes only one kind of proposition and one kind of logical subject for propositions that have singular or general terms in subject position.

The Fregean and scholastic doctrines differ then in several respects:

(1) The scholastic holds that a logical subject is an expression with a sign of quantity. Frege holds that a logical subject must be simple. In consequence, he holds that only singular propositions are of subject-predicate form.

(2) The scholastic holds that every logical subject contains a term and that the subject term of a proposition is interchangeable syntactically with the predicate term. Frege holds that the subject of a singular proposition, being simple, has no syntactical part that can serve in predicate position and, generally, that subjects and predicates have no common syntactical parts.

(3) The scholastic distinguishes subjects and predicates as expressions that have different logical (syncategorematic) elements. The subject is an expression of form 'some x' or 'every x' and it has a sign of quantity; the predicate is an expression of form 'is y' or 'isn't y' and it has a sign of quality. In Frege, the distinction between subjects and predicates is not due to any difference of syncategorematic elements since the basic subject-predicate propositions are *devoid* of such elements. In Frege, the difference between subject and predicate is a primitive difference between two kinds of categorematic expressions.

(4) The scholastic does not recognize a difference of logical form for singular and general propositions. Frege does.

Russell was well-acquainted with the scholastic doctrine and he saw the significance of the step that Frege had taken in giving singular propositions their special syntactical status:

The first serious advance in real logic since the time of the Greeks was made independently by Peano and Frege—both mathematicians. Traditional logic regarded the two propositions 'Socrates is mortal' and 'All men are mortal' as being of the same form; Peano and Frege showed that they are utterly different in form. Peano and Frege, who pointed out the error did so for technical reasons . . . but the philosophical importance of the advance which they made is impossible to exaggerate.[4]

In this connection, it is worth quoting the passage from Leibniz in which he argues that singular propositions have the logical form of general propositions, their only distinction being that they have 'wild' quantity.

How is it that opposition is valid in the case of singular propositions . . . since elsewhere a universal affirmative and a particular negative are opposed. Should we say that a singular proposition is equivalent to a particular and to a universal proposition? Yes, we should. So also when it is objected that a singular proposition is equivalent to a particular proposition, since the conclusion in the third figure must be particular, and can nevertheless be singular; e.g., 'Every writer is a man, some writer is the Apostle Peter, therefore the Apostle Peter is a man', I reply that here also the conclusion is really particular and it is as if we had drawn the conclusion 'Some Apostle Peter is a man'. For 'Some Apostle Peter' and 'Every Apostle Peter' coincide, since the term is singular.[5]

According to Leibniz's theory 'Peter envies John' could be assigned the same form as 'everybody envies somebody' by reading it as 'every Peter envies some John'. Referring to the Fregean analysis of 'everybody envies somebody' Dummett asks:

Why is this conception, under which the sentence was constructed in stages, more illuminating than the more natural idea according to which it was formed simultaneously out of its three constituents 'everybody' 'envies' and 'somebody' in exactly the same way that 'Peter envies John' is constructed out of its three components?[6]

Leibniz would here put Dummett's question the other way round asking why we cannot think of 'Peter envies John' as

[4] Bertrand Russell, *Our Knowledge of the External World* (A Mentor Book Edition, New York, 1960), p. 40.

[5] *Leibniz Logical Papers*, ed. G. H. R. Parkinson (Oxford, 1966), p. 115.

[6] Dummett, *Frege*, p. 11.

having the same form as 'everybody envies somebody'. To this, Leibniz's answer is: Indeed we *can* although strictly speaking 'Peter envies John' parses as 'some Peter envies some John', a proposition that entails 'every Peter envies some John'.

Of course, Dummett's question presupposes Frege's thesis of atomicity; it assumes the syntactical gap between 'Peter envies John' and 'everybody envies somebody'. The question then is not whether these two are distinct but why they are. In his answer, Dummett exploits the different conditions for the truth of the two sentences. Genrally, a singular sentence is true just in case its predicate is true of the individuals that are named by its proper names. For example, 'Socrates is mortal' is true if an only if 'is mortal' is true of Socrates. The rules for assigning truth to general sentences are somewhat more complicated. For example, the general sentence 'somebody is mortal' is true just in case some one singular sentence 'Socrates is mortal', 'Plato is mortal', 'Gabriel is mortal', etc., is true. The general sentence 'everybody is mortal' is true just in case each and every sentence 'Socrates is mortal', 'Plato is mortal', 'Gabriel is mortal', is true. In this way, the rules for assigning truth values to 'something is P' and 'everything is P' refer us back to the truth conditions of the basic sentences of form 'a is P'. We assign a constructional analysis to 'everybody envies somebody' because (says Dummett):

Once we know the constructional history of a sentence involving multiple generality, we can from these simple rules, determine the truth conditions of the sentence provided only that we already know the truth conditions of every sentence containing proper names in places the signs of generality stand. Thus 'everybody envies somebody' is true just in case each of the sentences 'Peter envies somebody,' 'James envies somebody,' . . . is true; and 'Peter envies somebody' is, in turn true just in case at least one of the sentences 'Peter envies John,' 'Peter envies James' . . . is true.[7]

In this explanation of the difference between 'Everybody envies somebody' and 'Peter envies John', we encounter the characteristically modern doctrine that the logical form of a sentence is an expression that exhibits its truth conditions. Specifically, the analysis of 'everybody envies somebody' as 'For anybody x

[7] Dummett, *Frege*, p. 11.

there is somebody y such that x envies y' is an acceptable 'translation' since the truth conditions of the 'translated' sentence have been made explicit. Speaking of the way truth conditons are related to the grammar of modern logic Quine remarks:

The grammar that we logicians tendentiously call standard is grammar designed with no other thought than to facilitate the tracing of truth conditions. And a very good thought this is.[8]

How good a thought it is we shall consider in due course. For the present, we take note of the Fregean doctrine that truth conditions of general propositions are to be traced recursively to the conditions for the truth of propositions that contain no signs of generality. For this is what Frege's version of general propositions enables us to do.

If we ask whether the standard Fregean account of 'everybody envies somebody' supports the atomicity thesis our answer must be that it does not. For that account makes use of atomic propositions and it must be rejected by anyone who agrees with Leibniz that even singular propositions are syntactically general. If Leibniz is right, there are no atomic sentences of the kind required for a recursive account of the truth conditions of general sentences. Put another way: If Leibniz is right, Dummett's constructional histories are semantic myths. For while it is certainly true that, say, 'everything is created' is true only if 'Socrates is created', 'Alaska is created' . . . are true, this is of little significance since each of the singular sentences is itself of the form 'every . . . is created' or 'some . . . is created'. To be sure, there may still be some point to observing that the truth of 'everything is created' is conditional on the truth of 'Socrates is created' but so, too, is it dependent on the truth of 'every Greek is created' and it is hard to see why 'every Socrates is created' is semantically more privileged just because the term in its subject is designed for unique application.

If on the other hand Frege is right about the existence of atomic propositions, then the recursive historical account of general sentences is a very attractive one. It may be thought that the very fact that atomic sentences can serve as ground in

[8] Quine, *Philosophy of Logic* (Prentice Hall, 1970), p. 35.

an elegant explanation of the truth conditions of general sentences is itself an argument in favour of their existence. If so, it is an unimpressive argument; unless the impossibility of a semantic explanation of general sentences that is not grounded in atomic sentences could be established, the appeal to the Fregean type of recursive model as a reason for accepting atomic propositions should be disregarded.[9]

3. We are beginning to face the intimidating prospect of deciding whether to accept or to reject Frege's atomicity thesis. And it is natural to wonder how one goes about deciding whether a certain class of propositions—in this case the class of atomic propositions—exists or fails to exist. The meaning of the question 'are there atomic propositions?' is however not necessarily affected by the fact that we are not clear on how to set about answering it. The Fregean thesis on the atomic character of singular propositions is clear enough and it is in sharp contrast to the scholastic theory. Moreover, the question of the existence of certain syntactical forms is something that we are learning to view in a scientific light. For we have, if only in principle, certain criteria for judging the adequacy of linguistic theories when they postulate the existence of some class of syntactical objects and even if it should be true that we are at present unable to judge the matter in the case of atomic propositions, we still have the right to expect that the question of their existence may admit of an empirical decision at some

---

[9] There is in fact a well-known alternative developed by Tarski. Fregean semantics takes the notion of the truth of *closed, atomic* sentences as primitive and defines the truth of quantified and truth-functionally compound sentences in terms of it. Tarskian semantics treats the notion of satisfaction of an *open* sentence by an individual or sequence of individuals as primitive and defines the truth of *closed* sentences, 'atomic', or quantified in terms of it. Thus, where a Fregean would say that '$(\exists x) Fx$' is true if and only if some atomic sentences 'Fa' is true, a Tarskian would say (roughly) that '$(\exists x) Fx$' is true if and only if some (unnamed) individual satisfies the open sentence 'Fx'. As Quine has shown, Tarskian (but not Fregean) semantics can be easily adapted for languages without individual constants and even without individual variables, such as his predicate functor version of MPL: the primitive notion in the latter case is the satisfaction not of an open sentence 'Fx' but of a predicate (or term) 'F' by individuals or sequences of individuals (*Ways of Paradox and Other Essays*, (Random House, rev. edn, 1976), Essay 29, especially section V, pp. 316—17). Tarskian semantics can also be adapted for a term logic such as TFL.

For an illuminating comparison of Fregean and Tarskian semantics (somewhat biased in Frege's favour), see G. Evans 'Pronouns, Quantifiers and Relative Clauses', *Canadian Journal of Philosophy*, 1977, volume III, number 3, section 2, pp. 471–7.

later date. In the meantime, there is a great deal we can do in examining the existing grounds for accepting or rejecting atomic propositions. Even an untested hypothesis can be judged plausible or implausible and we are in a position to do this much for the case of atomic propositions. What is more intimidating is the fact that Frege's thesis has been so overwhelmingly accepted by philosophers and linguists. Indeed the alternative doctrine is only rarely mentioned as a buried mistake and even then it is never set up as a denial of Frege's thesis but is only mentioned as a curious way of parsing singular propositions that does not somehow affect the question of the existence of atomic propositions.

The Fregean thesis is thus unchallenged and unnoticed against the background of its classical rival. In part, this came about because the traditional scholastic theory never explicitly denied the existence of atomic propositions. Which is not surprising: no one before Frege had clearly postulated a class of sentences whose characteristic feature was to be altogether lacking in 'syncategorematic' elements and the question of the existence of sentences of this kind simply did not arise.

After the triumph of Russell's popularization of Frege's logic, the situation was completely reversed; atomic propositions were essential to the new logic and it was natural to take them for granted. Epistemological considerations undoubtedly played a part in this. But in fact the logistic advantages of using Frege's logical language were of greater significance. Frege's logical grammar became canonical because of its inference power; the main reason for distinguishing the logical forms of 'Socrates is mortal' and 'every man is mortal' is the technical one that Russell alluded to: the power and scope of modern predicate logic in which the atomic proposition figures as the element of logical analysis. The rules of formation for the most effective logical languages that have ever been devised begin with atomic forms and proceed with the construction of non-atomic sentences by the addition of sentence forming operators (the signs of generality and the truth functions). It was felt that the traditional doctrine of the singular proposition must be wrong and that it could be safely ignored; had it been right, it should have been possible to construct a logic as powerful as Frege's in which singular propositions and general propositions have the logical form of an assertion or denial of a universal or particular proposition (i.e., a proposition of form 'every S . . .' or 'some S . . .').

Now this reason for accepting Frege over his scholastic opponents is an excellent one. It is surely legitimate to require of a logical syntax that it be logically effective and, in this crucial respect, the traditional formal logic failed dismally. If then we compare the logical syntax of Frege with the logical syntax of his predecessors and, in particular, if we compare the two logical grammars in their representation of singular propositions, the question whether there are atomic propositions appears to be idle. There is only one caveat: if it could be shown that a traditional representation of singular propositions is as logically effective (e.g., for reckoning with multiply general propositions) as Frege's atomic propositions have proved to be, then one might be prepared to reopen the matter. But here the burden of argument is upon the proponent of the older discarded theory and not upon Frege and his successors.

We shall presently accept the logistic challenge on behalf of the traditional doctrine. It is commonly assumed that Frege's spectacular success with inferences that the traditional logician failed to handle is a proof that traditional logic is, in principle as well as in fact, inferior to modern predicate logic in inference power. But this is unwarranted; Frege's success, while decisive, was never, in this sense, definitive. Pending a re-examination of the potentialities of the syntax of traditional logic, we shall keep the question of the truth of the thesis of atomicity alive even while acknowledging that, as matters stand, the logistic evidence is strongly in its favor.

Frege's successors did not challenge the atomicity thesis but neither did they neglect it. On the contrary, although we find no real scepticism about the thesis itself, there is a considerable literature devoted to explaining why singular propositions are as Frege said them to be. Some of the main arguments in support of Frege's account of singular sentences are examined in the next chapter. They are apologetic in character, being propounded in the conviction that Frege's account needs to be rationalized and clarified rather than proved; in particular, the following theses are dogmatically maintained:

(i) Logical subjects are always singular and the sole vehicle of predication is the singular sentence.

(ii) The most primitive kind of singular sentence consists of a designating subject (or subjects) and a characterizing predicate. The subject-expression and the predicate expression are of different syntactical types but they are not distinguished syncategorematically. The syntactic difference is due solely to the semantic difference of role: the subject designates, the predicate characterizes.

(iii) Singular sentences are syntactically and semantically more primitive than general sentences.

2

The Two Term Theory

1. In an inaugural lecture entitled 'History of the Corruption of Logic', P.T. Geach praises Aristotle's *de Interpretatione* for its 'analysis of the simplest kind of proposition' into name and predicable.

Aristotle like Plato, clearly intended these two classes—*onoma* and *rhema*, name and predicable—to be mutually exclusive. For one thing, in explaining the terms he tells us that predicables have tenses and names do not . . . Later in his exposition Aristotle brings out a more general and fundamental distinction; in order to negate a proposition we can negate the predicative part but not the name that stands in subject position.[1]

Geach also commends Aristotle for saying that a name is simple, 'a spoken sound significant by convention none of whose parts is significant in separation' which Geach takes to be evidence that Aristotle thought of logical subjects as syntactically simple. Geach expresses his agreement with these doctrines and he reminds the audience that he has argued for them at length in published works. He then goes on to describe a catastrophic event in the history of logic which he places some time after the completion of *de Interpretatione* and before the beginning of the *Prior Analytics*. This event Geach dubs 'Aristotle's Fall'. For, says Geach, 'Aristotle's logic is from first to last mainly a theory of the subject-predicate relation' and the view of predication he finally developed was not the view he began with:

He lost the Platonic insight that any predicative proposition splits up into two heterogeneous parts; instead he treats predication as an attachment of one term (*horos*) to another term. Whereas the *rhema*

---

[1] P. T. Geach, *Logic Matters* (Basil Blackwell, 1972), p. 45, hereafter referred to as *LM*.

was regarded as essentially predicative, 'always a sign of what is said of something else' it is impossible on the new doctrine for any term to be essentially predicative; on the contrary, any term that occurs in a proposition predicatively may be made into the subject term of another predication. I shall call this 'Aristotle's thesis of interchangeability'; his adoption of it marked a transition from the original name and predicable theory to a *two term theory* . . . Aristotle's going over to the two term theory was a disaster comparable only to the Fall of Adam.[2]

I find Geach's reading of Aristotle more fascinating than faithful; the 'two term theory' is already present in the *de Interpretatione* and there is no textual evidence to support a radical doctrinal change from an earlier period of innocent rectitude. Nevertheless Geach's main point is unexceptionable: Aristotle is the father of the doctrine that subjects and predicates have terms as common syntactical parts and he is responsible for formally treating general propositions as subject-predicate propositions on a par with singular propositions. Since Aristotle was the first logician his 'sin' and its consequences are momentous. 'Aristotle's fall into the two term theory was only the beginning of a long degeneration' and 'the restitution of genuine logic' had to await the Coming of Frege:

To Frege we owe it that modern logicians almost universally accept an absolute category-difference between names and predicables; this comes out graphically in the choice of letters from different founts of type for the schematic letters or variables answering to these two categories.[3]

2. After Frege, a sentence like 'Jeff is a mutt' is represented as Mj with 'j' as the logical subject. This use of a Mutt and Jeff script (tall Mutt letters for predicates and short Jeff letters for subjects), helps to keep us from temptation: one is not so ready to think of 'some dogs' as the logical subject of 'some dogs are mutts'.

In *Reference and Generality*, Geach argues against the 'corrupt' Aristotelian legacy that views the referring phrases of general categorical propositions 'some S' and 'every S' as their

---

[2] Geach, *LM*, p. 47.
[3] Geach, *LM*, p. 59.

logical subjects. He points out that contradictory predicables 'F' and '-F' will give us contradictory propositions when attached to a proper name 'a' but not when attached to a referring phrase of form 'some S' or 'every S'. For example, 'Jack can laugh' and 'Jack can't laugh' are contradictories but 'some men can laugh' and 'some men can't laugh' are both true. Thus we cannot regard 'some men' as a genuine subject to which contradictory predicates are attachable to get contradictory propositions.

This argument against allowing logical-subject status to 'some men' deploys the following Fregean criterion for genuine subjecthood:

An expression E is a logical subject relative to an expression F in a proposition 'EF' if and only if changing F to not-F yields a proposition that is contradictory to 'EF'.

I shall refer to this as the negatability criterion. That Frege used it is clear from the following passage:

We may say, taking subject and predicate in a linguistic sense: a concept is the reference of a predicate; an object is something . . . that can be the reference of a subject. It must be here remarked that the words 'all', 'any', 'no', 'some' are prefixed to concept words. In universal and particular affirmative and negative sentences, we are expressing relations between concepts; we use these words to indicate the special kind of relation. They are thus, logically speaking, not to be more closely associated with the concept words that follow them, but are to be related to the sentence as a whole. It is easy to see this in the case of negation. If in the sentence 'all mammals are land-dwellers' the phrase 'all mammals' expressed the logical subject of the predicate 'are land-dwellers' then in order to negate the whole sentence we should have to negate the predicate: 'are not land-dwellers.' Instead we must put the 'not' in front of 'all'; from which it follows that 'all' logically belongs with the predicate. On the other hand we do negate the sentence 'the concept mammal is subordinate to the concept land-dweller' by negating the predicate: 'is not subordinate to the concept land-dweller'.[4]

In saying that 'all' belongs to the predicate Frege assumes that a categorical proposition consists of a subject and a predicate without remainder; the predicate is that part which is

[4] *Frege—Philosophical Writings*, ed. Max Black and P. T. Geach (Cornell University Press, 1962), pp. 47–48. Hereafter referred to as Black & Geach.

negatable, the rest being the subject. In this case, '(not) all . . . are land-dwellers' is the predicate and 'mammals' is the subject. His rejection of 'all mammals' as the logical subject is responsible for the 'only if' in my formulation of the negatability criterion; the 'if' is due to his saying that it follows that 'all' is part of the predicate.[5]

Geach suggests that we can satisfy the negatability criterion another way. On Frege's view a first level predicate like 'is a land-dweller' stands for a concept and a pair of propositions 'every man is P', 'not every man is P' could be understood as contradictory predications about the concept for which the predicate stood. 'It thus seems natural to regard "every man . . ." and "not every man . . ." as being likewise predicables . . . a contradictory pair of second level predicables, by means of which we make contradictory predications about a concept.'[6]

Geach offers this as an acceptable alternative to the Fregean analysis which has 'man' as the subject and 'any . . . is P' as the predicate. But both Frege and Geach are at one in rejecting the view that 'every man' is the subject of 'every man is P'. Speaking of his own suggestion Geach says: 'Of course this is radically different from the sort of theory by which "every man" has a sort of reference to individual men as a *quasi* subject to which first level predicates are attached.' Geach is right when he says, in effect, that Frege's negatability criterion can be satisfied by treating 'every S' and 'not every S' as predicates respectively of the contradictory pair 'every S is P' and 'not every S is P'. But far from regarding it as natural to think of 'every S' as a predicate of the propositon 'every S is P', I find it more natural to think of it as the subject. Admittedly 'every S' does not satisfy the negatability criterion for logical subject-hood; but this need not mean that Geach is closer to nature than I am; for it may mean instead that something is amiss with the negatability criterion.

[5] Frege's view that logical words always have sentential scope will receive more serious attention later in this chapter. *Strictly* speaking, 'not' does not qualify the predicate of a proposition. But Frege is here pointing out that 'taking subject and predicate in a linguistic sense' we do conventionally form negative predicates to effect contradiction in the case of singular sentences. See also the discussion at the beginning of chapter 13.

[6] P. T. Geach, *Reference and Generality* (Cornell University Press, 1962), p. 58. Hereafter referred to as *R & G*.

The fact that the negation of 'a is P' is equivalent to 'a is not-P' was already observed by Aristotle in the *de Interpretatione*.

It is clear too that, with regard to particulars, if it is true when asked something, to deny it, then it is also true to affirm something. For instance: 'Is Socrates wise? No. Then Socrates is not-wise.' With universals on the other hand the corresponding affirmation is not true. For instance: 'Is every man wise? No. Then every man is not-wise.' This is false, but 'Then not every man is wise' is true; this is the opposite statement, the other is the contrary.[7]

Here we have Frege's contrast:

not: a is P = a is not-P
not: every S is P ≠ every S is not-P

The word 'not' distributes into the predicate in the case of 'a is P' but not in the case of 'every S is P'. Of course, one *could* distribute 'not' into a general proposition by changing the quantity of the subject as well as the quality of the predicate. We then have:

not: every S is P = some S is not-P
not: some S is P = every S is not-P

Let us call this the Principle of Not-Distribution. Are singular propositions exceptions to the Principle of Not-Distribution? *There is no reason to think so.* Assume, for the sake of argument, that the traditional view of singular propositions is correct. And, to fix matters more precisely, assume that Leibniz's version is correct and that singular propositions have wild quantity leaving us free to choose the quantity of a singular proposition and that the reason we do not bother to specify the quantity of 'a is P' is precisely because either one will do. Nevertheless, in exposing the transformation of subject and predicate under negation, it will be necessary to choose one or the other quantity and see what happens when this proposition is negated. There are two possibilities:

(i) 'not: every a is P' is transformed into 'some a is not-P'
(ii) 'not: some a is P' is transformed into 'every a is not-P'

It is clear that the traditional logician can in this way explain the *apparent* immunity of singular propositions to a change of

[7] Aristotle, *De Interpretatione*, ch. 10.

subject under negation. The change does take place, but neither quantity appears in actual discourse since in general, for singular 'a' the propositions 'every a is P' and 'some a is P' are equivalent. Because of this, the negation of 'Socrates is wise' will appear as 'Socrates is not-wise (unwise)' and the transformation of the subject will be hidden.

It is by now clear the Frege's negatability criterion cannot be deployed against the traditional doctrine which holds that 'every S' is the logical subject of 'every S is P'. To get his contrast between 'every S is P' and 'a is P', Frege must assume that the latter is an unquantified sentence. This is just what he does assume but precisely this is at issue between him and the traditional logician who takes 'Socrates' and 'every man' to be logical subjects of '. . . is wise'. Put another way: the traditional logician denies that a mere change in the predicate can ever achieve more than contrariety. For contradiction, we must change the subject as well as the predicate. Traditional logic thus holds that the negatability thesis is grounded in a logical mistake.

3. I shall take a brief look at a closely related argument for rejecting the idea that the referring phrases of general sentences ('some S', 'every S') are genuine logical subjects.

There is yet another difference between referring phrases and genuine logical subjects. Connectives that join propositions may also be used to join predicables; and the very meaning they have in the latter use is that by attaching a complex predicable so formed to a logical subject we get the same result as we should by first attaching the several predicables to that subject, and then using the connectives to join the propositions thus formed precisely as the respective predicables were joined by that connective . . . For referring phrases it is quite otherwise.[8]

Geach is here pointing to another difference between singular and general sentences. For we have:

a is P and Q = a is P and a is Q

but not

some A is P and Q = some A is P and some A is Q

[8] Geach, *R & G*, p. 59.

Similarly we have:

a is P or Q = a is P or a is P

but not:

every A is P or Q = every A is P or every A is Q.

If these facts are to constitute an argument against the idea of referring phrases as genuine logical subjects, it surely cannot be assumed that 'a is P' is different in logical form from 'every S is P' or from 'some S is P'. But if that assumption is removed, we can easily explain the difference of equivalences. It is a logical truism that any universal sentence distributes a conjunction in its predicate and every particular sentence distributes a disjunction in its predicate. Thus we have:

(every) a is P and Q = (every) a is P and (every) a is Q
every A is P and Q = every A is P and every A is Q
(some) a is P or Q = (some) a is P or (some) a is Q
some A is P or Q = some A is P or some A is Q.

Note that the wild quantity of 'a is P' accounts for the fact that the distribution is valid in both cases. One may even say that the traditional doctrine is in this respect superior to the standard doctrine. The latter merely points to a difference between 'a is P' and 'every S is P'; the former explains that the difference is due to the wild quantity of 'a is P'. The difference between 'a is P' and 'every S is P' or 'some S is P' is the difference between a proposition of wild or indifferent quantity and one of fixed quantity. The wild quantity of singular propositions gives them logical powers that are lacking in propositions of fixed quantity. The power to distribute conjunctions and disjunctions of predicates is only one example of the logical powers peculiar to propositions with definite singular subjects. It would perhaps be more accurate to call such propositions doubly general since they combine the powers of universal and particular propositions.

4. The next argument for Frege's atomicity thesis that I shall examine has achieved a considerable currency in recent years. Anyone who believes with Frege in a basic class of propositions devoid of syncategorematic elements must sooner or later take on the task of explaining the difference of subject and predicate which are for Frege the two categorematic elements that between them exhaust the atomic sentence. For it is not enough to insist on the absoluteness of the distinction and Fregean philosophers like Geach and Strawson have responded to the need for saying how and why the difference is absolute. In following their endeavours, it is easy to forget that this need is peculiar to the Fregean; before Frege, subject and predicate are distinguished by the difference of the *syncategorematic* elements: a subject contains a sign of quantity, a predicate contains a sign of quality. The Fregean could not avail himself of this simple recourse; predication for him takes place in atomic sentences and in those sentences the Fregean must signal the difference of subject and predicate by some convention that represents them with signs of different appearance (the Mutt and Jeff script being the most popular way of distinguishing predicate letters from subject letters). The convention itself marks a difference between two syntactical categories and argument in justification of the convention is needed.

The argument we now consider is found in a number of contemporary philosophers, the most prominent of whom are Geach, Anscombe, Dummett, and Strawson, all of whom accept it. Geach says that he appeals to it in order 'to show that names and predicables are necessarily different in category, and that we must reject the traditional idea of a term that can shift from predicate to subject position without change of sense'. In aid of this, Geach presents the following consideration:

A pair of contradictory predicates 'Fa' and '-Fa,' may legitimately be taken as the results of attaching contradictory predicates to a common subject; but if we re-wrote this pair as 'aF' and '-aF,' we could not regard them as the results of attaching a common predicate to a pair of contradictory subjects, 'a' and '-a.'[9]

In an earlier paper (*Analysis*, January, 1965) Anscombe says the same thing:

What signally distinguishes names from expressions for predicates is that expressions for predicates can be negated, names not. I mean

[9] Geach, *LM*, p. 70.

that negation, attached to a predicate yields a new predicate, but when attached to a name it does not yield any name.

More recently, Dummett holds that negatability distinguishes the logical predicate from the logical subject and he makes heavy weather of 'Aristotle's dictum that a quality has a contrary but a substance does not', replacing Aristotle's 'substance' by Frege's 'object' and urging us 'to recognize the correctness of the Aristotelian thesis that an object has no contrary'. Aristotle to the side, the original of these occurs in *Reference and Generality*:

Predicables always occur in contradictory pairs; and by attaching such a pair to a common subject, we get a contradictory pair of propositions. But we never have a pair of names so related that by attaching the same predicates to both we always get a pair of contradictory propositions.[10]

Strawson dubs this the 'thesis of asymmetry for subjects and predicates with respect to negation' or, for short, 'the asymmetry thesis'. Strawson too accepts the thesis and he undertakes to explain why it is true. I shall have no quarrel with Strawson's explanation as a way of understanding atomic sentences. Indeed I shall provisionally allow that the asymmetry thesis and Strawson's justification of it are unexceptionable to anyone who has already accepted the Fregean syntax of logical subjects and predicates.[11] In allowing this, I do not concede much since the point of the asymmetry thesis is to 'show that names and predicables are necessarily different in category' and thereby to justify the Fregean syntax and to reject its rival, the two term theory. But we shall find that without the prior dogmatic commitment to atomicity, the asymmetry thesis is either incoherent, false, or irrelevant to the question of Frege vs. Leibniz (I choose Leibniz as a typical representative of the two term theory).

We note first that Geach, Anscombe and Dummett persist in assuming that contradictory predicates of a common subject yield a contradictory pair of sentences. But the two term theorist holds that 'a is P' is implicitly quantified and that its

[10] Geach, *R & G*, p. 32.
[11] The concession is only provisional. I shall argue below that the thesis of asymmetry with respect to negation is quite unacceptable on Fregean grounds.

contradictory must have opposite quantity. If 'a is not P' has the same subject as 'a is P' then according to the traditional doctrine, it will be contrary to but not contradictory to 'a is P'. Of course, we could avoid this complication by assuming that the subject of both sentences is syntactically simple. But if the asymmetry thesis is based on *this* assumption, it cannot be used in an argument for rejecting the two term theory.

We could avoid begging the question by exhibiting the asymmetry of the subject and predicate with respect to contrariety. Thus we can suppose that there is no change in the subject and that only the predicate is changed. We still have an asymmetry since 'a is P' and 'a is not P' are contraries in contrast with the pair 'a is P' and 'not-a is P'. This fact may then be taken to suggest an 'absolute category difference' between subject and predicate expressions. I think it does reveal a category difference between subject and predicate expressions but not necessarily one that has anything to do with the difference between proper names and predicables. For suppose the two term theorist is right and we consider two sentences 'every A is P' and 'not every A is P' (where 'A' *may* be a proper name but need not be). The second of these would be more perspicuously represented as 'not: every A is P' which exhibits the scope of the word 'not' as clearly propositional. There is, of course, no syntactical device for negating a whole subject phrase; there are no subject phrases of form 'not every S' or 'not some S'; if the scope of the negative particle is non-propositional, these phrases are ill-formed. This, in any case, is how the traditional theory would view the non-negatability of the subject of categorical propositions. There is here no question of non-negatable names but a common garden variety matter of an ill-formed expression. (If, however, we *assume* that logical subjects are syntactically simple, then it appears we do have the 'Aristotelian' phenomenon of non-negatable names and Strawson's explanations seem very much in order.)

There is another possibility. Instead of speaking of negating the whole subject, we could restrict ourselves to negating the subject term, leaving it open whether the subject term *is* the whole subject (as Frege believes) or whether the subject term is preceded by an implicit sign of quantity as the two term theorist believes. In either case, we should be dealing with a syntactically negatable expression and we can then present an asymmetry of contrariety (or subcontrariety) to justify a category difference of subject and predicate. We should then have the contrast between the pair

a is P; a is not P

and the pair

a is P; not-a is P

where 'not-a' is the negation of a categorematic element that may or not be preceded by an implicity sign of quantity depending on whether Frege or the traditional theory is preferred. The contrast would now consist in the fact—if it is a fact—that this latter pair is not a contrary or subcontrary pair of propositions.

Suppose, however, that the traditional analysis is correct and that the form of the latter two sentences is either

some a is P; some not-a is P

or

every a is P; every not-a is P.

A moment's reflection reveals that each of these is in fact a contrary or subcontrary pair of propositions. For the first is equivalent to the pair of subcontraries

some P is a; some P is not-a

and the second is equivalent to the pair of contraries

every not-P is not-a; every not-p is a.

Since this is so, there is *no* asymmetry of contrariety or subcontrariety distinguishing subject from predicate terms; we got contrariety or subcontrariety by negating subject terms as well as by negating predicate terms. We see that this version of asymmetry is altogether useless as a critical instrument against the two term theory. For if the two term theory is right, there is no asymmetry of subject and predicate with respect to the contrarieties.[12]

[12] See *LM*, p. 71 where Geach acknowledges the symmetry of subject and predicate terms with respect to contrariety. The 'friendly critic' who pointed it out to him in correspondence is myself.

Perhaps enough has been said to indicate that the attempt to use a subject-predicate asymmetry of negation against the two term theory is doomed. We have so far found that the asymmetry thesis is either false or incoherent unless of course one already assumes that Frege's analysis of singular sentences is correct. This does not mean that subjects and predicates are symmetrical on the two term theory. For the traditional logician recognizes that logical subjects and logical predicates are differently affected by negation. We have, in fact, two competing theories of the logical form of 'Socrates is wise' and its contradictory.

In Frege, the asymmetry of subject and predicate is evidenced in the fact that we may contradict 'Socrates is wise' by changing the predicate but not by changing the subject so, for example, 'non-Socrates is wise', in contrast to 'Socrates is non-wise', is not a contradictory form. In Leibniz both subject and predicate are changed in contradiction but the asymmetry consists in the fact that the subject must change in quantity, the predicate in quality. Thus the form that contradicts '(every) Socrates is wise' cannot be '(every) non-Socrates is non-wise' but must instead be '(some) Socrates is non-wise'.

5. We turn now to consider some other ways of justifying the standard account of the logical syntax of singular propositions like 'Socrates is wise'. For Frege the syntactic distinction between a proper name and a predicate goes hand in hand with the ontological distinction between objects and concepts. In Frege's theory of language the terms 'proper name' and 'object' are correlatives. An object is what is named or nameable by a proper name; a proper name is an expression that names an object. Predicates and concepts are similarly correlative.

Geach and Dummett differ over the priorities. According to Geach, Frege held that we can recognize an object and distinguish it from a concept; our ability to recognize and distinguish objects enables us to determine the class of expressions that can serve as names: a name is an expression that stands for an object. It is easy to see that we could here have an independent way of grounding the difference between subject and predicate. Dummett, however, maintains that Frege thought of objects as the references of proper names and that the class of proper names could be distinguished by independent tests. If so, objects would be defined as the referents of the class of expressions that could serve as logical subjects in the atomic propositions. Dummett's arguments for this interpretation of Frege seem to me to be convincing:

> To say that someone has a general conception of a certain ontological category, but was uncertain whether what a given expression stood for belonged to that category or not . . . would mean he was uncertain about the way in which the expression functions in our language . . . He could not then possibly be said to know what it was that the expression stood for.[13]

The class of proper names is the class of expressions that can serve as logical subjects in Frege's symbolic language.

> It is therefore essential, if Frege's whole philosophy of language and the ontology which depends on it are to be even viable, that it should be possible to give clear and exact criteria, relating to their functioning within language, for discriminating proper names from expressions of other kinds; and, if we are to obtain a clear grasp of the way natural language could be reconstructed so as to take on the logically perspicuous form of Frege's symbolic language, it must be possible to give such criteria as they apply to proper names of natural language.[14]

Frege himself paid very little attention to the task of distinguishing proper names from other expressions. As Dummett says: 'It is to be presumed, not that he thought it unnecessary, but that he thought it unlikely that anyone would seriously challenge the claim that it could be accomplished'.

Dummett takes on the job of adducing criteria for the class of possible logical subjects and we shall take a moment to watch him at it. We cannot pretend to be disinterested. For if it should turn out that there are plausible criteria for the logical subject that cannot be satisfied by a certain kind of expression, this must mean that the expression is a poor candidate for being a logical subject. In particular, we must be concerned to see whether the tests are plausible and whether any plausible test is better satisfied by simple subjects of the Fregean kind or by the logical subjects of the Leibnizian kind; i.e., singular subjects with wild quantity.

[13] Dummett, *Frege*, p. 57.
[14] Dummett, *Frege*, p. 58.

Bearing in mind that 'Socrates is wise' is the raw material for 'x is wise' from which in turn we construct general sentences ('somebody/everybody is wise', 'if somebody is wise, he is fortunate'), Dummett pays special attention to certain simple patterns of inference that connect singular sentences to general sentences. These patterns of inference provide the ground for distinguishing proper names from other types of expressions. The recognition of their validity is taken as a fact 'that may be left at the intuitive level'.

The patterns in question furnish tests for proper names: it is, for example, 'a necessary condition for an expression "a" to be a proper name that it should be possible to infer from a sentence containing it the result of replacing in that sentence the expression "a" by "something"'. Thus, 'Mars' is a proper name only if 'something is a planet' follows from 'Mars is a planet'; this test excludes 'nothing' as a proper name since 'something is a planet' does not follow from 'nothing is a planet'. However, the test does not exclude the word 'something' itself. So Dummett makes it a further requirement that from two sentences 'a is P' and 'a is Q' we can infer 'something is P and it is Q' or 'some P is Q'. For example, we can infer 'some planet is red' from 'Mars is red' and 'Mars is a planet' but we cannot infer this conclusion from 'something is red', and 'something is a planet'. The word 'everything' can pass both of these tests so Dummett adds a third requirement: the disjunction of 'a is P' and 'a is Q' must be inferrable from 'a is P or Q'.

Dummett claims that the criteria he has given can be applied to 'separate proper names from other substantial phrases plural or indefinite involving in one way or another the expression of generality'. Now this means that expressions of form 'every S' and 'some S' will fail his tests; this claim is obviously important to Dummett and we shall begin to examine it in the next paragraph. Dummett has emphasized the crucial importance for Frege of being able to apply these tests and presumably the two generalization tests and the test of distribution with respect to disjunction of predicates are intended to be practibly applicable. But while it is certainly true that 'a' cannot be a proper name unless 'something is P' follows from 'a is P', this is of little use to anyone who does not know whether 'a' is functioning as a proper name in the sentence. Surely he who is in doubt about the syntactical status of 'Mars' in 'Mars is a planet' ought not to be credited with an intuitive recognition of the validity of the inference to 'something is a planet'. More generally, it is very doubtful that an inference pattern like existential generalization has a more primitive status in intuition than the ability to recognize proper names.

It is, nonetheless, true that existential generalization formally imposes a necessary condition on proper namehood; according to Dummett, this works to exclude expressions of form 'some S' and 'every S' from the class of proper names. Since we are not convinced that this is what happens, we shall put the matter in the form of a question: Is it in fact the case that existential generalization favours one or the other side of the controversy concerning the syntactical form of a subject consisting of a proper name? To this question the answer is yes; for it favours the *traditional* view that a proper name in subject position has an implicit sign of quantity.

This is so because existential generalization is for the Fregean a primitive rule of inference whose validity is left to the intuitive level. Not so for the Leibnizian: *he* can show that 'something is a planet' follows *syllogistically* from 'Mars is a planet'. The argument in question has a truistic tacit premiss 'Mars is a thing'. We then have:

(every/some) Mars is a planet
(some/every) Mars is a thing

so some thing is a planet

Thus the view that 'Mars' in subject position is an expression of form 'every S' or 'some S' explains why 'something is a planet' follows from 'Mars is a planet'. But if Frege is right, the subject of 'Mars is a planet' is syntactically simple and we can do no better than invoke a primitive principle of inference as an 'explanation'. Similar considerations apply to Dummett's second generalization requirement for proper names. The inference from 'Mars is a planet and Mars is red' to 'some planet is red' is syllogistic if we recognize the (wild) quantity of 'Mars is . . .' and there is no need to add primitive principle of existential generalization to our logic in order to account for inferences like these.

In any case, generalization does not single out singular subjects as the only genuine logical subjects. For 'existential generalization' works also in cases where the premisses are general: the inference to 'something is a planet' from 'some physical bodies are planets' has the same form as the inference 'something is a planet' from '(some) Mars is a planet'. The first inference can be validated by the addition of 'every physical body is a thing', the second by the addition of 'every Mars is a thing'.

The third requirement that 'a is P or a is Q' follows from 'a is P or A' is treated by Geach and Dummett as a primitive logical fact peculiar to singular subjects. We have already seen that this is not so. The equivalence of 'a is P or Q' and 'a is P or a is Q' falls under the general rule for particular propositions: some S is P or Q = some S is P or some S is Q. The principle holds for general as well as singular terms.

To sum up: Dummett's conditions have little to do with proper names in Dummett's sense and much to do with logical subjects in general. It is indeed the case that singular subjects have logical powers that set them apart from logical subjects of fixed quantity. But all the differences can be explained by the single hypothesis of the doubly quantified definite subject. Far from being a primitive subject without a sign of generality, the definite singular subject is saturated with quantity. This is the conception of a proper name in subject position that is attested to by the satisfaction of Dummett's requirements.

6. The need for criteria for an expression being a logical subject is critical for modern predicate logic (MPL) but has no parallel in traditional formal logic (TFL). The latter counts as a logical subject any expression of form 'some X' or 'every X', but the former offers no such simple linguistic clue for distinguishing its logical subjects. Since the logical subjects of the basic sentences of MPL are proper names, Dummett's project of formulating criteria for proper names is wholly appropriate and necessary. Proper names are 'object words' but one cannot rely on an independently determined class of objects to determine the class of proper names. For, according to Dummett, 'for Frege the application of the ontological category term "object" is dependent upon the linguistic category term "proper name" and not conversely'. Although Dummett wrongly believes that he has already ruled out 'some X' and 'every X' from the class of logical subjects, he goes further in the direction of ruling out other expressions that are not proper names but which seem to him to pass the tests for proper namehood that we have been discussing. One expression that is not ruled out by any of the aforementioned tests is 'wise' in 'Socrates is wise'. It might appear that we need not worry about predicate terms like this for surely in 'Socrates is wise' the term 'wise' does not locate what the proposition is about. Here Dummett reminds us of Ramsey's observation that 'Socrates is wise' *could* be about wisdom. For we might understand the proposition to say something about what Socrates is (viz., wise) and then 'wise' would locate what the proposition is about. Dummett is right in seeing Ramsey as a threat to Frege's analysis of 'Socrates is wise' as being about the thing named by its object word and not about the thing referred to by its concept word. Ramsey's point was made in objection to Russell's use of standard subject-predicate analysis to support the distinction between a particular like Socrates and a universal like wisdom. Ramsey would similarly object to exploiting the standard analysis as a way of discriminating objects from concepts. It would, however, be a mistake to confine the significance of Ramsey's argument to criticism of these ontological distinctions. For he is making a general claim that the grammatical subjects of a sentence are never a sure guide to what the sentence is being used to talk about. And this point is valid for general sentences as well. Thus 'a creature did stir' may be about a creature or about what a creature did depending on how we cut it:

a creature/ did stir
a creature did/ stir

If Ramsey is right, the correlation of a predicate and a subject with what we say and what we talk about is always arbitrary. Now this suggestion is tolerable to TFL which does not discriminate subject from predicate on semantic grounds. But it cannot be acceptable to the Fregean who must think of the logical subject as the referring expression and the logical predicate as the characterizing expression. So Ramsey must be answered, for 'wise' cannot be permitted to locate the subject matter of the proposition.

It is here that Dummett appeals to Aristotle's doctrine of contrariety, pointing out that predicates, unlike subjects, come in contrary pairs:

For any predicate there is another predicate which is true of just those objects of which the original predicate is false, and false of just those objects of which the original predicate is true. This is therefore the simplest case of the formation of a complex predicate: if 'Fx' is a predicate then 'It is not the case that Fx' is likewise a predicate . . . To say that an object does not have a contrary is to say that, in general, we cannot assume that, given any object, there is another object of which just those predicates are true which were false of the original object, and conversely. We may put this in terms of the legitimacy or otherwise of certain forms of definition . . . Given the predicate 'wise' we may introduce a new predicate 'foolish' by stipulating that, for every proper name 'a', 'a is foolish' is to have the same truth value as 'it is not the case that a is wise'; but we cannot, given the name 'Socrates,' legitimately introduce a new name, say 'Nonsocrates' by the stipulation that for every predicate 'Fx,' 'F(Nonsocrates)' is to have the same truth value as it is not the case that 'F(Socrates)' —however severely we restrict the range of predicates to which this stipulation is to be applied.[15]

I have quoted Dummett at some length because one finds variants of this way of dealing with Ramsey in other British Fregeans, notably Strawson and Geach. And if we waive the question begging assumptions implicit in Dummett's analysis of 'Socrates is wise' as an atomic sentence with a syntactically simple subject, the answer seems plausible as a way of justifying the radical distinction of subject and predicate. For in a standard language of MPL, predicates like 'is wise' and 'is unwise' are used in contradictory sentences whose subject is the same but subject expressions like 'Socrates' are not opposed to other subject expressions like 'non-Socrates' for use in contradictory sentences with the same predicate. But even if we grant this and proceed on purely Fregean grounds, Dummett's argument is open to a fatal objection. In MPL, negation is always sentential in scope and a predicate like 'is unwise' is not an expression in its own right. Dummett quotes Aristotle to the

15 Dummett, *Frege*, pp. 63–4.

effect that predicates have contraries but subjects do not. But the idea of predicate contrariety belongs to Aristotle and is foreign to Frege. Dummett's version of a predicate that is contrary to '. . . x . . .' is '− . . . x . . .' Now this doctrine is Fregean but it has little to do with Aristotle's. If '. . . x . . .' and '− . . . x . . .' are contrary predicates, then there is nothing to stop us from forming a contrary pair of subjects ' . . . F . . .' and '− . . . F . . .' But then there is no difference at all between subject and predicate that could distinguish them in the manner required by Dummett, Geach and Strawson. What Dummett, Geach and Strawson *need* is an opposition that is peculiar to the predicate and inapplicable to the subject. What they *have* is sentential negation which can be applied to both. Strictly speaking, the word 'not' applies to *neither* the subject *nor* the predicate. And strictly speaking, one cannot talk of contrary predicates in the system of MPL. Of course, we may define 'unwise' or 'foolish' as 'contrary' to 'wise'. But the consistent and careful Fregean (Quine is one) knows better than to talk of negative terms; coming across 'unwise' he notes that the negative particle does not really belong to the predicate and gives it its proper sentential scope. It must again be emphasized that just as the subject of the atomic sentence is without quantity so is the predicate without quality. And where there is a negative particle, its proper scope is always sentential and the sentence is non-atomic. So if we define 'x is foolish' as 'not x is wise' then 'Socrates is foolish' is a molecular sentence, a stylistic variant of 'not Socrates is wise'. It should not be thought that Frege's talk of negative predicates compromises this matter. Frege is explicit about prohibiting any notion of contrariety that is not derivative and reducible to sentence negation. And when he talks about negating a sentence by negating its predicate, he should be understood *literally*; one *way* of negating 'Socrates is wise' is by inserting the sign of propositional negation (and there is no other kind of negation sign in Frege) in the predicate. Another *way* is to prefix the negation sign to 'Socrates is wise'. Both are ways of negating the sentence. And negation in both is propositional. There is, in fact, no reason why one could not have another style of negating a sentence. For just as we define 'Socrates is foolish' as a negation of 'Socrates is wise' so too could we define 'non-Socrates is wise' as a negation of 'Socrates is wise'. We should then have another way of expressing negation. Of course, we do not do so in practice. That we do not is a problem for the Fregean. For why should we not do so?

One who believes that predicates come in contrary pairs, while subjects do not, must recognize a style of negation peculiar to predicates, one that is not reducible to negation. But this is precisely what Frege warns against in his late paper 'Negation'. For negation is a truth function and has no place inside the proposition, not in the subject and not in the predicate. In brief, Dummett's Aristotelianism would not be tolerated by Frege. And Strawson's thesis of an asymmetry of subject and predicate with respect to negation would similarly be rejected by Frege. If the differential use of negation as a way of rationalizing the distinction between subject and predicate is un-Fregean, then we are forced to the conclusion that Frege himself thought of the distinction in ontological terms. I suspect that Geach's interpretation of Frege's view of object and concept words as determined by the ontological distinction between object and concept is more faithful to Frege than is Dummett's contrary view. If that is correct, then Frege would not have viewed with sympathy Dummett's attempt to find independent linguistic criteria for proper names. But one must agree with Dummett that an ontologically independent grounding of the subject–predicate distinction is untenable.[16]

Finally, it should be remarked that Ramsey remains unanswered. Moreover, he would remain so even if we allowed the British Fregeans their illicit flirtation with Aristotle. Ramsey suggested that we could read 'Socrates is wise' with the

---

[16] The connection between the thesis of atomicity and the modern theory of negation in which the traditional oppositions of term contrariety and propositional contractoriness are absorbed in the truth function analysis is not hard to trace. Begin with propositions that have no logico-syntactical parts and construct new propositions by adding logical operators on these atomic forms and which serve to combine them with one another. It is then evident that what the traditional logician looked upon as term contrariety is really to be understood as a truth functional propositional opposition. Since all opposition is truth functional it is also evident that opposed forms cannot both be atomic. The characteristic absence, in modern logical theory, of contrariety as a distinct form of correlative opposition is responsible for a number of distinctively modern problems some of which are discussed below in chapters 13 and 14. Here it is important to see how the move away from the traditional oppositions is related to the thesis that the most elementary propositions are atomic.

copula to the left ('Socrates is/wise') in which case it is about what Socrates is and not about Socrates. If we allow this reading, then it would not matter that predicate terms have contraries but subject terms do not. To see why, consider the following two pairs of contradictories:

(A1) Socrates/is wise   (B1) Socrates is/wise
(A2) Socrates/isn't wise   (B2) Socrates isn't/wise

(B1) is about what Socrates is. But then (B2) is about what Socrates isn't! Both are about wisdom, (B1) claiming that Socrates has it, (B2) claiming that Socrates hasn't got it. Note that the presumed inability to get a contradiction by defining terms like 'non-Socrates' is irrelevant to the challenge offered by the B-readings to the assumption that an atomic proposition is about the object named by its object word.

7. I have, in this chapter, examined and rejected a number of apologetic arguments for the radical distinction between the parts of the atomic proposition. If successful, these arguments would justify the Fregean prohibition against forming a predicate whose term is a proper name; if 'Socrates' is a proper name, it is a logical subject and 'is Socrates' cannot be a (monadic) predicate on a par with 'is wise'. The last such argument that I shall examine has recently been given by Strawson. It is, he says, suggested by the schemata for atomic sentences which exhibit a progression starting with monadic and dyadic forms and going on to the predications of higher 'adicity':

Sentences exemplifying these schemata may contain more than one subject term but only one predicate term. So the subject terms are distinguished from the predicate terms by the fact that more than one of them may appear in some forms of such sentences. Our knowledge of the grammar of syntax of logical languages enables us to say more than this. Any term functioning as a predicate term is restricted as regards to its appearance in a complete sentence to just one of the listed forms; it is restricted to a form with just *one* place for the subject-term *or* to a form with just *two* places *or* to a form with just *three* places . . . and so on. But no subject-term is so restricted. One and the same subject-term may appear in a form with any number of subject places.[17]

[17] P. F. Strawson, *Subject and Predicate in Logic and Grammar* (Methuen, 1974), p. 4. Hereafter referred to as *SPLG*.

Strawson here observes that while a dyadic expression like 'father of' can only appear as predicate term in sentences with two subjects, 'Socrates' can appear as subject-term in sentences of any 'adicity'. Here then we have a significant difference between subject and predicate terms. Predicate terms have 'adicity', subject terms do not.

In evaluating this argument for the radical difference between subject expressions and predicate expressions of the basic sentences of a logical language, we must again guard against an appeal to 'facts' that are mere epiphenomena of the thesis on behalf of which the appeal is made. If Strawson's adicity argument is meant to show that an alternative analysis of the basic sentences which is free of the strictures of the syntax of MPL is implausible, it sadly fails. If, on the other hand, it is merely brought to exhibit some of the features peculiar to Fregean syntax and to show how these attest to the assumption that subject and predicate expressions of atomic sentences are radically distinct then it ought not to be taken as an argument for the difference that Strawson is anxious to justify between terms like 'Socrates' and expressions like 'wise' or 'wiser than.'

To get clear of parochial assumptions, we will again contrast the Fregean standpoint with the standpoint of traditional formal logic (TFL). A term of TFL is an expression X or Y in a proposition 'some/every X is Y'. Thus 'Socrates' and 'wise' are terms but 'father of' and 'between' are not terms. *A fortiori*, these latter expressions are not predicate terms. Instead TFL regards them as relational expressions that enter into terms. The rules for forming sentences in TFL allow for the incorporation of relational expressions in terms in the following way. If R is an n-place relational expression and $X_1, \ldots, X_{n-1}$, are terms, then 'R to some/every $X_1, \ldots,$ some/every X_{n-1}' is a term.[18] A term that contains a relational expression may be called a relational term (which is not to say that the relational expression is itself a term; it is not). Examples of sentences with relational terms are:

every *tail of a horse* is a *tail of an animal*
Socrates was *acquainted with Gorgias*
the action was *urged on Tom by everyone*.

[18] The formation rules for TFL are given below in chapter 9.

The TFL analysis recognizes 'adicity' in relational expressions but it distinguishes these from (predicate) terms. In the basic sentences of TFL, there is one subject and one predicate. Thus the predicate of 'some sailor gave every child a toy' is 'gave every child a toy', and the subject of this proposition is 'some sailor'. The subject expressions inside the predicate need not be thought of as subjects of the sentence. Instead the term 'one who gave every child a toy' is on all fours with 'sailor' as an expression that may serve as a subject or·predicate term of a sentence. Similarly, 'Gorgias' need not be treated as a subject of 'Socrates was acquainted with Gorgias' although it is the subject of 'Gorgias was an acquaintance of Socrates'. This is not incompatible with the observation made by Ramsey that the subject of a proposition does not necessarily locate what that proposition is about. The observation may in fact be generalized for the n-adic case: an n-adic proposition (i.e., one whose predicate term begins with an n-adic relational expression) can be read in $n + 1$ ways corresponding to $n + 1$ different things it could be about. For example, 'Pythagoras/did/lecture on/politics' could be read as being about Pythagoras, about what he did, or about politics. But only the first way corresponds to the subject of the proposition. In thus dissociating what a proposition is about from its logical subject, Ramsey's point is therapeutic in its effect. For it here challenges the doctrine that the only proper analysis is one that takes 'Pythagoras' and 'politics' to be the object words locating the subject matter and 'lectured on' to be the concept word or predicate that is said to hold of the ordered pair {Pythagoras, politics}.

In TFL the form of a dyadic sentence is 'some/every X is R to some/every Y'. The terms X and Y will, in the simplest case be themselves non-relational. There could be singular terms like 'Socrates' or general terms like 'philosopher' and TFL provides no evidence for restricting 'Socrates' to subject position. Strawson's appeal to the evidence provided by the syntax of MPL is merely self-serving. In MPL, the assymmetry between individual symbols and predicate letters is written into the formation rules and any evidence of asymmetry that assumes the canonical status of the forms of MPL must be dismissed as planted evidence.

This latest argument, by Strawson, like those that preceded it, by Geach and by Dummett, is characterized by the same inadmissible technique. The traditional rival is simply ignored and all efforts are apologetic attempts to explain the form of a basic proposition assumed to have no logical elements. The fact that philosophers of the calibre of Strawson and Dummett are enmeshed in the same question-begging procedures is proof, if any were needed, of the hold of the doctrine of atomicity on contemporary logical theory. I have said nothing of the profound influence of the doctrine of atomicity on other areas of philosophy. The *Tractatus* Wittgenstein is only one example of a major philosopher in the thrall of its dogmatic embrace.

8. In this chapter I have been concerned to show that the thesis of atomicity *is* a dogma. But dogmas are not necessarily false and the thesis of atomicity is subject to confirmation or disconfirmation in a developed linguistic science. The subordinate thesis of MPL that 'a wise man' does not belong with 'Socrates' but belongs rather to a class of expressions that includes 'taller than', 'donor of . . . to . . .' and other expressions of higher 'adicity' is equally subject to evaluation by the linguist. To date, linguistics by and large has conservatively stayed with the standpoint of traditional formal logic in treating 'Socrates' and 'a wise man' as expressions of the same grammatical equivalence class. Also TFL begins the series of n-adic expressions with n = 2; like the grammarian TFL does not consider 'a wise man' to belong to the same class as 'taller than' since the former but not the latter is a noun phrase that can serve as a subject. Nevertheless, at the present stage, the linguistic evidence is perhaps not decisive; it may be that this science is at an initial stage of development and one must allow for the possibility of a shift that could favour the logical syntax of MPL over TFL. The question is, moreover, not purely one of linguistic evidence for one thesis over its rival because the line of linguistic development is itself influenced by the logic that linguists take to be canonical. In constructing a theory of deep structure or in taking a position of the relations of syntax to semantics, the linguist is sensitive to what the logician tells him about logical form. One may hope and expect that the linguists will do some shopping for more options than are now on the market. And one of the purposes of the present essay is to offer TFL as a respectable alternative to the popular product now on the shelves.

3
Indefinite Reference

1. We have criticized a number of arguments for rejecting the traditional view that 'some S' and 'every S' are genuine logical subjects, arguments that exploit the disanalogies between the logical powers of 'a is P' and 'some S is P' (or 'every S is P'). Often the logical disanalogies are accompanied by a semantic appeal, contrasting the referential character of 'a' with the non-referential character of 'some S'. David Kaplan makes such an appeal. Arguing against those who might think of 'a is P' and 'some S is P' as having the same logical form he says:

> You can quickly disabuse yourself (of this idea) by comparing (1) a senator from New York is supporting Rockefeller and a senator from New York is not supporting Rockefeller; and (2) Jacob Javitz is supporting Rockefeller and Jacob Javitz is not supporting Rockefeller.
>
> (2) is a contradiction but (1) is true. In fact isn't it obvious that indefinite descriptions do not even purport to denote a unique object as names do? Accordingly Russel's theory of indefinite descriptions asserts that the logical form of a paradigm sentence like 'a such and such is so and so' is represented by an equivalent sentence 'something is both a such and such and a so and so' . . . Although grammatically, at least from the point of view of what is now called surface grammar, indefinite descriptions are terms and function like proper names, sentences that contain indefinite descriptions and appear to have subject predicate form should be treated as idioms and expanded as in the paradigm. Russell's theory of indefinite descriptions seems to me to be both correct and natural.[1]

Kaplan's point that 'a such and such' does not purport to denote a unique object, denies to it even unsuccessful reference.

---

[1] David Kaplan, 'What is Russell's Theory of Descriptions?', in *Physics, Logic and History*, ed. Wolfgang Yourgrau and Allen D. Breck (New York, Plenum Press, 1970), p. 280.

For it is sometimes said that a definite description like 'the present king of France' fails to refer. But the trouble with thinking of 'some S' as a referring expression is not only that there may be no S's but that 'some S' is not an expression whose role is to pick out an object by definitely describing it or naming it. Keith Donnellan thinks that Russell denied genuine referentiality even to definite descriptions:

Russell thought, I believe, that whenever we use descriptions as opposed to proper names, we introduce an element of generality which ought to be absent if what we are doing is referring to some particular thing . . . One of the conclusions we aré supposed to draw . . . is that such sentences (containing definite descriptions) express what are in reality completely general propositions . . . If there is anything which might be identified as reference here, it is reference in a very weak sense—namely reference to *whatever* is the one and only one, if there is any such. Now this is something we might well say about the attributive use of definite descriptions . . . But this lack of particularity is absent for the referential use of definite descriptions precisely because the description is here merely a device for getting one's audience to pick out or think of the thing to be spoken about, a device which may serve its referential use as opposed to the attributive, there is a *right* thing to be picked out and its being the right thing is not simply a function of its fitting the description.[2]

The qualification 'if there is any such' is sensitive to the consideration that a referring expression that fails to refer is still a referring expression. In the case where we do not, by hypothesis, have a genuine referential use, in Donnellan's sense, we may still have an identification of a single object. So Donnellan concedes a weak sense of reference.

It is important to be clear about the conditions for genuine reference and more particularly within the framework of a Fregean philosophy of language. The logical subjects of atomic propositions are distinguished by their semantic role of referring and anyone who mistakes a non-referring expression for a referring one is in danger of taking a non-atomic proposition for an atomic one. The danger is considerable: much depends on our presumed ability to distinguish the class of atomic propositions. Dummett, for example, holds that the

---

[2] Keith Donnellan, 'Reference and Definite Descriptions', in *Naming, Necessity, and Natural Kinds*, ed. S.P. Schwartz (Cornell University Press, 1977), p. 65.

class of logical words is distinguished by non-appearance in atomic propositions from the class of extra-logical words. And philosophers like Russell and Wittgenstein relied on their ability to discriminate the class of atomic propositions for certain of their metaphysical views. The role of a paradigm of genuine reference is not as central in a philosophy of language developed along traditional lines; first because the logical subjects of TFL are syntactically discriminated and second because the distinctions crucial to MPL between subject expressions like 'Socrates' and 'denoting phrases' like 'a senator' are not crucial in TFL. It is, therefore, natural to tolerate a sense of reference that would not be tolerated by the Fregeans. For if both 'Socrates' and 'a senator' have the form 'some S' then we will *generally* say that 'some S' refers to an S. And perhaps it may be acknowledged that only those who think of reference in a tendentiously Fregean way will find anything really odd about this. In any case, *we* shall not assume that the paradigm of reference is to be found in the role of individual constants of atomic sentences. Instead we shall want to tolerate a sense of reference that is even weaker than the one conceded by Donnellan to 'the S'. For we shall want to allow that 'a senator' genuinely refers in 'a senator is on the phone' and we shall reject as arbitrary, the conditions imposed on reference by most contemporary philosophers of language. There is, after all, nothing unnatural in saying that 'an S' in 'an S is P' refers to an S. This non-identifying kind of reference or 'supposition' is allowed for by Russell when he calls 'some S' a denoting phrase and it was extensively analysed by scholastic philosophers.

The idea of a reference to some S by a subject expression 'some S' is a ground of the distinction, made by pre-Fregean logicians, between distributed and undistributed occurrences of the subject terms of categorical propositions. Attending simply to the denotation of the subject term 'S' we may say that both 'some S is P' and 'every S is P' are about all of the S's. But the particular proposition says of the S's that some of them are P and its subject is said to refer to some and not necessarily to all of the S's; in contrast, the universal proposition says of the S's that all of them are P and its subject is said to refer to all of the S's. In 'some S is P' the reference of the subject is not coincident with the donotation of the subject term and the subject term is said to be undistributed; in 'every S is P' the reference of the subject is coincident with the denotation of the subject term and the term is said to be distributed.

In attending to indefinite reference one must keep clear of the notion of referring appropriate to the role of the subjects of the atomic proposition. In the atomic proposition the subject is complete in the sense that it does its job of referring in independence of the predicate. One may reasonably regard the semantic roles of the subject and predicate of the simplest atomic propositions as being enacted one after the other: the subject first refers to an object that may or not be P; the predicate 'is P' then characterizes the object referred to by the subject. For 'some S is P' this picture may be altogether inappropriate: one cannot coherently think of 'some man' in 'some man will land on Mars in the eighties' as referring to a man that may or may not land on Mars in the eighties followed by the predicate which characterizes the man in question as landing on Mars in the eighties. Rather one must think of 'some S' in 'some S is P' as referring to an S that is P so that the subject is understood to refer to the kind of thing specified by the predicate. It helps here to keep in mind Aristotle's way of formulating the truth conditions of the categorical proposition in its relation to the reference of its subject:

Saying of what is (P) that it is (P) is (saying what is) true.

If we may apply this to a particular proposition, one who says that some S is P has said what is true only if he has said of an S-that-is-P *that* it is P. This takes seriously the idea that only in the context of the whole proposition may we speak of the reference of its subject since the predicate enters essentially into the specification of its reference. It would perhaps be better to avoid talk of reference by the subject and to speak instead of a reference to an S that is P by the whole proposition. But this matter is partly one of terminological preference and tradition is on the side of associating reference with the subject expression. Moreover there is the consideration that the subject contains the term that focuses on the sort of thing the proposition is about: it is about S's and says of all or some of them that they are P. Since it is the subject term that serves to present a class of things concerning which a truth claim is being made it is not unnatural to speak of the subject as referring to some or all of the things that satisfy the truth claim. And perhaps only those who think that genuine reference belongs exclusively to the subjects of atomic propositions will continue to insist that there is something essentially misleading about characterizing the reference of 'some S' as a reference to certain things that could make 'some S is P' true.

That we cannot think of a reference to some S as other than a reference to such S as are P may also be seen from the following argument. Suppose that 'some S' refers to an S that may or may not be P and that we then think of the predicate as characterizing the S in question truly or falsely as the case may be. It is now open to us to suppose that the S referred to is not P and the predicate 'is P' will then not be true of the referent. Now this would mean that 'some S is P' could be false even if there happened to be an S that is P provided that no such S was referred to by 'some S'. We shall see that this is indeed so for certain contexts of utterance. But the truth condition for 'some S is P' is generally weaker than this; for 'some S is P' is very often true just in case *any* S is P. This being so 'some S', if it refers at all, refers to an S that is P. Back reference provides additional evidence for this. In most cases, where 'some S is P' is followed by 'it is also Q' the pronoun 'it' is equivalent to 'the S that is P' which indicates that what was referred to in the antecedent proposition is an S that is P.

The contemporary philosopher of language may find this doctrine somewhat paradoxical. For he holds that a referring expression identifies its referent in a manner that is independent of the predicate and so he tends to reject as anomalous a notion of reference that involves the predicate in a specification of the reference of the subject. We shall soon discuss Geach's argument that the predicate cannot be involved in this way. And one reason that Geach and other friends of MPL seem to be in a strong position comes to the fore when we consider the case where there are no S that are P. In that case one must surely say that 'some S is P' is false. But this appears to be inconsistent with saying that 'some S' has referred to an S that is P. For where there are no such S's there will be a failure to refer. And to most contemporary philosophers a failure to refer is tantamount to 'a truth-value gap'. If 'some S is P' is without truth value, it is not false, which contradicts our hypothesis that the dearth of S that are P renders 'some S is P' false.

I shall have more to say about the position of TFL on subjects that fail to refer. Here I am concerned to do no more than to urge the avoidance of current assumptions. If one is accustomed to think of logical subjects as 'object words' of atomic sentences then it is indeed natural to view them as semantically complete in their role of identifying expressions that present objects for characterization by the predicate of the sentence. It is then also natural to hold that a condition for a proposition having a truth value is that its logical subject refers to an object. We may call this the referring condition for having a truth value: unless its object word actually refers to objects the atomic sentence cannot be used to make a statement and one who utters the sentence is said not to have asserted a proposition. It is however clear that no such condition need govern the valuation of a sentence whose subject is indefinite. With the recognition that (the subject of) 'some S is P' purports to refer to an S that is P, comes the recognition that failure to refer to one is no worse than a failure to satisfy the truth conditions of the proposition. For where it is the case that no S is P and I say that some S is P I have not said of an S that is P that it is P so what I have said is false. I should here point out that Aristotle's well-known formulation of the falsity condition in Book IV of the *Metaphysics* (chapter 7) is stricter than this. That passage appears to be concerned with propositions that have (definite singular) non-vacuous subjects; for example, saying of Socrates who is wise that he is not wise is false. In other places however Aristotle is not loathe to assign falsity to propositions that have vacuous subjects. In chapter 10 of *Categories*, Book I, he maintains that 'Socrates is (un-) well' would be false if it were the case that Socrates did not exist.

It may serve to clear up certain misunderstandings to say something about the way I speak of reference and 'aboutness'. Success and failure to refer ranges over speech acts. I can neither succeed nor fail to refer to an S that is P without saying that an S is P. In saying that an S is a P I purport to refer to an S that is P and I can only purport to refer by saying that an S is a P. (To be silent is not to fail to refer; I cannot fail to refer unless I have purported to refer but have not succeeded to refer.) Reference is corrigible; I can fail to refer. On the other hand purporting to refer is an incorrigible speech act; having said that an S is P I cannot have failed to purport to refer to an S that is P. In this sense saying something *about* something is incorrigible. One may say that 'an S is P' is about an S that is P and *just mean* that it purports to refer to one. This use of 'about' is 'intentional' and incorrigible; what I say is about an S that is P whether one exists or not. Similarly when we say that 'some S' is about S's, we make use of an intentional sense of 'about'. Thus, purporting to refer and being about are not tied to truth conditions in the way that referring is.

We shall presently focus attention on another kind of reference that is independent of truth. If I mistake a rhinoceros in my garden for a unicorn in my garden then in saying that there is a unicorn in my garden I will not have succeeded to refer to what I have purported to refer. On the other hand, in one sense of referring, it can be said I have referred to the rhinoceros that I took to be a unicorn. This sense of 'epistemic' reference comes into play when my companion corrects me by pointing out that *it* ('what you referred to') is really a rhinoceros. Given the epistemic situation in which I have taken or mistaken something for an S, I can incorrigibly refer to it. Still this differs from being about; 'a unicorn is in the garden' is about unicorns or about a unicorn in the garden but in no sense of reference does it refer to a unicorn in the garden. Reference—even in this incorrigible sense—is to what exists.[3]

2. The notions of reference appropriate to 'some S is P' possess the first of two features that most contemporary philosophers of language require of genuine reference. But the second feature is missing and its possession will not be taken by us to be a condition of genuine reference. Typically it is stipulated that

   (i) Whatever is referred to must exist
   (ii) the utterance of a referring expression must (a) contain a

---

[3] Contrast 'it's a rhinoceros' with 'it's your imagination'. In the first but not the second 'it' refers to what you took to be a unicorn. The second has reference to the reason you made a mistake, not the object concerning which a mistake was made.

descriptive term uniquely true of the object referred to, (b) present the object demonstrably, or (c) provide some combination of demostrative presentation or description sufficient to identify it alone.

In the absence of an expression of the kind specified in (ii) the speaker must be prepared to substitute one of them on demand. This formulation of the conditions for successful reference is taken from Searle who calls them conditions of reference for singular definite referring expressions. Somewhat untypically, Searle is prepared to allow that expressions 'beginning with the indefinite article, such as "a man" as in "a man came" might be said to refer to a particular man' but his admission of a sense of referring for indefinite expressions is grudging:

There is a case for refusing to call such utterances instances of reference at all. I do not discuss the problem, as my present purpose is only to contrast singular definite referring expressions with other kinds of expressions.[4]

Searle sticks to that purpose; a sense of reference appropriate to indefinite subjects is never heard of again.

Geach is among those who are opposed to any serious sense of 'referring' for 'some S'. He, too, recognizes that many philosophers and linguists think it natural to say that 'a man' refers to a man. He is, therefore, concerned to 'rob this view of the simplicity and straightforwardness that makes it intuitively acceptable'.

. . . And what about 'some man'? Certainly this is not some man's name but it causes us no shock (many of us) if we read that at least in some of its uses this phrase refers to some man. If we turn from recent 'philosophical logic' to recent grammar, things are not much better . . . indeed Chomsky has expressly said that 'by and large the traditional views are correct as far as they go'. Proper names and phrases like 'some man' are alike called Noun Phrases—whatever virtues there may be in the capitals—and are regarded as belonging to the same substitution class.[5]

The interested reader will find details of Geach's criticism of

---

[4] John Searle, *Speech Acts* (Cambridge University Press, 1969), p. 27n. Hereafter referred to as *SA*.

[5] Geach, *LM*, pp. 115–16.

the idea of non-identificatory reference in chapter 3 of *Reference and Generality*.[6]

We feel the hankering after a looser sense of reference in Searle's remark that 'a man' might be taken to refer to a particular man. (Evidently Searle thinks that 'a man' does not do this actually.) And Geach takes the failure to identify a particular man to count against the idea that 'some man' is a genuine referring expression and he calls 'some S' and 'every S' quasi-referring expressions, constrasting them with proper names which he calls genuine referring expressions. I might, says Geach, say that a man has reached the top of Everest and not know who he is. In that case, I cannot be said to have referred to a particular man and if I haven't referred to a particular man I haven't referred at all. (If I *have* referred to someone, who—demands Geach—is he?) For Geach the paradigm logical subject is a proper name, or definite description, a paradigm he uses to impose an illegitimate requirement of identifiability of reference for 'some S'. For there is no presumption, in non-identifying reference, to be able to pick out the thing or things non-identifyingly referred to.

2.1 If we acknowledge a sense of reference for 'some S', we drop the usual identification requirements for reference; it is then but a small step to recognize a sense of genuine reference that does not require a reference to an S. I may, for example, credulously say that a ghost is making a noise in the attic and what I have said is false but although I fail to refer to what I purport to refer my actual reference is not necessarily vacuous or unsuccessful. For having said that a ghost made a noise, I might be told that it (the thing to which I referred by the referring phrase 'a ghost') was not a ghost but the upstairs maid or a cat. To be told this is to be told that *what I took to be a ghost* was not a ghost. Thus, the lack of a referent, as described by the referring phrase, prevents reference to a thing of that description but is no bar to reference to something that was taken to be a thing of that description. Let us call the kind of reference in which I take something to be so and so 'epistemic reference'.

---

[6] The topic of non-identificatory reference to some S is more fully dealt with below, chapter 5.

If we use '{S}' for whatever was taken for (or mistaken for) an S, then the existence condition for indefinite reference by 'some S' is weakened: what 'some S' epistemically refers to need not be an S; it need only be an {S}. For a reference can be made to what is taken for an S and if it should turn out that there are no S's, then the back-up epistemic reference to what was misdescribed as an S remains in force.

One who says that some S is P when in fact there are no S's will not have referred at all unless he has taken something to be an S in which case he will have referred to an {S}. He will, in any case, not have referred to an S that is P so what he has said in false. But the back up epistemic reference to an {S} is not tied to the truth conditions of the statement he has made. In this sense, epistemic reference is incorrigible.

It is not always open to us to say that the utterer of 'some S is P' has *made* an epistemic reference. One who hears a ghost-like noise is in the epistemic situation of taking something for something when he says that a ghost is in the attic.[7] But someone who says he is convinced that somewhere a ghost is in some attic is not taking anything to be ghost and his reference will succeed or fail with the success or failure of his truth claim. Similarly, while we attribute epistemic reference to one who chides us about a 'lady I saw you with last night' and may correct him with 'that was no lady, that was my wife', we cannot allow that a current utterer of 'Wilde admired some sententious ladies' has made an epistemic reference to anyone. For he will not by hypothesis have taken or mistaken anyone for a lady admired by Oscar Wilde, and he could make little sense of an objection to the effect that what he took for sententious ladies were really handsome young lords or Wilde's wives etc.

2.2 It may seem that indefinite reference is hardly worthy of the name and that even if we tolerate a use of 'reference' for it, it is not 'genuine', i.e., definite reference. I do not concede that

---

[7] Not everything is mistakable for a ghost. Thus one cannot mistake a theorem for a ghost and when someone says that a ghost is in the attic it is not possible for him to have epistemic reference to a theorem. Let |S| be the category of things that are or fail to be S's. Then being an |S| is a necessary condition for being an {S}. The relations of |S| and |P| for a theory of categories are explored by the author in a number of papers. See especially *Types and Ontology* and chapter 13 below.

definite reference is somehow more genuine than non-identify-ing reference. On the contrary, as I shall be arguing later, definite reference to an individual begins with and is semanti-cally dependent on an indefinite epistemic reference to that individual. If that is right, the fundamental form of reference is to be located in 'some S is P' and not in 'the S is P' or in 'a is P'. It is, therefore, important that the sense of reference which restricts it to definite reference be exposed as tendentious. It can hardly be doubted that talk of genuine reference to the exclusion of reference by 'some S' relies heavily on the assumption of atomicity according to which the only genuine logical subjects are the individual constants of the atomic propositions. When the Fregean is not allowed this assumption, his arguments against any sense of genuine reference for 'some S' are usually easy to dismiss. This will presently be illustrated when we consider some further objec-tions to allowing a sense of reference for 'some S'.

Expressions of form 'some S' are the primary referring expressions of traditional formal logic. But not all expressions of this form refer to an S or even purport to refer to one. When 'some S' purports to refer to some S, it occurs in a proposition a condition of whose truth is the existence of an S (in the domain under consideration). For example in 'I stepped on a snail', 'a snail' purports to refer to a snail; the existence of a snail is a truth condition of this proposition. The same expression does not play the role of a referring expression in 'no penguin has ever eaten a snail' or in 'I'd hate to step on a snail' since the existence of a snail is not a condition of truth for either of these propositions.

There are propositions whose truth conditions concern objects that may be thought of as members of some non-actual domain. If we use the term 'exists' in a way that permits us to say that a flying horse exists in the domain of Greek mythology, then we could modify the existential truth con-dition for purported reference to accommodate reference to such things. 'A flying horse was captured by Bellerophon' would then count as true and as actually (not merely 'purportedly') referring to a flying horse since its truth requires the existence of a flying horse in the realm of Greek myth and that condition happens to be satisfied. (Problems of reference to actual and non-actual things are discussed below in chapters 10 and 12.) To be allowed to speak of the existence of a thing in a non-actual domain is one thing. To say that in 'a ghost is in the attic' a ghost refers 'intentionally' to a ghost is another. Any proposition of form 'an S is P' specifies a state of affairs that obtains if the proposition is true and the state of affairs in question contains an S. One may say that 'a ghost' refers to a ghost in the state of affairs that would obtain if the proposition were true. This sense of intentional reference would make all reference incorrigibly successful. There would be no distinction between successfully referring and merely purporting to refer. I think that this sense of reference ought to be avoided; in any case, I shall avoid it. In the case of reference to flying horses, there could be failure. Thus, if I say that Bellerophon captured a flying kangaroo, there will be failure of reference since there is nothing like this in the realm of Greek mythology. So I think a sense of reference which preserves the distinction between actual and purported reference is to be preferred even if one wishes to allow reference to non-existent things. On the other hand, one may be permitted to use the word 'refers' loosely to cover 'purports to refer'. Thus the traditional logician often says that 'an S' refers to an S without bothering to specify that an S exists. In this usage, the friends of 'distribution' pointed out that S is undistributed in 'some S is P'; while 'S' denotes every S, 'some S' refers only to some S. I think that the license to use 'refers' in this loose way does little harm and I shall sometimes avail myself of it.

2.3 I have been urging that we withhold assent from the modern doctrine that 'a is P' and 'some S is P' differ in logical form. If we do so, the reference conditions for 'some S' can be applied in a manner that comprehends reference by '(some) a'. This suggests that, for purely logical concerns, we could altogether avoid recourse to the strong identificatory sense of reference. Speaking of reference in the strong identificatory sense, Searle makes an analogous point:

Reference is—in one sense of 'logical'—of no *logical* interest whatsoever. For each proposition containing a reference we can substitute an existential proposition which has the same truth conditions as the original. This, it seems to me, is the real discovery behind the theory of definite descriptions.[8]

Searle is here alluding to the theories of Russell and Quine who have shown how to analyse definite singular propositions as complex general propositions. We have seen that the traditional philosophers unencumbered by Fregean syntax can do this in another and simpler way by assigning wild quantity to 'a is P'. It is clear that whether with Frege we leave 'Socrates is mortal' as it stands, taking 'Socrates' as a simple name, or whether with Quine we reparse it as a general quantified proposition, with 'Socrates' as one of the predicates and with the uniqueness conditions that are a feature of Russell's theory of descriptions, or whether with Leibniz we read the proposition as a particular categorical proposition that entails its universal generalization, the circumstances under which the proposition is taken as true are the same. Leibniz, no less than Quine, holds that an adequate analysis of 'Socrates is mortal' as a general proposition will incorporate the pre-analytical truth conditions of the original 'unparsed' sentence. This is not to say that Quine or Russell could just as easily have taken a Leibnizian line in analysing singular propositions. For they remain committed to the syntax of atomic propositions even as they are programmatically replacing individual constants with bound individual variables. Despite this, the move to turn proper names into general terms is a move back to when logicians like Venn and Whately were teaching students how to put 'Socrates is a man' into a first figure syllogism, and back further to when Leibniz could make his almost incidental remark that 'the Apostle Peter is a writer' should be construed as a doubly general proposition. On the traditional view, all elementary propositions are general in form, and reference is primarily a function of subjects of form 'some S'.[9] When Quine

---

[8] Searle, *SA*, p. 94.

[9] We shall argue below (chapters 13, 14) that propositions of form 'every S is/isn't P' are defined by propositions of form 'not: some S isn't/is P' so that the so-called universal proposition begining with 'every S' are not primitive forms on a par with propositions beginning with 'some S'. There is a good reason to hold that reference by 'some S' is *primary* reference and that the sense in which we speak of 'every S' as a referring expression is secondary or derivative. For the present we nominally defer to tradition in treating 'every S' as a referring expression on a par with 'some S'. See chapter 13.

traces the source of reference to the existential quantifier, which binds the individual variables, he too is well within the Scholastic tradition which sees in 'some S' or 'something' the vehicle of determinate (albeit non-identificatory) *suppositio*.

3. In saying that 'some S' refers to some S, we speak of referring in a way that distinguishes it from denoting (although not from the way that Russell used the term in speaking of denoting phrases). We shall say that the *term* 'S' denotes the things in its extension. The word 'refers' has been reserved for the whole subject. In the case of 'some S' the reference and the denotation differ: 'some S' doesn't refer to every S but 'S' denotes every S. In the case of 'every S' we do have a coincidence of reference and denotation; 'every S' refers to all the things that 'S' denotes.

We have noted that the distinction between reference by the subject and denotation by the subject term was used by traditional logicians for explaining the difference between distributed and undistributed terms. The latter difference was already known independently because of its role in conditions of validity for syllogistic arguments. But the traditional logician saw a convenient way to explain the distinction for terms in subject position; a term in subject position was distributed just in case its denotation coincided with the reference of the subject and undistributed just in case its denotation did not coincide with the reference of the subject. In the case of singular subjects, the principle of tolerance continues to hold: the subject term is distributed or undistributed depending on the quantity we assign to the subject.

The assignment of distribution value to terms (including singular terms) presupposes the syntactical complexity of the logical subject. Frege's logical subjects are syntactically simple and so leave no room for a distinction between the reference of the 'whole' subject and the denotation of the subject term. Because the distinction between the reference of a subject and denotation of a subject term has no meaning in Frege's syntax, one may expect that a benighted Fregean like Geach will accuse the traditional theory of using an 'incoherent' distinction to explain the doctrine of distribution. And indeed this is the ground from which Geach launches his attack on the traditional doctrine of distribution.[10] Geach does not see that the distinction is only incoherent to those who hold that logical subjects are syntactically simple. I have criticized Geach for this elsewhere and shall not pause to do so here. My present concern is with Geach's criticisms as they bear directly on the thesis that 'some S' is a genuine referring expression. The following one is fairly thematic. Geach has just said that there is no meaning to referring apart from denoting. He goes on to say:

Even if we knew what 'referring' was, how could we say that 'some man' refers to some man. The question at once arises: who can be the man or men reffered to? When I say 'some men are P,' does the subject-term refer to just such men as the predicate term is true of? But then which men will the subject-term refer to if a predication of this sort is false? . . . If in the sentence represented by 'some men are P' the subject-term is meant to refer to some men, but fails to do so—then the sentence does not convey a false statement about some men, which contradicts our hypothesis.[11]

Geach here is dealing with a case where 'some man is P' is not uttered with reference to a given man that the speaker has in mind. Tacitly appealing to the paradigm of identificatory reference by a definite subject he argues that a reference by 'some man' to a man is conditional on the ability to give an informative answer to the question 'who can the man in question be?' Elsewhere Geach insists that even in an epistemic context of utterance, where the speaker has a certain man in mind, the speaker's reference cannot be pinned to that man since the truth conditions of 'some man is P' may be satisfied by *any* man that is P. In the non-epistemic context of utterance Geach's position seems stronger and it may appear that his demand for an identification of the man is not unreasonable. Moreover Geach rejects the view that the man in question referred to by 'some man' may be specified, if not identified, as the man that 'is P' is true of. That is Geach rejects the view we attributed to Aristotle in interpreting his formulation of the truth conditions of a predication '. . . is P' to say what is true is to refer to a thing that is P and say of it *that* it is P. Essentially,

---

[10] See *R & G*, chap. 1.
[11] Geach, *R & G*, p. 6.

he rejects this view because of the danger of failing to satisfy the condition that the right sort of thing be there so that we may refer to it in an identifying way, a condition we have seen to be more appropriate to Frege's names.

Taking 'some men are P', Geach's question is 'who can the men referred to be?' We have argued that an informative answer to this question need not be forthcoming. When Geach asks 'who can the men referred to be?', he must make use of the pronominal phrase 'the men' which is replaceable by 'they': who can they be, these men? So Geach's question concedes a sense of reference to 'some men'. It is, of course, legitimate for Geach or anyone else to want *more information* about the things or persons referred to in a proposition. An inability to supply this information should not be regarded as impugning the reference.

The determinateness of the reference of an indefinite referring expression of the form 'some S' need not be a matter of dispute between the traditionalists who grant 'some S' the status of logical subject and contemporaries who hold that predication can only take place between a definite singular term and a predicate. 'Predicates and singular terms are what predication joins'. The remark is Quine's. But so is the following:

'It' [is] a definite singular term whether its antecedent is or not. 'He', 'she', and 'it' are definite singular terms on a par with 'that lion' and 'the lion' . . . . The three compound sentences 'I saw a lion and you saw that lion', 'I saw a lion and you saw the lion', and 'I saw a lion and you saw it' are interchangeable. Such use of a definite singular term dependently upon an indefinite antecedent . . . makes no distinction between a prounoun such as 'it' and a singular description such as 'the lion'.[12]

This much, then, all can agree on. The indefinite expression 'a man' has a definite pronominalization: 'a man' pronominalizes as 'the man' or as 'he'. And it is merely tendentious to deny reference by 'a man' because neither 'a man' nor 'he' is an identifying expression. It is evident that Geach believes that a quantificationalist analysis avoids the idea of indefinite

---

[12] Quine, *WO*, p. 113.

reference. Perhaps, on some interpretations of the quantifier, it does. But Geach applauds Quine's idea that the binding of a variable in quantification is similar to the pronominalization that occurs in the move from 'someone' to 'he', or from 'something' to 'that thing' ('it'). Admittedly, the pronoun does not refer in an identifying way. For Quine, however, pronominal reference, based on the indefinite and non-identifying reference of the quantifier antecedent, is primary reference. The referential role of even proper names is to be understood in terms of pronominalization. Thus Quine says: 'what distinguishes a name is that it can stand coherently in place of a variable'. Or again—speaking of the atomic form 'Fa'—Quine says: 'our recognition of an "a" part . . . turns strictly on our use of variables in quantification'.

4. Scholastic philosophers aptly characterized the reference or *suppositio* of 'some S' as determinate. We have seen that the determinate character of 'some S' may be understood in terms of the license we have to refer to the S in question forming expressions like 'that S', 'the S', or 'it'. Further evidence of the potential determinateness of 'some S' is provided by the fact that we can infer 'a is P' from 'some S is P' where 'a' is a definite singular term, a non-identifying name that we have adopted for one of the S's referred to by 'some S'. (It should go without saying that the question 'who (what) is a?' is out of place.) Pronominalization and instantiation alike provide good hindsight into the determinate *suppositio* of 'some S'.

The really interesting question raised by pronominalization is *how* the pronoun achieves definite (albeit non-identifying) reference to the thing or things indefinitely referred to by the antecedent. For most contemporary philosophers the relation between an antecedent and a relative pronoun is understood in terms of an operator and the variable it binds. But the apparatus of quantifiers and variables belongs to the syntax of modern predicate logic. More specifically, a pronoun concenived of as a bound variable has the syntactic simplicity that fits it for its role in atomic sentences. None of this can figure in a traditional account of pronouns. So we face the questions for traditional logic: what are pronouns and how do they work?

Clearly, any viable theory of logical syntax must be able to answer these questions. We shall see (in chapter 5) that the two term theory is in this respect viable and that a traditional account of pronouns has certain advantages over the bound variable account.

4

Pronominalization

1. The logical syntax of TFL assigns quantities to all subject expressions. This gives our first insight into pronouns: a pronominal subject is an expression consisting of a sign of quantity and a term. The term of the pronominal subject will be called the proterm. The word 'pronoun' is ambiguous and we shall use it ambiguously. 'Pronoun' sometimes signifies the proterm of the pronominal subject; more often it signifies the whole subject including its sign of quantity. The traditional theory of pronouns views them as syntactically complex. I shall refer to this theory as the proterm theory to contrast it with the currently popular theory that pronouns are syntactically simple subject expressions (individual variables) bound by antecedent quantifiers.

For further insight into pronouns we inquire into the denotations of their proterms and into their quantities. Quite generally the proterm of a pronoun is designed to denote what was antecedently referred to. In this sense the pronoun is semantically bound to the antecedent sentence. But a syntactic binding is unnecessary and in this respect the proterm theory differs from the bound variable theory. It differs as well in accommodating different kinds of antecedent references and allowing for their denotation by different kinds of proterms. Thus where the antecedent is of form 'some S is (are) P' and the pronominal sentence of form 'it (they) is (are) Q' the bound variable theory invariably translates the conjuction of the antecedent and pronominal sentences by treating the pronoun as a bound variable. But this sort of translation is, as often as not, inappropriate as we find when we look at several familiar types of contexts of pronominalization.

We consider first those cases where the antecedent sentence is uttered by a speaker who is referring to a certain thing or things that he takes to be (an) S. The things to which the speaker has made reference exist but there is of course no guarantee that the things in question are S. We may speak here of the epistemic context of reference; some things are being referred to and the later pronominal subject will also refer to them. The back reference is achieved by the introduction of a proterm specifically designed to denote the things in question antecedently referred to by the speaker in the epistemic context of reference. For example the speaker may say that some children are at the door and follow this by 'they want to speak to Tam'. Let 'Js' be the proterm of the pronoun. Then 'Js' is introduced as a term for denoting the children in question. And one way of parsing 'they want to speak to Tam' is as '*Js want to speak to Tam' where the asterisk indicates that the pronominal subject has wild quantity. This is justified by the fact that 'some Js are Q' here entails 'all Js are Q' because the pronominal sentence refers to all of the things antecedently referred to and not merely to some of them. Where, as in this case, the antecedent reference is to some particular object or objects, the subsequent pronouns will have wild quantity and since they too will refer to those objects we shall call such pronouns referential pronouns.

Normally a referential pronoun is descriptive. Given 'some S are P; they are Q' the pronoun 'they' is equivalent to the descriptive expression 'the S in question'. But there are contexts where what is subsequently referred to is not a purported S-thing. Thus where 'some S are P' is followed by 'they are not S at all . . .' the pronoun is not equivalent to 'the S in question'. Instead the proterm must here be understood to denote what was antecedently taken (perhaps mistakenly) to be S. The pronoun is then equivalent to what may be called a definite ascription. Here we have another illustration of the way the predicate of a sentence may help to determine the reference of its subject. In the normal case 'they are Q' is equivalent to 'the S in question are Q' but in a context like 'some S are P; well I could be mistaken . . . they may not be S' the pronominal sentence is equivalent to 'the things in question that I take to be S may not be S'. Where the predicate of the pronominal sentence gainsays the descriptive content of the antecedent sentence the pronoun will still be referential; it refers to the thing in question to which the speaker of the antecedent sentence is epistemically related but it is then an *ascriptive* and not a descriptive pronoun.

Pronouns whose antecedent sentences are uttered by speakers who are not referring to some particular thing are non-referential. When, for example, a speaker ventures to say that (somewhere) some cat is on some mat adding that it is probably lying on the mat in question there is no reference to a particular cat or mat. Nor, clearly, can it be appropriate to object to what the speaker says with something like 'it is not a cat (but a dog that looks like a cat)'. So while the pronominal in 'it is probably lying on the mat' is interchangeable with 'the cat' (or even with 'the cat in question') there is in fact no particular thing under consideration that is being taken for a cat.

Suppose then that 'an S is a P' has been asserted in some non-epistemic context and that it is followed by 'and it is Q'. Let 'J' be the proterm of the pronominal sentence. Then one way of parsing the pronominal sentence is as 'some J is Q' where 'J' denotes things that are both S and P. The pronominal sentence is then equivalent to 'some S that is P is Q'. This way of parsing 'it is Q' removes the appearance of particular reference by the definite pronominal subject 'it' to some given thing that has presumably been referred to. Also the parsing is compatible with the standard treatment given to non-epistemic contexts. For the contemporary analysis of the sequence 'some S is P and it is Q' parses the pronoun as a bound variable. Note that proterm analysis unpacks the pronoun as a subject expression consisting of a sign of quantity followed by a term formed by compounding the subject and predicate terms of the antecedent sentence—'some S & P is Q'. In this respect the proterms of non-referential pronouns differ from the proterms of referential pronouns. In using a referential pronoun one creates a term for the specific job of denoting the thing under consideration. Note also that the quantity of the non-referential pronouns need not be wild. In the case of 'it is probably lying on the mat', the quantity of 'it' is the same as the quantity of its antecedent sentence. We shall refer to pronouns that may be parsed with compound terms and with quantities that are in accord with the antecedent sentence as B-type pronouns. This will serve to remind us that such pronouns correspond to the bound variables that translate them in the language of modern logic.

Not all non-referential pronouns are B-type. Gareth Evans has recently called attention to a type of non-referential pronoun—which he calls 'E-type'—for which a bound variable translation is inappropriate.[1] Though I shall follow him in referring to them as E-type pronouns I do not mean to suggest that Evans would agree to analysing E-type pronouns as subject expressions with quantities and proterms. Indeed such a suggestion is quite foreign to Evans' approach to definite subjects like proper names and pronouns. Nevertheless Evans does view E-type pronouns as descriptive expressions for which it is appropriate to substitute definite descriptions; to this extent he recognizes their syntactical complexity. More to the point, Evans rejects any approach that would require us to bind an E-type pronoun syntactically to its antecedent sentence. In any case, by an E-type pronoun I shall mean a non-referential pronominal subject expression whose proterm denotes the things that verify an antecedent sentence of form 'some S is/are P' *and whose quantity is wild.*

An example given by Gareth Evans is

(1) Tom owned some sheep and Harry vaccinated them

which not only informs us that Harry vaccinated some sheep that Tom owned but that he vaccinated all of the sheep that Tom owned. In effect (1) unpacks as 'Tom owned some sheep and Harry vaccinated some sheep owned by Tom, and Harry vaccinated all sheep owned by Tom'. Using a star to indicate wild quantity and letting 'Js' be the proterm that denotes sheep owned by Tom we represent (1) as

Tom owned some sheep and Harry vaccinated *Js

When does a non-referential pronoun take particular quantity and when does it take wild quantity? Linguists could tell us more about this perhaps. Consider

(2) some Hondurans are very rich; they keep mistresses; they have yachts

There is no presumption here that all rich Hondurans keep mistresses. On the other hand in

[1] Gareth Evans, 'Pronouns, Quantifiers and Relative Clauses', *Canadian Journal of Philosophy*, vol. III, 3, section 2, pp. 471—7.

(3) some Hondurans are very rich; *they* can afford Perrier at seventy nine cents a bottle, I can't!

'they' is an E-type pronoun. Similarly in

(4) some children are allergic to cats; cats have an adverse effect on them

'them' is an E-type pronoun equivalent to '*children who are allergic to cats'.

Evans holds that a pronoun has E-type status if it occurs in a sentence that is syntactically independent of its antecedent. Thus he holds that in the form 'some S is/are P; it/they is/are Q' the pronouns will be E-type. The Honduran mistresses sentence shows that this view is untenable. One consequence of Evans' position is that in the singular case there will be a presumption of uniqueness. Thus Evans argues that in

(5) Socrates owns a dog and it bit him

'it' is E-type and refers to every dog Socrates owns there being only one. I shall discuss this example later when we take up the question of the syntactic relations that pronouns have to their antecedents.

We have then distinguished between referential and non-referential pronouns and between two kinds of referential and two kinds of non-referential pronouns. Non-referential pronouns are descriptive and, as we now construe them, their proterms may be analysed as compounds of the terms of their antecedent sentences. But non-referential pronouns are themselves distinguished according to whether their quantities are in accord with the quantities of their antecedents, B-type pronouns having the same quantities as their antecedents and E-type pronouns having wild quantities. Referential pronouns may be descriptive (D-type) or ascriptive (A-type) depending on whether the pronominal subject is interpreted as referring to the thing in question that was taken to be an S by the utterer of the antecedent sentence. In either case the referential pronoun makes use of a proterm that has been introduced to denote just that thing or those things that the speaker of the antecedent sentence had referred to.

Our use of the label 'referential pronoun' to refer to pronouns with an epistemic background is tendentious. For we noted lately the reluctance to think of 'some S' as a genuinely referring expression. Even if, out of respect to the Fregean who appears to have de facto custody of 'referring', we restrict its application to definite subjects like proper names, we still have to justify its use for pronouns. For although pronouns are definite subjects they may have indefinite antecedents. Since an antecedent of form 'some S is P' has an indefinite subject, there may be doubt about the ability of 'it' in 'it is Q' to do a job of referring. Peter Geach has gone into this matter with some thoroughness. And because he continues to be our most careful and watchful authority for the orthodox position we shall gratefully examine his views. It can come as no surprise that the orthodox Fregean will resist the idea that relative pronouns can do a job of referring.

Geach first shows that a sentence like 'you cannot have a cake and eat it' does not embody a referring occurrence of a pronoun, not even if we replace 'it' by the quasi-demonstrative phrase 'that cake'.

What makes this exercise futile is that the demonstrative pronoun 'that' does not here serve to point to some cake in the physical context of utterance.[2]

One may agree with Geach about this and generally agree that where it is *appropriate* to interpret a pronominal expression as a B-type pronoun, there the pronominal expression is no more (and no less) a referring expression than is any other subject of form 'some S'. But Geach himself is aware of other less tractable kinds of back reference to indefinite antecedents. He asks:

If I begin a story with
  (1) a man was wearily walking along the main road from London to York
and continue the story by speaking of 'the man,' then am I not keeping on with references to one man . . . no less than if I had repeatedly used a proper name?[3]

This way of understanding subsequent references to 'the man' could open the door to the proscribed view that 'some

---

[2] P. T. Geach, *Back Reference*, Essays in Memory of Yohoshua Bar-Hillel, ed. Asa Kasher, (D. Reidel, *Language in Focus*, 1976), pp. 30—1. Hereafter referred to as *BR*.
[3] Geach, *BR*, p. 31.

man' may refer to a particular man. The temptation to think that pronouns genuinely refer must therefore be weakened. In aid of this Geach asks us to picture a situation in which B and C are talking about B's Cambridge days:

(2) C. I suppose that philosophy lecturers were all non-smokers and total abstainers.

(3) B. What an odd thing to suppose. A philosophy lecturer of my time was a heavy pipe smoker—I'm certain of that.

(4) C. Did he drink alcohol as well?

(5) B. He? Who?

(6) C. The man you were talking about.

(7) B. All I know is that after the meetings of the Moral Science Faculty Board the room reeked of pipe tobacco. So at least one of them must have been a heavy smoker.[4]

Concerning B's last remark Geach says

It would be rankly absurd for C to go on to ask whether 'he' also drank alcohol. For it is clear that when B uttered (3) he was not using 'a philosophy lecturer' to refer to any one philosophy lecturer.[5]

Geach then considers the possibility that the dialogue might have gone on differently. For B's rejoinder to (4) might have been (5a) 'I really don't know but I can well remember him puffing away at his old pipe during supervisions'. And Geach asks:

In that case would not B after all have been referring to some definite person—a reference picked by 'he' in C's (4) and again by 'him' in B's (5a)?[6]

Geach's answer to this betrays a common recognition of epistemic reference by 'some S' to an individual or individuals taken or mistaken for an S or for S's, and incidentally illustrates the lengths that the bound variable proponent will go to ignore this phenomenon or to allow it no logical importance. Here is his answer:

I reply that we must not confuse the questions whom B was referring

[4] Geach, BR, pp. 31—2.
[5] Geach, BR, p. 32.
[6] Geach, BR, p. 32.

to in uttering (3)—whom he had in mind and was alluding to—and whom B's utterance referred to. The former considerations do not touch the truth of what B said, . . . neither do they touch the reference made by B's phrase 'a philosophy lecturer'. So we must still say that this phrase as used by B in (3) does not make any reference to a definite person concerning whom C could then ask whether *he* drank alcohol and this holds regardless of whether B's response to (4) was (5) (7) or (5a).[7]

Even if one allowed that (3) could be true although the individual that B had in mind was no pipe smoker it would still not follow that speaker reference has no effect on truth values. For there are two kinds of reference to consider here and while speaker reference might be considered irrelevant to the truth value of (3), it is clearly relevant to the truth value of the pronominal sentence (5a). Geach is evidently worried about this for he continues

the difficulty is however not removed. For surely if C had heard B utter (5a) he would have understood it and how could he do this without catching on to the reference of 'him' in (5a)? The best I can do about this for the moment is to say that 'him' in C's *acceptation* of (5a) must be regarded as a pronoun of laziness—an abbreviation (in B's mouth) for 'that philosophy lecturer whom I now have in mind'. And what B had in mind when he uttered (3) is then irrelevant.[8]

I don't see how the laziness of the pronouns in (4) and (5a) can help Geach. For he is conceding that what B had in mind is the subject of C's question and that C is referring to that. Had C said instead 'Let me guess: he was also an alcoholic wasn't he?' it would certainly matter that 'he' referred to what B had in mind when asserting (3). Similarly, even if (3) is counted as true just because there was some pipe-smoking philosopher at Cambridge in the old days, (5a) will be false if B was mistaken in thinking that the man he had in mind as smoking a pipe was really smoking a cigar. Geach's suggestion that 'he' and 'him' are 'lazy pronouns going proxy for a demonstrative subject in B's mouth', 'the philosophy lecturer and heavy smoker whom I now have in mind', is puzzling. When was this (tacit) demonstrative act supposed to have taken place? Geach himself

---

[7] Geach, *BR*, p. 32.
[8] Geach, *BR*, p. 33.

seems to waver between thinking of it as concomitant with the assertion of (3) and thinking of it as having taken place after that. The suggestion that some tacit act took place between the assertion of (3) and (5a) is altogether ad hoc. On the other hand the assumption that in uttering (3) B was also performing a demonstrative act of referring to a certain individual is gratuitous; why not just relax and admit that 'a philosopher' can by itself do the job of referring to someone B has in mind and that the later pronouns can pick up the reference to the individual so referred to?

Geach's hypothetical conversation about the old Cambridge days has some of the elements of the following incident which took place at my university. Some years ago the secretary of the Philosophy Department told me that someone had several times tried to reach me the previous day but had not left his name. She added that he had a gravel voice. It later turned out that the man she spoke to had been trying to reach another Professor Sommers whose mail sometimes got mixed with mine and that the man in question, whose name I have forgotten if I ever knew it, did not have a gravel voice—a mistake that was possibly due to a bad phone connection. As it happened however an old friend of mine—a Dr Avivi—had more than once on that day tried to get in touch with me through my secretary but had found the lines busy. My friend Avivi does have a gravel voice but the secretary never spoke to him. Let us now consider the two statements made by the secretary

(i) a man tried several times to reach you yesterday
(ii) he had a gravel voice

There are three views concerning the truth values we may assign to (i) and (ii).

I Both are false since the man the secretary had in mind was not in fact trying to reach me and did not in fact have a gravel voice.

II (i) is true but (ii) is false because 'he' is here interchangeable with 'the man I spoke to' or some similar phrase that would specify the referent of (ii) as the man who was trying to reach my namesake.

III Both are true since there was in fact a man who was

trying to reach me that day and who has a gravel voice.

Of these three views the secretary took the first. At the time I inclined to the second. Geach would prefer the third. I think however that the third is incompatible with the idea that 'he' and 'the man I'm talking about' (or 'the man in question' or 'the man I'm referring to') are interchangeable. I now think that (i) and (ii) are both false, (i) being equivalent to 'a *certain* man tried several times to reach you' and 'he' picking up the reference to the man in question, in this case the man who spoke to the secretary. We have here a pronoun that picks up an epistemic reference to an individual referred to by an indefinite subject. It is just this sort of antecedent reference that Geach is concerned to deny. Nevertheless the straightforward account is that 'a man' here refers to a certain man and that 'he' picks this up. 'The man I am referring to' is evidence that 'a man' does so refer. To save his theory that 'a man' cannot do a job of referring, Geach would be forced to put into the mouth of the secretary a demonstrative subject 'that man', and to assume that a demonstrative act of reference has taken place sometime before the use of 'he' (which then goes proxy for the demonstrative). Though Geach is prepared to do this, he recognizes it as a temporary shift ('the best I can do about this for the moment') and we may regard this move as unthreatening to the naive theory that 'he' is a relative pronoun whose proterm denotes what was epistemically referred to by 'a man' in the antecedent sentence.

2. We have called attention to the effort to force referential pronouns into the procrustean bed of the bound variable theory. The effort continues for non-referential pronouns of the sort distinguished by Evans as E-type. Evans holds that a pronoun is E-type whenever the pronominal sentence is syntactically separate from its antecedent. Thus where Geach would translate 'some Hondurans are very rich; they can afford yachts' as 'some Hondurans are such that they are very rich and they can afford yachts' Evans would insist that 'they' in the pronominal sentence is syntactically independent of its antecedent and is to be understood as '(all) the very rich Hondurans'. While we may agree with Evans about this we cannot agree that the occurrence of a pronoun in a syntactically independent sentence is evidence of E-type status. Thus Geach and Evans are divided on how to construe 'it' in 'Socrates owned a dog and it bit him', Evans holding that it is E-type and syntactically free of its antecedent, Geach holding that it is B-type and syntactically bound. Neither view appears to me to be acceptable. Evans reads. (11) as equivalent to 'Socrates owned a dog and every dog that Socrates owned bit him', it being understood that Socrates owned no more than one dog. He is forced to this understanding by his theory that 'it' is an E-type pronoun and so not equivalent to '*some* dog owned by Socrates'. It is however not at all clear that one cannot say of someone who owned many dogs that he owned a dog and that it bit him. So the reasonable interpretation of (11) is weaker than Evans would have it, with the pronominal sentence being equivalent to 'some dog that Socrates owned bit Socrates'. My quarrel with Geach is less substantive but more serious. For Geach does not allow that the sentence 'it bit him' is a conjunct grammatically independent of 'Socrates owned a dog', insisting that 'it' is syntactically bound by an antecedent quantifier. Geach's view contrasts with the proterm analysis of B-type pronouns and I shall examine Geach's main argument for it. The argument, which is typical and generally accepted, does heavy duty in support of the bound variable theory of pronouns.

Geach says:

Pronouns whose antecedents are applicatival phrases correspond strictly in their syntax to variables bound by quantifiers . . . For lack of this light, the medievals who discussed relative-pronouns with antecedents—were groping in the dark despite all their ingenuity. Let us consider how such puzzles as theirs arise:

(15) Socrates owned a dog, and it bit Socrates

A medieval would treat this as a conjunctive proposition, and enquire after the reference (*suppositio*) of the pronoun 'it'; I have seen modern discussions that make the same mistake. For mistake it is. If we may legitimately symbolize (15) as 'p & q', then a contradictory of (15) . . . would be

(16) Socrates did not own a dog or else: Socrates owned a dog and it did not bite Socrates.

But (15) and (16) are not contradictories; a moment's thought shows that both could be true . . .

Compare what we get using restricted quantification:

(17) (∃x) dog (Socrates owned x & x bit Socrates)

In (17) the unfortunate appearance of there being a proposition 'Socrates owned a dog' as one conjunct has quite disappeared.[9]

of (15) Geach also says:

It makes not a farthing of difference if we substitute 'the dog' or 'that dog' for 'it'. For no definite dog is before the readers' eyes, or is brought by the sentence before the mind's eye, to supply a reference for this subject-term. And 'the' and 'that' must be parsed like 'it,' not as demonstratives but as *relativa* looking to 'a dog'.[10]

The objection that 'a dog' and 'it' can have no reference because they are not identificatory expressions is familiar. But it is quite irrelevant here for we are agreed that the antecedent of (15) is not asserted in an epistemic context and that 'it' is not a referential pronoun. But the matter of a contradictory to (15) is new, as is the claim that (15) and its like cannot be construed as conjunctions. This latter claim is of course tied up with the 'right solution': the canonical expression of (15) with 'it' as variable bound by the restricted quantifier 'some dog' within a single sentence, (17).

In examining Geach's argument it will be convenient to remove some of the irrelevant constructions brought in by the relational character of the two propositions in (15). Let D be 'a dog', O be 'owned by Socrates' and B be 'biter of Socrates'. Then (15) becomes:

(15*) a D is O and it is B

which Geach tentatively treats as of form 'p & q'. Now one unexceptionable way to contradict (15*) is

(18) if a D is O then it isn't B

for 'p & q' and 'p → − q' are contradictories. Geach offers, in effect,

(16*) no D is O or else: a D is O and it isn't B

which is, *prima facie*, not a contradictory of (15*) despite its form ' − pv (p&q)'.

[9] Geach, *LM*, pp. 118–19.
[10] Geach, *LM*, p. 119.

(16*) appears to be compatible with (15*) and Geach takes this to be fatal to any analysis that treats (15*) as a conjunction 'p & q' of 'some D is O' and 'it is B'. To answer Geach we will remind him that even the simple form 'p & − p' is contradictory only where it is assumed that 'p' recurs univocally. If, for example, 'Tom' refers to Tom Swift in 'Tom is hungry' and to Tom Sawyer in 'Tom isn't hungry' we couldn't represent their conjunction as 'p & − p'. We do need here to achieve something like the effect of 'that dog' or 'the dog in question' in order to justify representing 'it is (isn't) B' with recurrent 'q'. Similarly, we need to make sure that 'a D is O' in (15) and (16*) does not have different truth conditions in its two occurrences if we are to justify its reappearance with recurrent 'p'. In its appearance in (15), 'a D is O' could be true if Socrates owns no more than one dog. But in (16*) *as Geach reads it*, it cannot be true unless Socrates owns a second dog which does not bite him. It looks as if Geach is not minding his p's and q's.

We here have a B-type pronominal. Making the proterm of the pronominals explicit, we can avoid Geach's error and guarantee the univocity of the recurrent propositions. So let us use 'J' as the proterm of the original pronominal with J denoting an individual that is both D and O and then use it again in the contradictory:

(15*) a D is O and some J is B
(16**) no D is O or a D is O and not: some J is B

The recurrent propositions in (15*) and (16**) have the same truth conditions and (16**) is the contradictory of (15*).

A common device for contradicting an anaphoric conjunction used in vernacular situations is illustrated by (18). (18) guarantees reference to 'the dog in question' by saying in effect that if any dog whatever is owned by Socrates then that dog does not bite him.

It is worth remarking that Geach's objection to the conjunctive interpretation and his doctrine that (15) should be analysed as (17) is inconsistent with what he says elsewhere about the meaning of 'such that' in contexts like 'there is an A such that p'. Russell had said that 'such that' is an indefinable notion not reducible to other logical notions. Geach acutely observes that 'such that' . . . is an all-purpose connective, a sort of universal joint which goes proxy for whichever connective—'and', 'if', 'only if', etc.—may be required by context. Applied to 'there is a dog such that Socrates owned him and he bit Socrates', the resolution of 'such that' yields 'there is a dog and Socrates owned him and he bit Socrates', a conjunction of the kind that Geach finds so objectionable. Moreover, the problem is quite general. Given 'some A is B' Geach would first translate it as 'there is an A and it is B', which certainly gives the appearance of having 'there is an A' as one conjunct and is presumably open to the objection that its denial 'either there is no A or else there is an A and it is not B' is not what it should be. The problem is easily avoided by anyone who is prepared to give up the bound variable theory of pronouns and to recognize that pronouns are like other subjects in having terms—in this case, terms that denote what an antecedent subject has referred to. Underlying the contemporary reluctance to think of 'an S is P and it is Q' as a conjunction whose conjuncts are semantically tied but syntactically seperable is the problem of what truth value to assign the pronominal sentence 'it is Q' when the antecedent sentence 'an S is P' is false. The correct answer from the traditional standpoint is 'false'. As for 'it isn't Q', that too is false. Here 'isn't Q' is read as equivalent to 'is non-Q'. The problem arises for those who reject Aristotle's distinction (in Catagories I, 10) between falsely asserting 'Socrates isn't well' and truly denying 'Socrates is well'. According to Aristotle if Socrates never existed then both contrary sentences 'Socrates is well' and 'Socrates isn't well (or is unwell)' are false and their negations true.

On this view, if Socretes never owned a dog then the pronominal sentences 'it bit him' and 'it didn't bite him' are both false. More generally, if p is an antecedent sentence and q and q' are contrary pronominal sentences whose pronouns both have reference to p then anyone who affirms or denies 'p & q' will accept as common ground the disjunction:

$$p \& q \& -q' \lor p \& q' \& -q \lor -p \& -q \& -q'.$$

We shall be arguing that a plausible interpretation of a proposition such as 'the present king of France is bald' or its contrary 'the present king of France isn't bald' will treat 'the present king of France' as a descriptive pronoun harking back to a tacit antecedent proposition such as 'France now has a king'. Since all such antecedent propositions are false the contrary pronominal propositions will both be false. The view that when the antecedent is false contrary pronominals are neither true nor false is held by those who hold the Fregean view that 'α is un-P' is a form of the negation of 'α is P'. This renders it impossible to hold that 'α is P' and 'α is un-P' could both be false.

According to Geach, (15) is a sentence consisting of a quantified expression and a matrix. The quantified expression ('a dog') is the operator that binds the variable in the matrix. In this solution, pronouns are bound variables and quantifiers are their antecedents; the relation of cross reference is the relation of being bound by a quantifier. Also in 'there is a dog such that Socrates owned it . . .' the expression 'such that' must be understood *sui genesis* and indefinable in the manner of Russell. We thereby remove 'the unfortunate appearance' that (15) has of being a conjunction of 'Socrates owned a dog' and 'he bit Socrates'. A similar analysis would remove the 'unfortunate appearance' that (18) has; for (18) looks like a conditional sentence. The dispersing of these illusions comes from the 'syntactical insight' that recent Fregeans offer into natural language that pronouns are variables bound by antecedents that are operators. This insight into pronominalization demands acceptance of the following thesis: pronominalization or cross reference *always takes place within a single sentence* not syntactically divisible into (closed) sentential parts. Contrary to all surface appearances pronominalization from one sentence containing the pronoun to another sentence containing the antecedent is impossible.

Now this is a very strong condition on pronominalization and it has been taken too much for granted by philosophers. Here perhaps the logistic success of Frege's syntax has seduced philosophers into an uncritical acceptance of a doctrine that 'saves' them from the tendency to give credence to their intuitions concerning pronouns. For we certainly think that pronominalization often picks up an earlier reference from a sentence already completed. But this, we have been persuaded, is an illusion. Sometimes the exorcism of this illusion requires some harsh measures. Geach who is committed to the orthodox thesis on pronominalization, and who is also more aware then most of how weak the flesh can be, comes up against the problem of reconciling the bound variable theory of pronouns of the vernacular with the fact that inferences in the vernacular often have a pronominal conclusion. The example Geach gives is a syllogism devised by Strawson. Because it is embarrassing for the bound variable theory Geach calls it a quasi-syllogism; it has the form of a dialogue:

> A: A man has just drunk a pint of sulphuric acid
> B: Nobody who has drunk a pint of sulphuric acid lives through the day
> A: Very well then, *he* won't live through the day

To this Geach says:

> It is very tempting to take 'he' in A's second remark as picking up the reference from 'a man' in A's first remark. But let us not forget the arguments in Chapter One against the view that 'a man' ever refers to a man. And if 'a man' makes no such reference, 'he' cannot pick up any such reference from 'a man'.[11]

We may safely snub this old herring; no one is pretending that an epistemic reference has been made to an identifiable (by A) man and the back reference of 'he' should not be made to sound as if it were dependent on such a reference. The problem facing Geach is simple enough. In A's second remark we have a pronoun that he normally handles as a bound variable but its antecedent is clearly a separate sentence. Now in the normal case the modern logician will fuse two sentences to get the pronoun within the scope of the quantifier, construing for example 'a man came; he is wet' as 'some man$_x$ is such that x came and x is wet'. But binding across an inference line is impossible and this threatens the bound variable theory of pronouns. To my mind this threat cannot be countered. Geach would like nothing better than that pronominalization across inference lines should never happen. So when it does happen we find him heatedly denying that it has happened. The offending premiss is brought down to the conclusion to form a part of it construing A's second remark as repeating his first and reading it as 'a man has just drunk a pint of sulphuric acid—he won't

---

[11] Geach, *RG*, pp. 126—7.

live through the day'. It is, says Geach, as if

A had on his writing tablet first of all the shorter proposition 'a man
has just drunk a pint of sulphuric acid' and then the longer
proposition 'a man has just drunk a pint of sulphuric acid—he won't
live through the day'; the particle 'very well then' expresses A's
inference of the longer proposition from the shorter one. The added
clause in the longer proposition is a mere fragment of a sentence, not a
conjunct in a conjunctive proposition; it has no truth-value, and 'he'
has here no reference.[12]

Contrast this 'explanation' with that of the proterm theorist
who would here regard 'he' as a pronoun referring back to A's
first remark. The inference is valid because A's remark is
equivalent to 'someone (J) is a man and he (*J) has drunk a pint
of sulphuric acid'.[13] Geach comes pretty close to seeing that the
conclusion is something like '*J won't live through the day'—
but he cannot bring himself to this without admitting that
pronominal sentences can occur as syntactically free sentences
whose anaphoric relation to the antecedent is entirely semantic.

Geach is prepared to say just about anything to make cross
reference over an inference line go away. But there are
innumerable cases which give the appearance of just such cross
reference. Consider:

A: A man is asking for you.
B: He must have been given my room number by the desk
   clerk.

Geach will read B thus: A man is asking for me; he must have
been given my room number by the desk clerk. On this reading,
'he' cross refers to 'a man' in B's long assertion but does not
refer to 'a man' in A's assertion. If so, there appears to be no
logical connection between what A says and what B says;
instead we understand the connection to be one of prompter to
repeater. A more plausible solution along the lines suggested by
Geach would be to drop the idea of an inference by reconstru-
ing B's assertion as an elliptical conditional:

(If a man is asking for me) then he must have given my name
by the room clerk.

---

[12] Geach, *RG*, p. 127.
[13] The explanation given here assigns wild quantity to the pronoun in accordance
with the account given in chapter 5, section 3.

If we adopt this solution, we must be prepared to reconstrue all arguments whose conclusion have a pronoun that appears to refer to some antecedent among the premises as non-inferences; in all such cases, the appearance of different sentences must be dispelled, the 'conclusion' becomes the consequent of a single conditional proposition whose antecedent is a conjunction of the 'premisses'. Perhaps Geach was prevented from taking this line because of the dialogical character of Strawson's syllogism. But there, too, it could be done by reading the conclusion itself if not the whole 'quasi-syllogism' as a conditional whose antecedent is the conjunction of the two premises. The price is not inconsiderable—after all, if we are not to be arbitrary it means the replacement of *all* inferences by conditional statements. But the price could be paid and, in many a case, would be willingly paid by the bound variable proponent.

I believe, however, that all such devices must prove futile: there are cases of cross reference where the sentence that contains the pronoun cannot be attached to the sentence that contains the antecedent by a truth-functional connective to form a single sentence. Take for example:

A: A man is at the door.
B: Is he a stranger?

Here even if we imagine both A and B to be deaf mutes and leave A's remark on the tablet for attachment to B's question, we will find no way to get the required binding of 'he' by 'a man'. We might try:

Some man, x, (x is at the door and is x armed?)

But how are we to read it? The conjunction is at least as peculiar as a non-truth-functional conjunctional reading for 'Socrates owned a dog and it bit Socrates' which Geach rejected. Of course, questions are not the only problem for the bound variable theory of pronouns. Consider:

A: A man is at the door.   B: Arm him
A: A man is at the door.   B: It is not a man but a woman!

These and similar examples are good evidence that pronominalization is not exclusively an intrasentential phenomenon. Nevertheless, the bound variable theory persists in the face of just such examples. Thus we find Searle parsing 'the king of France exists. Is he bald?' à la Russell as

(i) $[(\exists x)(fx \cdot (y)(fy = y = x))] \cdot ? [Gx]?$

In a footnote to this suggested translation of (i) (which is rejected for reasons not relevant to our discussion), Searle remarks:

(i) assumes that quantifiers can sometimes reach across ilocutionary force indicators. This seems to be a reasonable assumption since pronouns do it in natural languages: e.g., 'A man came. Did you see him?'[14]

I have seen Grice assume the same thing in more complicated cases. But I have not seen any explanation of this alleged phenomenon.[15] How does a quantifier bind into a question, an objection, a promise, a command, an entreaty, etc., to absorb it into a single syntactical unit? This question is especially pressing when neither sentence is indicative, for example:

Bring me a muffin! Don't you think I'll eat it?

But it is also embarrassing in the case of two indicative statements made by different persons when the antecedent is epistemic.

A: A man is on the roof.   B: It is not a man.

There seems no way to construe 'it' as a syntactically bound variable and again the single sentence constraint is the culprit.

2.1 In the absence of any coherent explanation of those matters, we must certainly give theoretical weight to the surface appearance that relative pronouns are, more often than not, not contained in the same sentence as their antecedents. This is far more reasonable than the course advocated by Searle, Geach

---

[14] Searle, *SA*, p. 161.
[15] Note that Searle precedes the question in (i) by a sign of conjunction. We can only wonder how to read it; certainly not as a truth-functional connective. Moreover, despite the stated assumption that quantifiers may reach across into questions, the existential quantifier of (i) falls short and the question is left dangling for lack of a right hand bracket tying it to the quantifier. Perhaps Searle's typesetter was uneasy about quantifying into the question. If so, his qualms were healthy ones.

and other Fregean philosophers. For theirs is the course of one who is committed to the theory of bound variables come what may. Surely the most attractive theory can demand too much in the way of cosmetic removal of disturbing surface appearances.

There is an alternative theory. Strawson relies on it when he says that the relative pronoun whose antecendent is 'a man' is taking up the reference to a definite person indefinitely made. This states the fact; it does not tell us how the pronoun accomplishes this. For an account that does justice to the facts, we must first of all turn with sympathy to the doctrine that logical subjects consist of a syncategorematic sign of quantity as well as a categorematic subject-term. We may then distinguish the reference of the whole subject from the denotation of the subject-term. This, in turn, makes it possible for us to see that a pronoun too has an implicit sign of quantity and that its term or 'proterm' can be understood to be especially designed to denote what some contextually given subject is referring to. Once we command the use of the proterm we are free to use it in new and independent sentences. Recall how this traditionalist theory views pronominalization in

(1) Some men are at the door. They are strangers.

The word 'they' is parsed as 'some persons unique in having just been referred to' where the context shows that the reference in question was made by 'some men' in the previous sentence. Pronouns are *definite* subjects and it is to be expected that the quantity of the pronominal sentence is wild; clearly 'some persons . . .' entails 'all persons unique in having been referred to are strangers'. Of course, the theory allows for cross reference between expressions of two syntactically independent sentences. So no difficulties arise if we give the second sentence the form of a question.

(1a) Some men are at the door. Are they strangers?

Similarly, the proterm theory allows for dialogical contradiction.

A: Some men are at the door.
B: They aren't men; they're women!

The kind of cross reference where the pronoun occurs in a

belief sentence while its antecedent occurs in a regular has received much attention in recent years. An example is:

(1) Some men are at the door. Fred believes they are friendly.

Problems arise when one attempts to handle the cross reference in the usual way by binding the pronoun from the non-belief sentence. These problems have been taken seriously if only because standard logic deals with indicative sentences and when a problem of cross reference arises for two indicative sentences it cannot be dismissed as irrelevant to logic in the way one might want to dismiss the problem (for the bound variable theory) of cross reference between a statement and a command or a question. I do not here propose to discuss pronominalization into belief sentences and other sentences with opaque verbs or operators. It is evident that the proterm theory of pronouns will put some old questions in a new light. In any case, for the proterm theory there are no difficulties of a *syntactical* kind to cross reference between belief and non-belief contexts.[16]

3. The doctrine that pronominalization must take place within the sentence is a requirement of the syntax of modern predicate logic. It gives bad insight into pronouns of natural language. Another example of the misuse of modern logical syntax to enforce a bad theory of pronouns is Geach's 'Latin Prose Theory' of relative pronouns. According to Geach, a phrase of form 'A that is P' (e.g., 'man that is poor') is not a genuine logical unit. Phrases of this sort (and also phrases like 'poor man' which is equivalent to a phrase of form 'A that is P') are said to be systematically ambiguous in:

(1) some Q is an A that is P
(2) every A that is P is Q
(3) only an A that is P is Q

These are respectively parsed by Geach as:

(1*) some Q is an A and it is P
(2*) every A, if it is P is Q
(3*) an(y) A is P only if it is Q

[16] For an ingenious quantificationalist solution to some of these difficulties see David Kaplan's 'Quantifying In', *Words and Objections*, ed. D. Davidson and J. Hintikka (D. Reidel, 1969) pp. 206—42.

Quine, too, accepts the Latin Prose Theory 'as a description of the accomplished grammatical fact' though he thinks that our acquisition of competence in handling compound terms proceeds along other lines. Geach gives two arguments for his theory. The first he rightly sees as inconclusive.

We could of course validly draw the conclusion 'Socrates is a donkey' from the premisses 'Socrates is an animal and he can bray' and 'any animal, if he can bray, is a donkey'; and these are respectively equivalent to 'Socrates is an animal that can bray' and 'any animal that can bray is a donkey'. This suggests that the phrase 'animal that can bray' is a systematically ambiguous one so that we must divine from the context which connective is packed up with 'he' into the portmanteau word 'that'. But we cannot count this as proved . . .
We may however confirm the suggestion of ambiguity by considering another sort of medieval example. In the pair of propositions:

(12) Any man who owns a donkey beats it.
(13) Some man who owns a donkey does not beat it.

'man who owns a donkey' has all the look of being a complex term replaceable by the single word 'donkey-owner'; yet if we do make this replacement (12) and (13) become unintelligible. It may seem as though this happened only because 'it' is deprived of an antecedent . . . if so, we might overcome the difficulty by rewording (12) and (13) so as to supply this sense without having a pronoun that refers back to part of the term 'man who owns a donkey'.

(14) Any man who owns a donkey owns a donkey and beats it.
(15) Some man who owns a donkey owns a donkey and does not beat it.

. . . It looks as though (12) and (14), (13) and (15) are equivalent pairs . . . but it is not so. Whereas (12) and (13) are contradictories, their supposed equivalents (14) and (15) are not; for both would be true if each donkey-owner has two donkeys and beat only one of them . . . We can surely see that the right rewording is got by our old dodge of splitting up a grammatically relative pronoun:

(18) Any man, if he owns a donkey, beats it.
(19) Some man owns a donkey and he does not beat it.

. . . now the ostensible complex term has upon analysis quite disappeared. I maintain that the complex term A that is P is a sort of logical mirage.[17]

[17] Geach, *RG*, p. 116.

Unsurprisingly, the Latin Prose Theory analyses propositions in just the manner that is familiar to those who translate (1) (2) and (3) into the notation of a standard language that uses restricted quantification (the kind favoured by Geach). We then have:

(1*) some A, x, (x is P and x is Q)
(2*) every A, x, (if x is P then x is Q)
(3*) every A, x, (x is Q only if x is P)

Nevertheless, the theory has intrinsic implausibility. In the first place, Geach has *not* shown that a univocal interpretation of 'A that is P' could not work in the three cases. To be sure, he does not consider his first argument to be decisive. But, in fact, the syllogism with the premisses 'Socrates is an animal that can bray' and 'any animal that can bray is a donkey' strongly suggests that 'animal that can bray' is a genuine logical unit. Geach's medieval straightman would correctly say that 'A that is P' is a conjunctive term 'A and P' (animal and brayer) and he would certainly object to the idea that 'animal that can bray' is not a logical unit in 'Socrates is an animal that can bray' and 'any animal that can bray is a donkey', rightly taking the fact that 'animal that can bray' serves univocally as the middle term in a valid syllogism to be an excellent indication of its logical integrity. He would, moreover, rightly reject (14) and (15) as not being candidates for equivalents to (12) and (13) because they too fail to specify the antecedent for the pronoun 'it'. The trouble with 'donkey-owner', as Geach saw, is that the antecedent of 'it' was removed. The trouble with (14) is that 'it' has too many antecedents which is just as bad as having none. On hearing that a man who owns a donkey owns a donkey and beats it, we rightly ask for the antecedent to 'it'. And if it is stipulated that 'it' refers to the second occurrence of 'a beats it, we rightly 'it' refers to the second occurrence of 'a donkey' and not to the first, then who would think of (14) as an equivalent of (12)? It should, in any case, be obvious that the failure of (14) and (15) to be equivalent to (12) and (13) has nothing at all to do with the logical unity of 'a man who owns a donkey'. There remains the simple and straightforward scholastic account of 'man who owns a donkey' as 'man and owner of a donkey'. And there is the similar account of 'poor man' as 'man and poor'. For remember that Geach would have us say that 'poor man' is not a middle term in 'every poor man is hungry' and 'some Spaniard is a poor man' (the first being parsed as 'every man, if he is poor . . .' the second being parsed as 'man and he is poor') even though from these two as premisses we can draw the conclusion 'some Spaniard is hungry'. Since the univocal treatment of compounds like 'man that is poor' and 'poor man' is far more plausible, one may well ask why Quine and Geach have taken the course of rejecting it. And the obvious answer is that there is no way of keeping 'man that is poor' intact in *quantificational* translations of 'some A that is P is . . .' and 'every A that is P . . .' Hence, the 'syntactical insight' that 'A that is P' is not univocal in those contexts. Here, at least, Quine has relaxed his fine policy of requiring incontestable proof from anyone who says of two different expressions that they mean the same thing and equally strong proof from anyone who says of a single recurrent expression that it means different things in different contexts.[18] We can set it up as an admirable Quinean maxim that an expresion is univocal until proven equivocal. Is showing that the requirements of canonical translation cannot be met by keeping 'A that is P' intact proof enough? Quine thinks so. And one might think so if the bound variable theory of pronouns were linguistically viable in other respects. As matters stand, there is little reason to impugn the univocity of 'poor man' or 'man that is poor' in 'every PM is . . . ' and 'some . . . is a PM'.

4. We have argued that the surface appearance of integrity for phrases of form 'S that is P' is to be trusted and also that one may trust that pronominalization may be intersentential despite the demands made by quantificationalist analysis of logical form. The constructionist idea that the relative pronoun must be syntactically bound to its antecedent has no place in a theory of logical syntax that presumes to give insights into the 'pronouns of the vernacular'.

There remains the semantic tie between the pronoun and the antecedent subject and some perspicuous way of indicating it is desirable. We shall use the device of indexing the subject expression of the antecedent sentence in a manner that

---

[18] See *Word and Object*, pp. 130—1.

anticipates it and ties it to the pronoun that follows. One way of doing this is use the same letter for the index as is later used to represent the proterm of the pronoun. For example suppose the pronominal sentence is 'it is asleep' and that the proterm of 'it' is 'J' and suppose also that the antecedent sentence is 'a cat is on the mat'. We index the antecedent subject 'a cat' with a subscript letter 'j' to anticipate the pronominalization. The conjunction of antecedent and pronominal may then be represented thus:

⌞A cat⌟$_j$ is on the mat and *J is asleep.

The bottom corners set off the subject expression to which the pronoun has cross reference; the use of the same letter renders the cross reference perspicuous; the star signifies wild quantity.

When a pronoun is in the same sentence as the antecedent subject to which it cross refers the same method or representing the cross reference may be used. For example the pronominalization in 'A man I know hates himself' could be represented as '⌞A man I know⌟$_r$ hates *R'. However pronominalization is also an intersentential phenomenon. So the more perspicuous analysis of the sentence is

I know ⌞a man⌟$_r$; *R hates *R.

To the practitioner of MPL whose policy with pronouns is opposed to an intersentential representation, this way of treating pronominalization is unduly perverse. Pending linguistic investigation into the question perhaps the reasonable policy is to trust surface appearance and to allow for pronominalization both within and across sentences. We may then represent a sentence like 'a boy who was fooling her kissed a girl who loved him' as '⌞a boy⌟$_j$ who was fooling *M kissed ⌞a girl⌟$_m$ who loved *J'. An intersentential analysis of the same sentence could be something like ⌞a boy⌟$_j$ kissed ⌞a girl⌟$_m$; *J was fooling *M; *M loved *J.

4.1 We have been representing pronouns like 'it' and 'they' by expressions like '*J' and '*K'. It is useful to have available some notational indicator that tells us when the pronominal expression represents a singular and when it represents a plural pronoun. To distinguish plural pronouns from singular ones we may affix to their proterm letters the letter 's'. Thus '*Ks' could be used to represent pronouns like 'they' 'them' 'those' and so on. Applied to 'some men are at the door; they could easily break it' our convention would give us something like:

⌐some men⌐ⱼ are at the door_k; '*Js could easily break *K'.

5. The use of proterms for analysing pronouns confers considerable syntactic latitude and considerable expressive power to the language of termist logic. The reader will recall that termist syntax allows for the formation of 'negative names' like 'nonSocrates'. Here the fact that 'Socrates' may be taken as a term makes it possible to form its contrary. (And of course the contrary of a name does not have a unique denotation and so is not itself a name.) The modern logician approaches an expression like 'nonSocrates' as a part of a relational predicate 'is not identical with Socrates'. We shall find (in chapter 6) that termist logic has no need for a sign for identity and indeed can do without the idea of such a relation altogether. In TFL 'nonSocrates' and 'nonShakespeare' are terms on a par with 'non-philosopher' and 'non-poet'; a sentence like 'Bacon is not Shakespeare' is a monadic sentence on all fours with 'Bacon is not a poet'. More generally, a sentence taken to assert that one thing is not identical with another can—in TFL—be understood as a non-relational sentence: instead of 'a $\neq$ b' the termist simply writes '*a is not b'. The ability to form the contrary of names and of proterms gives to termist logic an expressive power not possessed by a standard first order system not equipped with axioms for handling inferences involving identity. As the termist interprets it a sequence like 'a man is at the door; only he can help us' has the form '⌐some M⌐ⱼ is D; *I is H; no (-I) is H'. The corresponding MPL analysis would involve identity with a part to the effect that something x is at the door and can help us and anything y that can help us is identical with x.

5.1 Using proterms one is also able to form 'propronouns', i.e. pronouns whose antecedents are themselves pronouns. Consider for example the following sentence

some clowns of my acquaintance were practicing in my yard
some of them were inexperienced; others were old hands
some of the latter were giving pointers to some of the former.

This could be analysed as of form

$_{\llcorner}$some S_{Jk} are P
$_{\llcorner}$some Js_{Jk} were Q; some $_{\llcorner}$Js that are not K_{Jm} were R
some Ms were giving some Z to some Ks.

The ability to form negative proterms and the ability to form propronouns is the kind of expressive power one wants from an account of pronouns that is adequate to some of the demands on a logical syntax of natural language. The next chapter will subject pronominalization to close scrutiny. We shall find it necessary to radically revise our view of the proterm. But its essential nature will remain unaffected: it is a term introduced for the special purpose of denoting what was antecedently referred to. As with any other term, one can form its contrary and it can serve as the subject term of an antecedent referring expression for further pronominalization.

6. We may summarize some of the discussion of this chapter. It began with the observation that a termist analysis parses the pronoun with quantity and a 'proterm'. We distinguished between those pronouns whose proterms denote an individual or individuals to which the speaker of the antecedent sentence stands in some epistemic relation (e.g. acquaintance), and those whose proterms are equivalent to compound terms whose term elements are taken from the antecedent sentence. The former we dubbed 'referential' the latter 'not referential'. In the next chapter we shall completely abandon the compound term analysis of the so-called non-referential pronouns going over to a view that treats B and E-type pronouns as weakly referential and syntactically very much like A and D-type pronouns. The distinction between epistemic strongly referential and non-epistemic and weakly referential pronouns will correspond to the present analysis as a distinction between two fundamental types of pronominalization. According to the proterm analysis of pronouns, intersentential pronominalization is primary. When pronominalization proceeds across sentences, the basic tie is semantic and not syntactical. We argued that most pronominal ties are of this nature and in particular we argued that syntactic binding in canonical translation is altogether inappropriate in the case of referential pronouns and in the case where sentences cannot be understood to be truth-functionally tied. We looked at some of the arguments for the bound variable theory of pronouns and found them unconvincing. Finally we introduced some notation for the proterm theory and showed how the abilities to represent the contraries of proterms and to form propronouns gives the language of a traditional termist logic a considerable advantage in expressive power.

5

Pronominal Reference

1. Termist logic has no place for the individual constants and variables that play the role of syntactic subjects in standard systems of MPL. A viable and adequate termist logic must therefore be capable of expressing what a modern predicate logic—using individual symbols—expresses. This applies more particularly to the pronouns that MPL translates as bound variables. We have, in chapter 4 suggested how these 'B-type' pronouns may be given a termist analysis in certain simple cases. But the more complicated and interesting problems arise when we consider pronouns flanking relational expressions, reflexive pronouns, pronominalizations from antecedents of conditionals to their consequents, and others to which the practitioner of MPL takes justifiable pride in giving canonical expression. The problem confronting us here is analytic. Every elementary sentence of TFL is of form 'some /every S is /isn't P.' If a sentence like 'it is P' is to be parsed as of this form, the pronoun will be analysed as an expression containing a word of quantity and a proterm. Our job is to make these explicit and to do this not only for such simple forms but for a variety of sentence forms that are successfully dealt with by MPL. Our discussion will be informal; the more formal development of TFL is not undertaken until chapter 9. For a more systematic account of procedures for translating between MPL and TFL the reader is referred to Appendix A.

One may doubt whether the resources of a language that lacks the apparatus of modern quantification could possibly be equal in expressive power to a standard logical language. However the findings of Schonfinkel, Quine and others who have worked on the problem of devising variable-free languages of adequate expressive power allay this worry; it has been shown that any sentence of a standard language can be translated as a sentence in a predicate functor type of language that is free of variables. This important result had been elaborated by Quine in two important but neglected papers and its significance for the theory of logical syntax has not yet been assessed.[1] Quine suggests that a predicate functor approach to logical form is 'somehow more basic' than a quantificational approach. This ought to give some pause to those who find the bound variable so indispensible for logical syntax. (Yet it is Quine more than anyone, who is responsible for the popularity of the thesis that the pronouns of natural language are really bound variables. Bound variables are eliminated in favor of operations on predicates. So they are somehow not so basic after all.)

In the next sections we shall pursue a predicate functor type of approach to pronouns that are usually translated as bound variables. We shall at the outset not attend to referential pronouns, concentrating instead on non-referential pronouns of the B-type variety. To these pronouns we shall initially apply the type of analysis given in the previous chapter. We there understood the proterms of B-type pronouns to be compound terms whose elements are the subject and predicate terms of the antecedent sentence. We shall very soon find that this approach is severely limited and unworkable. A more adequate functor approach will then be offered. This second approach does not suffer from some of the limitations of the first but it too proves unacceptable. We shall then scrap the compound term approach to the parsing of pronouns in natural languages. A third and final account of the proterms of B-type pronouns is presented in the later sections of this chapter.

The form of B-type pronominalization that we have been discussing has antecedents of form 'some S'. We have ignored pronouns whose antecedents are of form 'every S' for the good reason that such pronouns may be readily construed as mere proxies for their antecedents. Consider for example the difference between the two pronouns in 'some boy kissed every girl at the party: I wonder why they let him'. The pronoun 'him' which has a particular antecedent cannot be replaced by that ante-

[1] W. V. O. Quine, Algebraic Logic and Predicate Functors (1970); 'The Variable' (1976). Both papers are available in Quine's *The Ways of Paradox and Other Essays* (Harvard University Press, 1976).

cedent without weakening the statement and changing its meaning. 'They' on the other hand could be replaced by its antecedent 'every girl at the party' and may indeed be treated as a conventional abbreviation for that antecedent. In general, pronouns of particular antecedents are genuine and 'creative' in contrast to the purely surrogative pronouns of universal antecedents.

Our tentative account has it that sequences of the form 'some S is / are P; it /they is /are Q' may be construed as 'some S is/are P; some S & P is/are Q'. In this way of construing the pronominal subject we give it the quantity of the antecedent subject and a proterm compounded of the terms in the antecedent sentence. Semantically the proterm denotes the members of the class of items that verify the antecedent sentence.

The compound term way of interpreting B-type pronouns works well enough for 'some S ... it ...'. But it becomes suspect when we consider pronominalizations of greater complexity. Indeed the suspicion that the approach is unworkable is confirmed as soon as we move away from the monadic cases. Consider, for example, 'a boy loved a girl and he kissed her'. Here the policy of compounding the subject term of the pronominal fails utterly. For it yields 'a boy who loved a girl kissed a girl who was loved by a boy', but we want something like 'a boy who loved a girl kissed the girl who was loved by the boy' which won't do since it reintroduces the pronominal expressions 'the girl' (or 'her') and 'the boy' ('him') in an unanalysed form. There is, moreover, no way of getting around this difficulty which arises whenever the antecedent sentence is relational. We conclude that the proposed analysis of B-type pronouns cannot be correct.

There is an alternative termist way of analysing pronominal sentences which I shall call the predicate functor way. It corresponds to the kind of analysis that Quine has proposed for a language that is free of pronouns (or bound variables). In the predicate functor way, a sequence of form 'some S is P and it is Q' is parsed as 'some S is P and some S is P and Q'. This contrasts with the subject functor way; instead of forming a compound subject term for the pronominal subject we form one for the predicate. The 'predicate way' can be extended to relational sentences as well. Thus the pronominal sentence in 'a boy loved a girl and he kissed her' would now be analysed as 'a boy loved and kissed a girl'.

A predicate functor analysis construes all pronominal subjects as mere abbreviations for the antecedent subjects. This loses the information provided by the predicate term of the antecedent sentence but the loss is made good by the appearance of this term in the compound predicate of the pronominal sentence. The pronominal predicate term is a compound term, a conjunction or disjunction, depending on whether the antecedent and pronominal sentences are conjoined or disjoined. Thus the form 'some S is P or it is Q' parses as 'some S is P or some S is P or Q' which i) treats the pronoun as simply standing in for the antecedent subject and ii) construes the pronominal predicate disjunctively since the antecedent and pronominal sentences are themselves disjoined.

Having achieved some initial success with the predicate way of giving a termist representation to pronominal sentences we could proceed to apply it to more complicated cases. We consider several examples:

   (a) if a man signs a contract he must honour it.

In treating (a) we have regard to its equivalence to 'any man doesn't sign a contract or he must honour it'. This becomes

   (a') any man doesn't sign or must honour any contract.

Here the predicate functor is a relational product of form 'not R or S' where 'R' and 'S' are two place relational expressions.

   (b) some painter loves himself
   (b') some painter is identical with and a lover of some painter
   (c) a boy who was fooling her kissed a girl who loved him
   (c') a boy was fooling and kissed and was loved by a girl
   (d) some critic admires every work collected by his father
   (d') some critic is fathered by and admires every work collected by some man
   (e) for any three persons, if the first is taller than the second and the second is taller than the third, then the first is taller than the third

(e) any man is taller than or (else) not taller than anyone taller than any man.

The compound relational expression tying 'any man' to 'any man' is of form 'R or not-R to everyone R to . . . '

These examples indicate how a termist logic is capable of dispensing with B-type pronouns in expressing what is usually expressed in quantificational idiom. It is in fact possible to go quite far in this direction using only operations on predicates and relations that are available in a language like English. For example we form converses of relations and relational products and we can crop a three place relational expression treating it as a two place relational expression as we do in tying 'some critic' to 'some man' by the 'two place' relation 'an admirer of every work collected by'. But after a while one finds it necessary to make use of functors that are unnatural and artificial. Indeed the programme cannot be carried through without the use of the kind of functors that Quine lists for a language capable of translating all the formulas of quantificational logic into a purely termist language that is free of individual variables. Nevertheless the predicate functor way is good theoretical evidence that a formal termist logician can contrive to say whatever the practitioner of MPL can say with the apparatus of quantifiers and variables.

It is clear, all the same, that this sort of analysis while semantically revealing is not syntactically adequate from a naturalist standpoint. A predicate functor equivalent that *eliminates* the pronouns of a pronominal sentence does not explain their syntactic structure; it is more accurate to say with Quine that it explains it away. In this one respect the subject functor way is superior to the predicate functor way: it at least adheres more closely to the idea that an analysis of the pronominal sentence should reveal the structure of the pronoun itself by giving it its proper quantity and giving its proterm its proper denotation. This one does—even if one does it badly—when 'it is Q' is parsed as 'some S that is P is Q'. One does not do this in parsing it as 'some S is P and Q'. So while the predicate functor way provides a semantically perspicuous equivalent for the pronominal sentence it does not provide the kind of analysis that explicates the pronoun itself as a subject expression. On the other hand we saw that an analysis of the subject that assigns to it a compound proterm will soon fail even to give an equivalent of the pronominal sentence to be analysed.

The trouble with functor approaches goes deeper still. Consider the non-relational case where the subject-type of analysis was successful. We there say that 'it is Q' may be construed as 'some S that is P is Q'. This account parses 'it' as 'some S that is P'. But this too is unsatisfactory since it does not capture the definiteness of 'it' as a subject expression. Clearly something vital is lost when a pronoun like 'it' or 'they' is analysed as an indefinite subject expression.

2. We need some way of capturing the quality of definiteness that even B-type pronouns have. Since the mark of a definite subject is wild quantity our analysis of the pronominal sentence must construe it as a particular sentence that entails its universal generalization. But this calls for a new way of understanding the proterm of the B-type pronoun; we must so construe the proterm that a wild quantity assignment to the pronominal subject makes good sense. Thus if 'ϕ' is the proterm, our account of 'ϕ' must explain how the pronominal sentence '. . . some ϕ . . .' entails '. . . every ϕ . . .'.

A particular sentence 'some ϕ is ψ' is said to have wild quantity when the denotation of 'ϕ' is such that 'some ϕ is ψ' semantically entails 'every ϕ is ψ'. Formally we then may represent the sentence as '*ϕ is ψ', the star being used to signify 'some' in the context that allows for its replacement by 'every'. In actual language 'ϕ' may be a proper name and a special mark of wildness will then be omitted. Since both speaker and hearer know that 'Cicero' uniquely denotes Cicero, it is known that 'some Cicero is eloquent' entails 'any Cicero is eloquent' and the use of either sign or, for that matter, the use of a sign with the force of the star—will add no information. On the other hand where 'ϕ' is a descriptive term as in '(the) present king of France' the definite article will partly function as a sign of wild quantity. See below, subsections 2.2 and 2.3.

It is easy to see why referential (A and D-type) pronouns have wild quantity: some individual or individuals have been antecedentally focused on and the proterm is introduced to denote just that individual or those individuals. Later reference by the pronoun is to all and not only to some of the individuals denoted by the proterm so wild quantity is in order. But in a sequence embodying a B-type pronoun there is no 'thing in question' being focused on. Thus in 'some man will reach Mars in the nineties; he will (probably) be a trained biologist' there is no antecedent reference to some particular man who will reach Mars; any man who reaches Mars in the nineties can serve to verify the prediction. But if in the manner of functor analysis we form a proterm denoting all men who reach Mars we cannot assign wild quantity to the pronoun 'he'. Clearly an interpretation of the pronominal sentence that has it entailing 'every man who reaches Mars in the nineties will be a trained biologist' is unacceptably strong.

Our problem is to seek for an interpretation of the proterm that makes sense of the pronoun's wild quantity and to do so in the face of the fact that no particular thing is being referred to in the case of non-referential pronouns. This problem has a familiar ring. We recall Geach's objections to speaking of reference for 'some S' and for the pronouns that have back reference to such indefinite phrases. The device of forming a proterm to denote 'the thing in question' does seem inappropriate for non-referential pronouns. Acknowledging this, we still refuse to blink the fact that 'it' and 'they' are always definite subjects interchangeable with phrases of form '*the* S (that is P)'. All this suggests that we take another look at the proterms of B-type pronouns. For we must see how to construe them in a manner that allows for assigning wild quantity to them even though the pronouns under consideration have not been used in situations where there is an epistemic focus on some particular individual or individuals which the proterm could be said to denote.

We shall henceforth assume that pronouns, being definite, have wild quantity and that B-type pronouns are no exceptions. In the case of B-type pronouns we have the problem of determining their proterms in a way that explains their wild quantity. However this problem is part of the more general problem of characterizing the subject terms of definite subjects. To what sort of subject term is it appropriate to prefix a wild quantity? When the term is a proper name the answer is clear enough: a name like 'Socrates' denotes no more than one thing so 'some Socrates is P' entails 'every Socrates is P'. The singularity of denotation is good reason for parsing 'Socrates is P' as '*Socrates is P'. But singularity is not the only reason to assign wild quantity. Consider for example, the referential pronoun in a sequence like 'some men are at the door; they want to speak to Leslie'. If 'Js' denotes the men in question then the pronominal subject '*Js' will refer to more than one J. Since singularity of application is not a condition for the assignment of wild quantity to a plural definite subject we shall want a more general condition. A proper characterization of sentences with definite subjects should explain in a general way why such sentences have wild quantity. This is one way that the termist logician finds himself facing the perennially teasing question of understanding definite subjects.

2.1 The purpose of the discussion that follows is the specification of the kinds of terms suitable for the position of subject term in definite subject expressions. In aid of this we shall examine some of the distinct ways that terms get to do their job of denoting the things in their extensions.

A term like 'round' is said to be defined by a set of things. If we take this way of defining 'round' seriously we cannot go on to say that the principle of construction of such a set is that we include all and only round things in it. On the other hand it is hardly illuminating to say that it just happens that all and only round things are in the set defining 'round'. Or if we do say this then we have given up the idea of explaining how to construct a set for defining 'round'.

We could give a non-questionbegging procedure for inclusion in the defining set if it is assumed that we are able to determine whether two things are very similar in shape. We may then think of the set as being constructed in something like the following way:

We define a term $\hat{P}_s$ by the set of objects whose only member is the sun. The caret is a sign for terms that have restricted application to some given individual under consideration. The subscript 's' here indicates that the thing uniquely denoted by the term is the sun. Other terms may be similarly defined, each denoting the sun. Let us suppose that $\hat{P}_s$, $\hat{Q}_s$, and $\hat{R}_s$ are so

defined. We shall refer to such terms as 'U-terms'.
Extensionally, the U-terms $\hat{P}_s$, $\hat{Q}_s$ and $\hat{R}_s$ are equivalent. They
may however be discriminated if each is associated with a
different determinable feature of the sun. For example we may
associate $\hat{P}_s$ with colour and $\hat{R}_s$ with shape and it would then
make sense to say that the sun is $\hat{P}_s$ in colour and $\hat{R}_s$ in shape
but not that the sun is $\hat{R}_s$ in colour or $\hat{P}_s$ in shape.[2] Also since
the terms denote uniquely, it will be necessarily true that the
sun is $\hat{P}_s$ and $\hat{R}_s$. Let us also suppose that the moon is $\hat{P}_m$ (in
colour) and $\hat{R}_m$ (in shape). By hypothesis we are able to
determine whether two things are similar or dissimilar in shape
so let us assume that we have determined that the sun and
moon are very similar in shape. Having noted this similarity we
may begin the construction of a set of objects mutually similar
in shape (or sufficiently so) and which contains the sun and the
moon as members. Let us suppose that the next object we
consider is a penny and that the penny satisfies the condition
for inclusion in the set. We may at this point pause and define a
term R* to denote whatever is either $\hat{R}_s$, $\hat{R}_m$ or $\hat{R}_p$ but nothing
else. As we have defined it R* is a plural U-term but not a
general term; its denotation, though not unique, is restricted
since it includes only certain objects mutually similar in shape
but not *all* such objects. Finally we may define a truly general
term R, by the set of all objects similar to those under
consideration. Because the set includes all and only objects that
would pass the tests for being sufficiently similar to the initial
object or objects, it defines a general term. The very idea of such
a set means we know how to go on to add to its membership: we
then stipulate that no object that could be found to be
sufficiently similar to those already included is excluded from
membership. A term so defined is a 'G-term' in contrast to 'U-
terms' that denote certain objects but which possibly exclude
other objects that may well be sufficiently similar to those
included in respect of some determinable feature under
consideration. We may take R to represent 'round' but
although 'round' applies to all and only objects that are round
we are not committed to the viewpoint that all of the objects in

---

[2] For discussion of 'features' see my paper 'Types & Ontology', reprinted in
Philosophical Logic, ed. P. F. Strawson (Oxford University Press, 1967), p. 162, and
chapter 13 below.

the set that defines it have the *same* shape. The view, that roundness is a common property possessed by all round objects is neither ruled out nor necessitated by the definition. One could, for example, think of 'round' as equivalent to a disjunction of U-terms associated with the same determinable, each one denoting an object in the maximal set. Any object in the maximal set defining 'round' is or could be characterized by its own U-term. Each object has its shape and however similar in shape it may be to some other object in the set nothing requires us to say that any two objects have a determinate property in common.

2.2 We are looking at U-terms with an eye to their suitability as subject terms in definite referring expressions. Although we can define U-terms that apply to pairs or larger n-tuples of things, our immediate purpose is better served by attending to U-terms that correspond to monadic G-terms like 'round' or 'planet'. 'Planet' differs from 'round' in being a sortal term. We have discussed the way U-terms denote the different objects in the class of round things and we shall now say something about U-terms that apply to things in the extensions of sortal G-terms. A sortal G-term like 'planet' denotes many objects that are similar to one another each of which is characterized by a U-term. However, 'planet' differs significantly from 'round' in the way that any two objects it denotes are similar to each other. Objects denoted by 'round' are similar to each other with respect to a *single* determinable feature (shape). Objects denoted by 'planet' are similar to each other with respect to *several* determinable features (motion and mass among others). Suppose then that the U-term '$\hat{P}_j$' applies to Jupiter in virtue of its type of motion, its shape, and its mass and that $\hat{P}_s$ applies uniquely to Saturn with respect to the very same determinables. We may find that Jupiter and Saturn are similar enough in their determinations of these determinables to warrant the construction of a set of mutually similar objects. Thus both are found to be roughly circular in their motions, both roughly spherical in shape, and both are found to have a very large mass (larger than that of the largest meteorite and smaller than the mass of the sun). Knowing how to go on to include other objects we define the G-term 'planet' by a maximal set of objects that includes Jupiter and Saturn and other objects that are similar to Jupiter and Saturn in their determinations of the aforementioned determinables. The definition of sortal terms by maximal sets of objects, similar in several respects, is therefore somewhat more complex than the definition of a simple adjectival term like 'round' or 'red' by objects similar in a *single* respect, but the complexity is fairly straightforward and may here be ignored.

According to strictures imposed by a termist logical syntax a definite referring expression must be of form '*S'. For instance the pronominal subject of 'I saw a planet; it (the planet) was red' must be parsed with wild quantity. We are however unable to parse 'the planet was red' by simply treating the definite article as a sign for wild quantity. And this means that, despite appearances, the G-term 'planet' is *not* the subject term of 'the planet' or of its pronominal equivalent, 'it'.

2.3 The question of the character of the term in a definite subject has been before us all along. And the answer we can now give is that, *pace* Russell, and despite appearances to the contrary, the subject-term in 'the planet' is not a G-term but a U-term. In the context of 'I saw a planet; the planet was red' the pronominal expression 'the planet' is referential and 'D-type'. The speaker is referring to a particular object and the proterm of 'the planet' or 'it' is a U-term that denotes this object in virtue of its shape, mass, and type of motion. Let this U-term be represented by '$\hat{P}$'. The move from 'a planet' to 'the planet' is a move from an indefinite referring expression to a definite referring expression. The definite article in 'the planet' thus performs *two* tasks: it signifies the wild quantity of the definite subject and it is a U-term indicator. It thus combines the roles of the '*' and the ' $\hat{}$ ' in the subject form '*$\hat{P}$'.

Just as 'the' operates on 'planet' to give the subject-term of 'the planet' U-term status, so too does 'certain' in 'a certain planet, often discussed by philosophers interested in identity statements, is being approached by a space vehicle recently launched by the Soviet Union'. Consider the difference between

if a girl comes to the party Harry will be very uncomfortable and

> if a certain girl comes to the party Harry will be very
> uncomfortable.

The former predicts that *any* girl's coming to the party will
occasion Harry's discomfort. The latter predicts this effect for
a particular girl that the speaker has not identified for us. In 'a
certain girl will come' the word 'certain' is a U-term indicator.
It is not part of the quantifier expression, but a syncategorematic part of the subject term in much the way that 'un-' in 'an
unwise man' is a syncategorematic part of the subject term
'unwise man.' Let 'ĝirl' be a U-term denoting the particular girl
I have in mind when I say that a certain girl will be coming.
Then 'a certain girl will be coming' parses as 'a ĝirl will be
coming' and its pronominal sequel 'she will make Harry
uncomfortable' parses as '*ĝirl will make Harry uncomfortable'.

The subject of 'a certain girl will be coming to the party' is
indefinite. Despite this the speaker is referring to a girl that he
could identify for us, and 'a certain girl' is here being used to
make an identifying reference to the girl in question. Let us
suppose that the speaker omits the word 'certain' but that
nevertheless he is referring to a certain girl. Then in the
sequence 'a girl will be coming to the party; she will make
Harry uncomfortable' the pronoun 'she' will again be parsed as
'*ĝirl' (the term 'ĝirl' U-denoting the girl in question). Here the
antecedent sentence lacks a U-term indicator and the question
arises whether to parse it as if it read 'a certain girl will be
coming to the party'. I believe that this question should be
answered affirmatively. For reasons given in our earlier
discussion of the secretary's remark ('a man has been trying to
reach you') the use of 'an S' is identificatory whenever the
speaker means to refer to a certain S. If so, and where the
epistemic context of assertion warrants it, 'a girl will be
coming' should be parsed with a U-term subject-term and
interpreted as making reference to a particular thing. Similarly
'I saw a planet' should be understood as 'I saw a certain planet'
and parsed as 'I saw a P̂'.

2.4 We have yet to give an account of pronominalization

between non-identificatory referring expressions. Consider again my prediction about space travel in the last decade of the twentieth century where I say:

Some man will land on Mars; he will be a biologist.

This has the form 'Some S is P; it is Q' where 'it' is a B-type pronoun. Nothing has been taken for as S so no particular S is under consideration; 'some S' weakly refers to an S that is not identified by the speaker. The reference of 'it' is also non-identificatory. Indeed, among definite subjects, only B-type pronouns have a weak mode of reference.

In chapter 4, B and E-type pronouns were dubbed 'non-referential' in deference to the usage which restricted referring to names and other identificatory expressions. In speaking now of the *weak* reference of B-type pronouns we revert to the more tolerant and less tendentious terminology of chapter 3. Definite pronouns that 'weakly' refer are anaphorically tied to indefinite antecedents. For a better grasp of them we must look more closely still at the antecedents.

Whenever a sentence of form 'some S is P' is uttered by a speaker who is not reffering to a particular individual, it can be verified by *any* individual that is both an S and a P. I shall say that 'some S is P' *comprehends* the set of S things that are P and speak of this set as the comprehension of 'some S is P'. In traditional logic 'comprehension' is not applied to sentences but to terms, the comprehension of a term being the set of attributes possessed by the individuals it denotes. Comprehension was seen as inverse to denotation: 'bald man', for example, comprehends more attributes and denotes fewer individuals than 'man'. With apologies to the Port Royal logicians, I am usurping 'comprehension' for the set of verifying individuals of a sentence. The new job that 'comprehension' does is related to the old; just as 'bald man' comprehends baldness and humanity so 'some man is bald' comprehends all and only individuals who have both. Nevertheless there is considerable violence to the traditional meaning for, as I use it, comprehension is an extensional notion; what is comprehended by a sentence is a set of things and not a set of attributes.

A sentence may be associated with more than one set of individuals that could verify it. Thus 'a boy loved a girl' is

verified by individuals from either of two comprehension sets;
boys who love girls and girls loved by boys. Not every sentence
is associated with a set of individuals that could verify it.
Indeed no universal sentence is. A sentence like 'every human
being is featherless' has no comprehension: an individual who
is both featherless and human may help to confirm it but no
individual could possibly verify it.

In predicting that a man will land of Mars in the nineties I
purport to refer to an individual in the comprehension of 'a
man will land on Mars in the nineties'. Reference is distinct
from comprehension. All men who land on Mars in the nineties
are comprehended by the prediction, but only one is being
weakly referred to. We distinguish then between the comprehension of a sentence, the denotations of its terms and the
reference of its subject. 'Some S is P' comprehends all SP
things, 'S' denotes all S things and 'some S' refers to an SP
thing.

The reader will recall why we say that 'some S' refers to an *S
that is P*. There is first the straightforward idea that 'some S'
refers to some S. This idea was not questioned by pre-Fregean
logicians who distinguished between reference by 'some S' and
'every S'. The former purports to refer to some S, the latter to
every S. The distinction between reference and denotation was
used to determine the distribution value of the term S. The term
itself denotes every S and when its denotation coincides with
the reference of its subject, the term is said to be distributed and
undistributed otherwise. Accepting the idea that 'some S'
purports to refer to some S we argued in chapter 3 that the S
purportedly referred to is an S *that is P*. For suppose that 'some
S' refers to an S that may or may not be P, and suppose it refers
to one that is not P. 'Some S is P' would then be false even if it
were true that some other S is P. But 'some S is P' is true just in
case *any* S is P. It follows that a reference to some S must
purport to be to an S that is P and that 'some S is P' is true just
in case 'some S' successfully refers. For in that case one has said
of some S that is P *that* it is P. In the Aristotelian formula: to
say truly that something is P is to say of what *is* (P) *that* it is (P).

Whenever 'some S is P' is followed by '(and) it is Q' the
proterm of the pronoun has the job of denoting what was
antecedentally referred to by 'some S'. In the case of epistemic

reference the proterm is a U-term introduced to denote the individual taken for an S. This does not apply to proterms in non-epistemic contexts of reference where the question 'which S does the proterm denote?' is quite inappropriate. Nevertheless we want to understand B-type pronouns within a general account of relative pronouns and so we want to say that even in the case of weak or non-epistemic reference to an S that is P the proterm is a U-term introduced to denote "the S in question". The next subsection aims to show how we may construe the proterm of B-type pronouns in a manner strictly analogous to the proterms of strongly referential pronouns.

2.5 Consider the two statements made by the same sentence in epistemic and non-epistemic contexts where I predict that a girl will come to the party and she will fascinate Harry:

(1a) a (certain) girl will come to the party and she will fascinate Harry

(1b) a girl will come to the party and (she) will fascinate Harry.

In asserting (1a) I refer to a particular girl. The antecedent does this in an indefinite manner. The pronominal does it in a definite manner (by means of the definite subject 'she'). The pronoun of (1a) is referential. More specifically 'she' is here a D-type pronoun whose proterm denotes the girl in question. In (1b) the context is non-epistemic and 'she' is a B-type pronoun. As such it is non-referential or 'quasi-referential'. Just here we may agree with Geach that the subject is a referring expression that gives the appearance of referring to an individual without doing so. For no particular girl is under consideration and the use of the definite pronominal subject in (1b) is not on a par with its genuinely referential use in (1a). Since B-type pronouns are dispensable and since they do not do a genuine job of referring, the function they serve is practical rather than theoretical. That their dispensability is tied to their secondary semantic status is recognized by Quine when he says of the functor forms that they are more basic than their pronominal equivalents. Thus despite Quine's exploitation of bound variables for ontological insights his recent researches into functor logic has led him to relegate the bound variable to a secondary semantic role giving pride of place to the predicate functors that systematically eliminate it. And indeed the semantic perspicuity of 'some S is P and Q' is not in question; it refers to and can be verified by an S that is P and Q. 'Some S is P and it is Q', on the other hand, is less clear cut. Quine has characterized the occurrence of the pronoun in non-opaque contexts as referential. But since the pronoun does not refer to any given individual, the characterization is not as transparent as Quine suggests.

Any B-type pronoun can be explained away but in practice the actual use of predicate functors for eliminating it is very often quite impractical. We do need some way of making quasi-reference to things that are identified only as satisfying certain conditions. I refer to a boy who loves a girl and later find it convenient to be able to refer to the boy and the girl 'in question' going on to say that he (the boy) kisses her (the girl). Consider again the difference between using pronouns and avoiding them in asserting that being taller than is a transitive relation between persons:

(2a) if any person is taller than another then anyone taller than the first is taller than the second

(2b) any person is *either taller than or else fails to be taller than anyone taller than* any person.

(2a) makes use of the pronominal expressions 'the first' and 'the second'. (2b) is a predicate functor equivalent of (2a). It contains no pronouns but at the price of connecting the two flanking subject expressions with the intricate (italicized) relational expression.

As often as not B-type pronouns cannot be eliminated without intolerable circumlocution. Moreover a pronoun-free formulation is not always possible in the natural languages. It is an empirical fact that the functor resources of a language like English are simply *not* equal to the demands of a full programme for eliminating B-type pronouns in favour of pronoun-free formulations. This does not mean that there are any B-type pronouns that are uneliminable in *principle*. But it does mean that we come to a point at which the introduction of functors needed for eliminating them is very artificial from the standpoint of English syntax. We shall see below that the logical syntax of natural language can be given a representation in a simple plus-minus algebra. Although any pronoun can be represented in the notation of this algebra the syntactic possibilities for forming functors are limited and it is not always possible to represent a functor equivalent for sentences with B-type pronouns without going beyond the combinatory resources of the plus-minus algebra. In effect the possibilities for B-type pronominalization in a natural language out-run the natural capacity of the language for eliminating them. The implications of this cannot be discussed here.

We have then an overriding practical need for quasi-reference to individuals identified only as satisfying certain conditions. The most plausible account of the structure of the subject expressions that serve this need is that, in adopting the fiction that we are referring to some given individual that satisfies the antecedently stated conditions, we go for verisimilitude by introducing a proterm to denote 'the individual in question'. That we pretend to refer to an individual as if one were before us for referential consideration, is suggested by the fact that very often the B-type pronoun is naturally replaceable by the referring phrase 'the individual in question'.[3]

The mock reference account of B-type pronouns sheds light on Quine's remark that functor pronoun-free formulations are somehow more basic than their pronominal equivalents so that for example

(A) some girl will come to the party and fascinate Harry

should be considered semantically more perspicuous than

(1b) some girl will come to the party and she will fascinate Harry.

The functor formula (A) weakly refers to a girl who will come to the party and fascinate Harry. The proterm of the pronoun in

---

[3] That even B-type pronouns refer accounts for pronominalization across inference lines as in Strawson's example (above, p. 82) where the proterm of 'he' denotes the man referred to in the major premise. Referentially understood B-type pronouns need not be viewed as defined by functors that explain them away. Some functors—the term and propositional connectives of chapter 9—*are* fundamental. Others such as the Self and Permutation functors can themselves be understood by way of pronominalization. For example, we may use ' Some S $_j$ existed and *J destroyed *J to explain 'Some S self-destructed'.

(1b) is introduced to denote the girl in question, achieving an effect of definite reference by trading on the indefinite reference made by (A) to a girl who satisfies the stated conditions. Seen in this light (A) will seem more basic than (1 b).

2.6 The mock reference account of B-type pronominalization is intuitively acceptable and it has the syntactic advantage of allowing us to parse B-type pronouns as we parse the pronouns of genuine reference. To see more clearly into the nature of the B-type proterm we shall take another look at the way a B-type pronominalization is related to its pronoun-free counterpart.

Let G be a pronominalization of form ⌐'Something$_{Jj}$ exists and . . J . .' and let H be its pronoun-free equivalent. (The reader may take as an example of G a proposition of form 'something exists and it is S' and as an example of H a proposition of form 'something is an S'. The simplicity of the example will not detract from the general argument.) As we construe 'J' it is a makeshift U-term introduced for the purpose of denoting an unidentified individual in the comprehension of H. We may now replace 'J' in the pronominal sentence '(. . J . .)' by 'J̇$_i$' and the result '(. . J̇$_i$ . .)' is true sentence. According to this account 'J' is to 'J̇$_i$' as a makeshift device is to its permanent (albeit arbitrary) replacement.

B-type pronouns are our present concern. Later chapters will present arguments for the more general thesis that all names for individuals are arbitrary U-terms introduced as permanent replacements for pronominal subject terms. In the present case the assignment of J̇$_i$ to the proterm position occupied by J corresponds to the familiar MPL move known as existential instantiation which consists of replacing an existentially bound variable (say the 'x' in the matrix of '($\exists$x)Sx') by an arbitrary individual constant.

We have applied to the proterms such terms as 'mock' or 'makeshift'. We shall also speak of them as 'instantial' proterms as a reminder of their B-type status and of their close kinship to the bound variables of MPL that figure in existential and universal instantiation. The correspondence of the instantial proterms of TFL to the bound variables of MPL comes into its own when the characteristic MPL instantiation technique for proving the validity of an argument are seen to have exact analogues in an improved system of traditional formal logic.

The mention of logical proofs reminds us that an acceptable account of B-type pronouns must be able to show how one may reckon logically with sentences that contain them. It must, for example, allow for going from 'some S is P; it is Q; it is R' to 'some R is Q'. Formally speaking one could rely on systematic procedures for eliminating the pronominal sentences with B-type pronouns in favour of pronoun-free sentences and apply the inference rules of a term-functor logic to the latter. But a more natural approach that applies directly to B-type pronominal sentences is available to the termist logician. In our example, he may take the sentences 'it is Q' and 'it is R' with wild quantity for the pronominal subjects and get 'every J is Q and some J is R' from which 'some R is Q' follows by ordinary rules of syllogistic. Trivial as it is, the example suggests how a traditional formal logic may handle inferences with B-type pronouns.

3. Our theory that B-type pronouns have instantial U-terms applies to pronominalizations with any number of antecedent subjects and it allows for both intersentential and intrasentential pronominalizations.

In the relational sentence 'a boy loved a girl', 'a boy' weakly refers to a boy who loved a girl in the comprehension set of boys who loved girls, and 'a girl' weakly refers to the girl loved by the boy in the comprehension set of girls loved by boys. The pronominal sentence 'he kissed her' is analysed accordingly and the whole pronominalization looks like this:

$$_{\iota}\text{a boy}_{\text{Jk}} \text{ loved } _{\iota}\text{a girl}_{\text{Jj}}; {}^{*}\text{K kissed } {}^{*}\text{J.}$$

In the standard treatment of predicate logic, pronominalization is invariably intrasentential taking place between a quantifier antecedent and the variable it binds. In term logic pronominalization may be syntactically intersentential; it connects the subject of the antecedent sentence to the subject-term of the pronominal sentence, the latter *denoting* what the former refers to. One consequence of this difference is the way predicate logic parses sentences that appear to be separate as parts of a single sentence (in treating, say, the form 'some S is P; it is Q'). The opposite holds for term logic which may give an intersentential analysis to what appears to be pronominalization within a single sentence. For example (1) 'a boy who was fooling her kissed a girl who loved him' could be analysed thus:

(1a) ˌa boyˌₖ kissed a ˌgirlˌⱼ
(1b) *K was fooling *J
(1c) *J loved *K.

A compressed and closer to the surface parsing of (1) is

A ˌboyˌₖ who was fooling *J kissed ˌa girlˌⱼ who loved *K.

Other examples where an intersentential analysis is appropriate for intrasentential surface pronominalization are

(2) some bald man shaved himself
(2a) ˌsome manˌᵢ is bald and *I shaved *I
(3) every bald man shaves himself
(3a) if ˌa manˌⱼ is bald then *J shaves *J.

(2a) and (3a) may be compressed and rendered, respectively, as (2a') 'ˌSome bald manˌᵢ shaved *I' and (3a') 'ˌevery bald manˌⱼ shaves *J'. If (3a) is true any U-term that is introduced to denote a bald man will denote a self-shaver. Thus (3a) entails sentences with dotted letters such as 'if $\dot{J}_i$ is a man and $\dot{J}_i$ is bald, then *$\dot{J}_i$ shaves *$\dot{J}$', if $\dot{K}$ is a man and $\dot{K}_i$ is bald then *$\dot{K}$ shaves *$\dot{K}_i$' and so forth. And generally since 'if an S is P than . . . it . . .' is the same as 'if *any* S is P then . . . it . . .'; a change of U-term does not affect the truth value of the instantiating conditional.[4]

4. So far it has been assumed that instantial proterms occur only in the definite subjects of B-type pronouns. But a very plausible case can be made out for saying that other subject-terms have an instantial character. Believing that a black swan must somewhere exist I may say that some swan is black. In the sentence,

(1) some swan is black

the term 'swan' is a G-term. But (1) clearly entails

(2) a certain swan is black

---

[4] For the rules governing 'any' and 'an' see appendix C.

and we have argued (section 2.3) that 'certain' is a U-term indicator. We should parse (2) with a U-term in subject position. Let 'U$_{(swan)}$' be a U-term denoting a swan. Then (2) parses as 'Some U$_{(swan)}$ is black'. By hypothesis we do not have an epistemic reference to any individual taken for a swan. The move from (1) to (2) is therefore analogous to the move made in a B-type pronominalization where one introduces an instantial U-term to denote an individual whose existence satisfies the truth conditions of a certain pronoun-free formula. The move from (1) to (2) is similar in this respect, for (2) introduces a U-term denoting an individual in the comprehension of (1) and its own comprehension as well. Here then we have an example of an instantial U-term occupying the position of subject-term in an *indefinite* non-pronominal subject.

The use of 'a certain S', even in a context where nothing has been taken for an S, raises expectations. On being told that a certain swan is black one waits to hear more, perhaps enough to be able to answer the question 'which one?' A similar effect may be got *retrospectively*. I may follow 'some swan is black' by 'and it will someday be observed and captured'. Although the antecedent is not of the tell-tale form 'a certain S', the effect of quasi-reference to a particular individual is the same. For I have gone *on* to talk of a certain S and he who hears the sequel is prepared to construe 'some swan' as 'a certain swan'.

That instantial U-terms may occupy subject positions in non-pronominal sentences thus suggests that antecedents of B-type pronouns may themselves be sentences of this kind. A pronominalized equivalent of 'some swan is black' is 'A (certain) swan exists and that swan (it) is black' which may we represent with a G-term and an index as

$_\lrcorner$some swan$_{\lrcorner j}$ exists and *J is black.

Alternatively we could represent it without an index but with recurrent instantial U-terms in *both* subject positions:

some U$_{(swan)}$ exists and *U$_{(swan)}$ is black

If we construe the antecedent with an instantial U-term in the subject position then 'some swan exists and it . . .' amounts to 'A *certain* swan exists and it . . .'.

Interpreting 'Some swan . . . that swan' as 'A *certain*

swan . . . that swan . . .' has several formal virtues:

(a) It formally represents B and E type pronominalizations in the way that A and D type pronominalizations may generally be represented, with antecedent pre-focused on 'the thing in question'.

(b) By introducing the U-term at once, it indicates how we may dispense with the need for using indices for the cross reference of antecedent and pronoun.

(c) It reads the antecedent as referring to a specific (if unspecified) individual about whom we are to get more information anon. And this seems right: in going on to talk about that thing we seem to be supplying information that satisfies expectations already raised by the antecedent.

Although the recurrent U-term interpretation has these important formal advantages it seems to me preferable to use the index subscript style of representing 'some S . . . it . . .'. One is then free to read the antecedent with a G-term in conformity with the vernacular surface; pronominalizations of form 'an S . . . that S . . .' are perhaps more usual than pronominalizations of form 'a certain S . . . that S . . .'. One is also free to hold that 'an S' tacitly gives way to 'a certain S' before we move on to 'that S'. And finally one is free to read the antecedent subject phrase '$_\llcorner$some$_{\lrcorner j}$' as 'a certain S' thereby treating the half-brackets and subscript as a U-term indicator and the subject-term of this phrase as an instantial U-term that later reappears as the proterm of the pronominal subject. The question of how to construe the antecedents of B-type pronouns thus remains open and unbegged by the index notation for pronominal cross-reference.

5. Though we take note of the correspondence between the U-terms of TFL and the individual variables and constants of MPL the difference between any term and any 'individual symbol' is crucial. Unlike the names that serve as subjects of atomic propositions a term can appear in both subject and predicate positions and a term can be negated to form its contrary. But a name suitable for being a logical subject in an atomic proposition cannot be negated nor can it appear as a term in predicate position. The differences between names and terms is responsible for very different treatments (by term logic and by predicate logic) of notions of identity and difference. In the next chapter we shall present the termist position on identity but here we remark that the ability to form the contrary of a U-term makes it easy for the termist logician to give a plausible account of phrases like 'someone else', 'everyone else' and 'no one else'. In these phrases the word 'else' is the contrary of a U-term. Consider

Lila talked; everyone else was silent
Lila talked; every (non-Lila) was silent

Harry didn't laugh; someone else did
Harry didn't laugh; some non-Harry did

a man from Kent protested; everyone else acquiesced
a $_\llcorner$man from Kent$_{\lrcorner i}$ protested; every $(-I)$ acquiesced

there's one Deity, at most
if $_\llcorner$a Deity$_{\lrcorner i}$ exists then no $(-I)$ is a Deity

certain initiates were allowed (to enter)
no one else was allowed
$_\llcorner$some initiates$_{\lrcorner i}$ were allowed; no non-Is were allowed.

The last sequence uses plural U-terms to effect a reference to the initiates in question.

In chapter 4 we remarked on the termist ability to form contraries of proterms and pronominal subject whose antecedent subjects are themselves pronouns. We now make the same observations with a clearer appreciation of the nature of the proterm. Consider again an example of propronominalization:

(1) Americans will land on Mars in the nineties
(2) some (of them) will be women
(3) some of the women will be cooks; the rest of them will be trained scientists.

This sequence has the following form:

(1) $_\llcorner$some A$_{\lrcorner i}$ are L
(2) $_\llcorner$some I$_{\lrcorner j}$ are W
(3) $_\llcorner$some J$_{\lrcorner k}$ are C; all J & not-K are S.

6. In this chapter we have pursued an examination of

pronominalization. Among the conclusions we have reached
are: i) a functor approach which parses the pronominal
sentence by means of operations on the terms of the antecedent
and the pronominal sentence does not give an adequate analysis
of pronouns as definite subjects; ii) pronouns in common with
other definite subjects must be construed with wild quantity; iii)
with the possible exception of E-type pronouns, the proterms
of pronouns are terms of restricted application or 'U-terms'.
The proterms of pronouns that translate as bound variables are
'instantial' U-terms; iv) in common with other terms, U-terms
have contraries. But the contrary of a U-term is not itself a U-
term.

Epistemic reference to a *certain* S by 'some S' is identificatory
reference. Pronominal reference to 'some S' is then 'referential'
in the strong sense. This last point about epistemic identificatory reference by an indefinite subject reminds us of what is
perhaps the most important feature that distinguishes the
language of term logic from any standard (Fregean) logical
language. The reader will recall Geach's insistence that even
when the speaker is referring to a *particular* thing and taking it
to be an S, 'an S is P' translates as '$(\exists x)(Sx \& Px)$' which may be
verified by *any* S that is P. And indeed, whenever he might be
tempted to think about the meaning or truth conditions of
statements made in context of epistemic reference to something
taken to be an S, the orthodox Fregean is in no position to allow
that 'an S is P' says more than what is conveyed by its canonical
translation as an existential sentence. In the language of
modern predicate logic the proper name is the only vehicle of
genuine reference so 'an S' cannot be represented as a genuine
referring expression. The lesson to be learnt by entertaining a
termist alternative is that the Fregean view of genuine reference
is imposed by formation rules that rule out all expressions,
except proper names, as subject expressions. When this lesson is
learned all the arguments for the privileged status of proper
names as the only genuine referring expressions are seen as
apologetic attempts to justify a theory of reference that is
appropriate to the rules of a particular logical language that has
been adopted. The more liberal alternatives to the theory of
reference are then seen as having been ruled out by the
formation rules of the preferred language.

These circumstances encourage *ignoratio elenchi* by faithful Fregeans who cannot see to the right or to the left of the positions they are occupying. We repeatedly observed in chapter 2 how those who argued for the atomicity thesis and against the two term theory were simply unaware of the syntactic resources of the latter theory. And in this and the preceding chapter we have been able to remark how these same philosophers with the blinker vision vouchsafed them by the syntactic limitations of 'standard languages' have been confidently able to say what genuine reference must be like by being unable to see what it could be like.

6
Do we need Identity?

1. We predicate, says Frege, a concept of an object. The ontological distinction between concept and object thus corresponds to the syntactical distinction between predicates and names which are the basic ingredients of the atomic proposition:

> The concept (as I understand the word) is predicative. It is, in fact, the reference of a grammatical predicate. On the other hand, a name of an object, the proper name, is quite incapable of being used as a grammatical predicate.[1]

This doctrine, that a name cannot appear as a term in predicate position, is almost universally accepted today. And, of course, it demands some analytical firmness in dealing with misleading surface appearances. Frege himself noted that the doctrine

> might appear false . . . Surely one can just as well assert of a thing that it is Alexander the Great, or is the number four, or is the planet Venus, as that it is green or is a mammal? If anyone thinks this he is not distinguishing the usages of the word 'is'. In the last two examples it serves as a copula, as mere verbal sign of predication. We are here saying that something falls under a concept, and the grammatical predicate stands for this concept. In the first three examples, on the other hand, 'is' is used like the 'equals' sign in arithmetic, to express an equation. I use the word 'equal' and the symbol ' = ' in the sense 'the same as', 'no other than', 'identical with'. In the sentence 'the morning star is Venus' we have two proper names, 'morning star' and 'Venus' for the same object. In the sentence 'the morning star is a planet' we have a proper name 'the morning star' and a concept-word, 'planet'. So far as language goes, no more has happened than that 'Venus' has been replaced by 'a planet'; but really the relation has

---

[1] Black and Geach, p. 43.

become wholly different. An equation is reversible; an object's falling under a concept is an irreversible relation. In the sentence 'the morning star is Venus' 'is' is obviously not a mere copula . . . one might say instead: 'the morning star is no other than Venus' . . . What is predicated here is thus not *Venus* but *no other than Venus*. These words stand for a concept, admittedly only one object falls under this, but such a concept must always be distinguished from the object. We have here the word 'Venus' that can never be a proper predicate, although it can form part of a predicate. The reference of this word is thus something that can never occur as a concept, but only as an object.[2]

In this classic passage, Frege distinguishes between the 'is' of predication in 'a is a planet' and the 'is' of identity, in 'a is Venus'. I do not know whether this distinction was definitely made before Frege. The distinction is sometimes attributed to Leibniz but I have not found in Leibniz's logical writings any passage that supports this. Frege says that the 'is' of identity occurs obviously in 'the morning star is Venus' or at any rate that it is obvious that the 'is' is there not the 'is' of predication. If this is right, then one wonders why logicians before Frege had not made more of the distinction. An appeal to obviousness is in any case not to be relied upon in a matter of such importance and re-reading of the passage shows that the 'is' of identity is made obvious to us only after we have accepted the logical syntax of concept-words and object-words. Frege would have been more candid if he had more openly appealed to his category distinction between names and predicates to enforce the distinction between the two kinds of 'is'. In effect, he does this. Let us agree that 'Venus' and 'the morning star' are proper names. If we rendered the two in logical notation, we might represent them by lower case letters, say 'b' for 'Venus' and 'a' for 'the morning star'. But now if we read the expression 'a is b' with the 'is' of predication, it is ill-formed: it lacks a predicate. It is *therefore* obvious that 'a is b' has the form 'F(a, b) where F is the grammatical predicate which represents 'is identical with' or 'is no other than'. Clearly, it is only after one has adopted the syntax that prohibits the predication of proper names that one is forced to read 'a is b' dyadically and to see in it a sign of identity.

[2] Black and Geach, p. 44.

It is then fair to say that Frege has yet to persuade us of the need for a new sense of 'is'. For we may take the course of refusing to accept the ill-formedness of 'a is b' when 'is' is read as the 'mere copula'. It might seem, however, that a sentence like '2 + 2 is 4' provides a clear instance of the 'is' of identity. For surely '2 + 2 is 4' says nothing different from '2 + 2 = 4'. But this consideration is two-edged: instead of arguing for an 'is' of identity in '2 + 2 is 4' it may argue for an 'equals' of copulation in '2 + 2 = 4'. It may sound contradictory to speak of sentences like '2 + 2 = 4' and 'the morning star is Venus' as identity sentences when we do not acknowledge that they contain a relational expression for identity. But not really: an identity proposition will now be defined as a monadic proposition that has proper names in *both* subject and predicate positions. Moreover, one who holds that identity propositions are non-relational will hold that 'is identical with' and 'is no other than' are merely stylistic variants of 'is' and 'isn't', typically used when the predicate term that follows them is a definite singular term. The non-relationalist would say that it makes no more sense to interpret 'is no other than' relationally (understanding, say, 'the morning star is no other than Venus' as the claim that being no other than holds true of the pair, the morning star and Venus, in that order) than it makes sense to interpret 'was hardly' relationally (understanding, say, 'Sam was hardly a criminal' as the claim that being hardly holds true of Sam and some criminal, in that order). So the linguistic evidence is, to say the least, inconclusive, as between a relational and non-relational view of identity propositions.

If we adopt the non-relationalist position—a traditional one as we shall see—we remove at one fell swoop all the paradoxes associated with the assumption that identity is a relation. For we are denying the need to talk of identity in this way, and *a fortiori*, we are denying the need for a logically new primitive sign, ' = ', to be added to those already recognized in traditional formal logic (these include 'not', 'some', 'and', but *not* ' = '). To be sure, we must eventually be able to show that we can handle inferences for which identity is characteristically needed in modern logic. But the fear of impending logistic weakness is far too often a cause of avoiding or ignoring any suggestion that is at odds with the currently standard logical grammar. And in the present instance, the shoe is on the other foot. For the monadic reading of 'identity' statements has the following two advantages over the Fregean dyadic reading:

(i) it avoids the need for a logically primitive relation.
(ii) it avoids the need for new axioms governing the relation of identity.

The two advantages are clearly related. We have already discussed the first; the second must now be shown.

2. The traditionalist theory holds that affirmative singular propositions have the form '*a is P' where '*a' is a singular subject with wild quantity. A singular sentence is an *identity* sentence when and only when its predicate term is also a definite singular term. Thus if 'b' is a definite singular term (what Frege calls a proper name) then '*a is b' is an identity sentence. We distinguish as before the expression '*a' which is complex from the simple expression 'a' which represents the subject-term of the proposition '*a is b'. In this case, the terms are designed to denote no more than one individual but this does not matter: syntactically either term can appear in subject or in predicate position. On the other hand, the expression '*a' cannot be predicated; a *normal* set of formation rules for the language of traditional formal logic would rule out 'predicate' expressions like 'is every S'.

Where Frege writes 'a = b' we shall write the monadic sentence '*a is b'. And we shall now prove the monadic counterparts of the standard identity principles of modern predicate logic with identity.

(i) One law of identity is that the identity relation is reflexive. The monadic counterpart of this is that '*a is a' is a logical truth. That this is so is evident if we give it the form of a universal proposition (which we are free to do). Then '*a is a' is an instance of 'every x is x' which is a logical truth in traditional logic. (It is known as *the* law of identity.)

(ii) Corresponding to the law which asserts the symmetry of the identity relation we have to show that '*b is a' follows from '*a is b'. Traditional logic needs no special principle for this since it is an instance of the general principle of conversion for propositions of form 'some x is y'. In this case, we read the identity propositions as particular propositions and we have

if *a is b then *b is a

as a special instance of

if some x is y, then some y is x.

(iii) If identity is a relation then we need to be told that it is transitive. But if identity is not a relation we can prove the corresponding law for monadic statements: if *a is b and *b is c then *a is c. To show this we merely write each of the monadic sentences as a universal sentence and the law becomes a variant of a syllogism in Barbara.

(iv) The monadic correspondence to the principle that identical things are indiscernible is the principle that from '*a is b' and '*b is P', '*a is P' follows. If all these propositions are assigned universal quantity, this is proved syllogistically:

(every) a is b
(every) b is P

(every) a is P

(v) The non-relational form of the principle of the identity of indiscernibles asserts that if '*a is P' always follows from '*b is P' then *a is b. To prove this we observe that by the hypothesis that a and b are indiscernible, then if '*b is b' is true, '*a is b' will be true. But (by the principle of 'reflexivity') '*b is b' *is* true. So *a is b.

These results of applying the monadic interpretation show that it is superior to Frege's dyadic interpretation in eliminating the need for special axioms governing a primitive relation of identity. The results cannot be achieved with a Fregean syntax. And this alone suggests the desirability of a sympathetic reappraisal and development of the syntax of traditional formal logic.

Dummett has correctly observed that 'it was Frege who first made identity a logical notion'. To which one may remark: no one before Frege had any need for a logic of identity; in traditional formal logic, the so-called laws of identity are neatly absorbed as special instances of familiar laws of term logic.

3. Scepticism about the logical syntax of Frege, with its absolute distinction between object-words and concept-words, has led to this scepticism about the need for a special logic of identity. It might be thought that sceptical attitudes toward Frege's syntax of names and predicates is natural to someone who is refusing to take seriously what Frege says about the difference between objects and concepts. But if objects and concepts are as different as Frege says they are, then it would seem entirely reasonable to hold that object-words and concept-words are as syntactically different as Frege makes them and the prohibition against predicating object-words is then also reasonable. I do not find much in this. In the first place to anyone who finds an alternative to the atomicity thesis, the object-concept distinction loses its syntactical authority and becomes a metaphysical distinction of no great interest to the logician or the grammarian. The strength of the object-concept distinction is precisely the strength of Frege's logical syntax; the former is dependent on the latter and not vice versa. (Here I agree with Dummett and disagree with Geach and Strawson who hold that Frege's category of proper names is defined by and grounded in the ontological category of objects or particulars. See above, chapter 2, section 6.) But even if we have independent reasons to accept the object-concept distinction, it does not follow that a singular proposition like 'Socrates is mortal' is made up of an object-word and a concept-word. For the traditionalist analysis may still be right and the proposition may have a complex subject consisting of a sign of quantity and an object-name. Simply to assume as Frege does, that logical subjects are simple object-names, is to beg this question.

It may still be said that this point merely concerns the subject of the allegedly atomic proposition. But we could give up atomicity and allow for the complexity of the subject without admitting that we can predicate object-names. The question of the predicability of proper names seems to be independent of our attitudes to the logical form of the subject of definite singular propositions. After all, even Aristotle, the arch term logician, opposed the predication of proper names. And Geach seems to be doing no more than echoing Aristotle when he says:

A proper name is never used predicatively—unless it ceases to be a proper name, as in 'he is a Napoleon of finance' or (Frege's example) 'Trieste is no Vienna'; in such cases the word alludes to certain attributes of the object customarily designated by the proper name. In statements of identity we may indeed say that the copula joining two proper names has a special role . . . In 'Tully is Cicero' the copula is no longer the trivial bit of grammatical form that it is in 'Socrates is a man'. On that very account however, our absolute distinction of names and predicables is inviolate; for the predicable (say) 'is the same man as Cicero' is totally different from the name 'Cicero'.[3]

Here again we see how the prohibition against predicating proper names leads to the relation theory of identity. Moreover, Geach's reasons for denying predicability to proper names seem *here* to be independent of the question of what the form of a logical subject is. To be sure, Geach does in the end tell us that proper names and predicables are utterly different but his examples have a force that is independent of this consideration. I think, however, that one may counter this by supplying common examples where a proper name does appear as the predicate term. 'Tully is Cicero', 'Istanbul is Constantinople', and 'the morning star is Venus' are examples of predicating proper names. Frege brought such examples and he explains them *away* by introducing the 'is' of identity. Geach does not do more than this. So his pronouncement that a proper name cannot be used predicatively is no more than a manifesto of the logical syntax which recognizes the 'absolute distinction' Geach finally appeals to. There may be any number of non-syntactical reasons why one does not predicate proper names. Aristotle's were metaphysical; he believed in a hierarchy which begins with individuals and goes up to genera and he held that the order of natural predication corresponds to the hierarchical order of individuals, species and genus. But Aristotle nowhere saw a syntactical prohibition against predicating proper names. If, for example, some one should say 'some animal is Socrates' then Aristotle called his predication 'unnatural' or 'accidental' but he never thought of impugning its well-formedness. He similarly objected to 'some white thing is a log'.

[3] Geach, *R & G*, p. 42.

At another place where Geach is criticizing the traditional doctrine of 'distribution' he tells us that 'a proper name cannot stand as a predicate term at all—it stands for an individual, not for something that does or does not hold good of individuals'. But how does Geach know that 'is Cicero' (with the good old 'is' of predication) does *not* 'hold good' of Tully? I see nothing but dogmatic fervor in this: and in the end this criticism of the traditional theory rests on the failure to view it with any clarity or sympathy. Over and over again, Geach fails to see that the traditional logician has an alternative syntax which is not under the constraints of Frege's logical grammar.

4. We have adopted the Leibnizian ('wild quantity') variant for the logical form of definite singular propositions and shown how to derive the analogues to the laws of identity within the framework of traditional formal logic. It is surely ironical that the relation of identity and the logic of this relation are so closely associated with 'Leibniz's Law'. For Leibniz has no need of the identity relation; if what I have been saying is correct and we assume that Leibniz is not internally inconsistent on a fundamental matter of logic then the so-called Leibniz Law of the substitutivity of identicals cannot, in any sense, be a Law that holds for things taken to be *related* by identity. In one customary formulation, Leibniz's Law is said to say that if a is identical with b, then whatever can be said of a can also be said of b and vice versa (Benson Mates). It is sometimes said that we can define identity in this way in any logic which permits quantification over properties (a second-order logic). There is, of course, no way for anyone to prove the law and in any first-order system of standard logic that includes identity, identity is viewed as a primitive relation governed by certain axioms. (Frege who adopted the second-order version of Leibniz's Law still considered identity to be primitive, refusing to use the law as a definition of the identity relation.)[4]

An examination of Leibniz's own formulations of the principle of substitutivity indicates that he never thought of it as stating a condition for the truth of 'a = b' if that is read as a dyadic statement. In most of his formulations, Leibniz says that when two *terms* (most often general terms) are the *same*

---

[4] See Dummett, *Frege*, pp. 542–3.

they are substitutible *salva veritate* in all contexts. And two terms 'A' and 'B' are 'the same' whenever every A is B and every B is A, i.e., whenever they have the same denotation.

If we reformulate Leibniz's 'axiom' in this way, then we give 'a = b' and 'b = a' monadic readings:

> If every a is b and every b is a then whatever is true of a is true of b and whatever is true of b is true of a.

Now *this* law is provable and Leibniz's own formulations of it were often accompanied by a proof which is usually syllogistic in character. For example, the paper 'A Specimen of the Universal Calculus' begins by saying that a universal proposition 'every a is b' will be expressed as 'a is b'. In an addendum to the specimen, we find this formulation and proof of Leibniz's Law:

> If a is b and b is a then a and b are said to b 'the same'. From this it can easily be proved that one can everywhere be substituted in place of the other without loss of truth; for if a is b and b is a, and b is c or d is a, then a is c or d is b.[5]

The proof is syllogistic for 'every a is b' and 'every b is c' entails 'every a is c' and 'every a is b and every d is a' entails 'every d is b'. Note that 'every b is a' doesn't even figure in the proof; the real point of the proof is that identity propositions are two-way universal propositions subject to the usual syllogistic laws. It is, in any case, evident that the principle of substitutivity is quite general and that it applies to general terms as well as to singular terms. In fact, Leibniz rarely uses singular terms in his examples.[6]

[5] Leibniz, *Logical Papers*, ed. G. H. R. Parkinson (Oxford, 1966), p. 71.

[6] The original version of 'Leibniz's Law' is found in Aristotle *Topics* Book 7; chapter 1, 152b, pp. 25–30. It is cited by Quine (*WO*, 116) with approval: 'For Aristotle had the matter straight: things are identical when 'whatever is predicated of one is also predicated of the other'. Quine omits the second half of this passage: 'and anything of which one is a predicate the other ought also to be a predicate'.

A recent writer actually brackets this part and advises: 'a modern reader may disregard the bracketed part of the test; the "a" and "b" of our rule of substitution, even if singular terms, could be regarded as predicates of some other subjects in the pre-Fregean "traditional" predication theory'.

The omission and the bracketing are both significant as is the acknowledgement that identity propositions cannot involve general terms in MPL. It is clear that Aristotle like Leibniz did not assume that identity was a relation and that he thought that 'A' and 'B' are 'the same' just in case every A is B and every B is A; from which it followed that

It is, in this connnection, worth taking a closer look at the place of the law of substitutivity of identicals (for singular terms) within the general logic of terms. The rule of inference for classical term logic is the *Dictum de Omni*:

What is true of every X is true of what is X.

The basic pattern of inference is:

$$\begin{array}{c} \text{every X is Y} \\ \dots \text{X} \dots \\ \hline \dots \text{Y} \dots \end{array}$$

The *Dictum de Omni* lays down two conditions on syllogistic inference:

(1) One premiss must be universal.
(2) The middle terms must have opposite distribution values.

The syllogistic pattern is one of substitution: given a universal proposition as the major premiss we can derive as conclusion the proposition substituting the major term for the middle term of the minor premiss. Now these two conditions will *always* be satisfied if the major premiss is an identity statement. For we can then automatically assign to the major premiss a universal quantity and we are subsequently free to assign whatever quantity we need in order to get opposed distribution values for the middle term. Thus we may be sure that the following inference pattern will satisfy the *Dictum*:

$$\begin{array}{c} \text{a is b} \\ \dots \text{a} \dots \\ \hline \dots \text{b} \dots \end{array}$$

Philosophers today usually think of the law of substitutivity in connection with identity statements. But if we read 'a = b'

---

whatever is an A is a B and whatever is a B is an A and what 'is A' is true of 'is B' will be true of and vice versa. The second part of Aristotle's formula shows clearly that we are here not dealing with 'individual constants' but with terms that can appear in either subject or predicate positions and that Aristotle did not think of 'A is the same as B' as predicating identity of A and B. cf. Ignacio Angelelli 'Friends and Opponents of the Substitutivity of Identicals'; *Studies on Frege II*, ed. M. Schirn (Frommann Holzboog, 43, 1976).

monadically (the ' = ' of predication) the law of substitutivity of identity is seen as a special case of the law of substitutivity once popularly known as the *Dictum de Omni*. To be sure, when the major premiss is 'a is b' (where a and b are both singular terms), we get the most impressive application of the *Dictum*, impressive because the conditions for substitutivity are *automatically* satisfied whenever the major premiss has two singular terms.

5. So much then for Leibniz's Law. It is a classical example of how to make a philosopher say something he never intended to say. In this case, Leibniz got credit for an axiom he doesn't need and which he probably would not even accept in the form it is usually stated (with identity as a relation).

If identity *is* thought of as a relation, then the most reasonable thing to say is that it is a relation a thing bears to itself. This is Frege's considered view and it leads him to the celebrated doctrine that a proper name has a sense as well as a reference. It is worth noting that the *semantic complexity* of proper names is the direct consequence of the doctrine of their *syntactic simplicity*. As we just saw, the syntactic simplicity of the logical subject leads to the doctrine that identity is a relation. And the relational theory of identity led Frege to his theory of sense and reference. Let us review Frege's explanation of why it is that the sentence 'the morning star is the evening star' is informative, although the sentence 'the morning star is the morning star' is not informative. Both are dyadic and both state a relation between the morning star and the evening star or between the evening star and the evening star. Since they are about the same things and say the same thing about them, we cannot but wonder why one is informative and the other not. The wonderment disappears as soon as we say that a proper name presents its reference by way of its sense. The information conveyed by saying that the morning star is the evening star is precisely that what is presented as the morning star is the same as what is presented as the evening star.

Let us see whether there is an analogue of the paradox of informativeness if identity is a pseudo-relation and identity sentences are construed as monadic. The existence of the morning star is not in question. We may then assign 'every a is a' as the form of 'the morning star is the morning star'. This sentence is uninformative since it is tautological. But we similarly assign 'every a is b' as the form of 'the morning star is the evening star'. This sentence is informative and there is no paradox in saying so. The paradox arises for the dyadic reading of 'a is b' and 'a is a' precisely because in both cases we *predicate* identity of two logical subjects where both subjects refer to the same things. But in the monadic reading, we have a single logical subject in both cases; in the one case, we tautologically predicate 'is a' of (every) a; in the other case, we informatively predicate 'is b' of every a. There is much to be said for Frege's solution to the paradox of identity. But it is on the whole preferable to avoid a problem even if one has an elegant solution for it at hand.

6. In recent literature, we find Geach criticizing Frege for not recognizing that we cannot predicate absolute identity of a thing with itself; according to Geach, all we can say is that 'a is the same T as b' where T is a substantive term. Since I do not agree that any form of a relational sentence of identity is involved in saying that 'a is b', I will not enter the lists for or against Geach's relative identity. I mention it here because of one curious development. If, Geach says, we accept relative identity, then we are in a position to define 'is P' as 'is the same P as itself'. That Geach or anyone else should think of this as a desirable thing to do is curious enough. But it comes close to getting us into another paradox of identity.[7] For when I say that Socrates is Socrates, what I am really saying is that Socrates is the same man as Socrates. But now if I say that Socrates is a man, I am saying that Socrates is the same man as Socrates. In the Frege paradox, we wondered how two propositions that said the same things about the same things could be different. Now—in the paradox of identity—we must wonder how two propositions that are so different could be saying the same thing. The proposal that 'Socrates is a man' is dyadic in form is, of course, altogether at odds with the traditional analyses which treat even identity propositions as monadic. The proposal is to my mind altogether unnatural but perhaps it is natural that it should come from one as

---

[7] For why Geach thinks it is a good thing, see *R & G*, p. 191.

passionately opposed as Geach is to 'the bad old logic' (as he calls it).

7. Discussion of identity has recently been augmented by the views of Saul Kripke on the modality of identity propositions. According to Kripke, an identity proposition 'a is identical with b' is, if true, necessarily true. For example, Kripke holds that 'Tully is Cicero' is necessarily true. One formal argument that he gives for this applies Leibniz's Law to the premiss 'a is identical with b' and the premiss 'a is necessarily identical with a' to conclude that 'a is necessarily identical with b'. Kripke says that he finds the suggestion that an object can contingently bear a relation of identity to itself a dark doctrine. But the philosopher who construes identity propositions non-relationally is not given light by being informed that a 'relation of identity' holds necessarily between any object and itself. For the non-relational theorist the doctrine that a true proposition such as 'Cicero is Cicero' or 'Tully is Cicero' makes a relation claim is a dark doctrine regardless of the modal status of the proposition. Let us therefore examine the fate of Kripke's thesis of necessary identities when identities are construed non-relationally. If Kripke's thesis is not peculiar to the relational interpretation there will be arguments, analogous to the ones Kripke gives, for the view that 'Tully is necessarily Cicero' is entailed by 'Tully is Cicero', when these are read as monadic propositions.

Where Kripke uses 'a is necessarily identical with b' we shall use the monadic form 'every A is necessarily B' in which 'A' and 'B' may be singular or general. We inquire into the non-relational fate of Kripke's thesis that Tully is necessarily Cicero by examining the truth conditions of the general forms 'every A is necessarily A'.

According to Kripke, 'every A is necessarily A' is true for any term A that applies essentially to the things it denotes. An example of a term of this kind is 'cat': whatever is a cat is necessarily a cat; if Felix is a cat there is no conceivable situation (possible world) in which Felix is not a cat. 'Philosopher', on the other hand, applies inessentially. Tom is a philosopher but in other circumstances he would not have been one and, generally, whoever is a philosopher is not necessarily a philosopher.

Kripke's view that Tully is necessarily Cicero is related to his thesis that proper names like 'Cicero' are rigid designators. As Kripke observes, we can never truly say that Cicero might not have been Cicero; in effect, Cicero is necessarily Cicero. Stated as a non-relational identity, we would formulate this as the universal proposition 'every Cicero is necessarily Cicero'. Continuing with the non-relational TFL treatment we see that 'Tully is Cicero' entails 'Tully is necessarily Cicero'. For from 'Tully is Cicero' and 'every Cicero is necessarily Cicero', we may conclude syllogistically that 'every Tully is necessarily Cicero'. And, generally, whenever a and b are proper names we have the syllogism:

every a is b
every b is necessarily b
--
every a is necessarily b

The same applies to general terms like 'cat' and 'mammal'; we may, for example, deduce 'any cat is necessarily a mammal' from 'any cat is a mammal' and 'any mammal is necessarily a mammal'. In its TFL version, the Kripke doctrine that 'is Cicero' is necessarily true of Tully and 'is a mammal' is necessarily true of any cat is seen to depend on the general assumption that certain terms necessarily apply to what they denote.

Using 'a is necessarily identical with a' as a self-evident premiss Kripke says that it follows by Leibniz's Law that if a is identical with b then a is necessarily identical with b. But Kripke's premiss is unacceptable as a logical truth if identity propositions are non-relational. In TFL 'every A is necessarily A' has no status as a logical truth; it is not in *general* true that every S is necessarily S, but only true for proper names and certain other terms that apply to whatever they apply without regard to the modalities. It is, therefore, not in general true that everything is necessarily identical with itself. (It is, in TFL, not even coherent to say this since there is no meaning to a relation of identity between a thing and itself.)

If 'every A is necessarily A' is not a logical truth then Kripke's thesis that true identity propositions whose terms are proper names are necessarily true cannot be made out by any argument analogous to Kripke's use of Leibniz's law. It may still be possible to give independent arguments for the necessity of true proper name identity propositions such as 'Tully is Cicero'. This question will be taken up again in chapters 11 and 12.

8. We saw how the monadic non-relational theory of identity yields laws that are the counterparts of the laws governing the identity relation in a standard logic and how the monadic theory is spared the paradoxes of identity, absolute and relative. Two areas of doubt concerning the viability of the monadic theory remain. There is first the problem of its expressive power. Can we, using a monadic notion of identity, say things like 'there are exactly two luminaries' or 'there is at most one Creator'? The second area of doubt concerns the ability of the monadic theory to cope with arguments involved in identity statements. I shall briefly comment on these two matters in turn.

The logical representation of numerical proportions like 'there is at most one creator' presents no difficulty for the monadic theory. The form of this proposition may be represented in a manner that parallels its translation in MPL with identity:

if ⌞a being⌟ᵢ is a creator and ⌞a being⌟ⱼ is a creator then *I is J.

Another way to say this will rely on the number of the antecedent:

if ⌞a being⌟ᵢ is a creator then no non-I is a creator.

These are equally acceptable ways of saying that there is at most one creator.

In the case of antecedents with plural subjects, the pronoun will be plural and we indicate this notationally. Thus

except for some children, no one is in the yard

would be represented as a conjunction of '⌞some children⌟ᵢ are in the yard' and 'no others are':

⌞some children⌟ᵢ are in the yard and no non-Is are in the yard

The propriety of the device for distinguishing singular from plural proterms is justified by our ability to translate a sentence like 'there is at most one creator' without reliance on the singularity of the antecedent. We could similarly indicate plurality by devices like '$_L$some S$_{Ji}$ is P and $_L$some S$_{Jj}$ is P and *I is not J'; since that can be done, we may use the plural 'I' to indicate the plurality of the proterm whose antecedent subject is an indefinite plural expression 'some S$_s$'.

It is, I hope, clear that the monadic theory is at no disadvantage when it comes to representing the logical form of propositions involving numerical expressions. A sentence like 'there were exactly four Beatles' is somewhat more complicated but it does not present any theoretical difficulties.

I turn now to the problem of the logical competence of the monadic theory. For one reaction to the foregoing might be: 'Very well, you have shown that the two term theory can have a notion of identity in which identity statements are monadic. One may even grant that the theorems are more elegant or economical in the traditional logic of terms than the corresponding theorems in a system of modern predicate logic. But MPL is an instrument of proven scope and adequacy and we are prepared for some inelegance within an efficient system. In any case, you cannot really mean to suggest that we give up the theory of atomic propositions which has led to the relational conception of identity just because we can do without it in traditional logic. That would mean giving up all the other advantages that predicate logic enjoys over traditional formal logic'.

I believe that this rejoinder has some force. And indeed I have not suggested that anyone should 'give up' modern predicate logic. Nevertheless, the rejoinder is based on the assumption that modern logic enjoys a fixed logistical advantage over any form of traditional formal logic. This assumption is false and the implications of its being false will engage us in later chapters. But even now we may see how the monadic theory of identity may account for inferences comprehended within a modern predicate logic with identity. An example is the valid argument:

Cicero envies everyone else
Tully is not envied by Cicero

Tully is Cicero

Regimented in the manner of traditional formal logic the first premiss becomes

every Cicero is envious of every non-Cicero

which is equivalent to

(1) every non-Cicero is envied by Cicero

The second premiss is equivalent to

(2) everyone envied by Cicero is non-Tully

(1) and (2) syllogistically yield

(3) every non-Cicero is non-Tully

which is equivalent by contraposition to

(every) Tully is Cicero

I have in this example anticipated some of the results of the next chapter concerning the ability of traditional logic to deal with relational propositions. Thus I have assumed that TFL can infer 'b' is envied by 'a' from 'a envies b'. But few philosophers would insist that modern logic holds the monopoly on such inferences and those who do have no grounds whatever for their bias.

7

Relations in Traditional Formal Logic

1. It is generally agreed that the logical conquest of arguments with relational expressions was one of Frege's greatest technical achievements. And it is thought that TFL's inability or unwillingness to see in 'Socrates is taller than Plato' a two-place predicate is the reason for its failure to formalize relational arguments. While it is true that here MPL succeeded where TFL failed, there is considerable confusion over the reasons for the failure. Arguments with relational expressions were not altogether neglected by earlier writers. We find William of Sherwood observing that 'every man sees some man' follows from 'some man is seen by every man'—an example of inference from determinate to confused *suppositio*. Before Frege, observations like this one were sporadic and unsystematic and it is quite correct to say that TFL was at its weakest when reckoning logically with relational propositions.

It is, however, a mistake to attribute this to the fact that TFL does not order predicates in accordance with the number of subjects they take. In William of Sherwood's example, it is clear that the relational expression 'seen by' is isolated for purposes of inference from the passive to the active voice which enables the move from the determinate occurrence of 'some man' to its confused occurrence in the conclusion. Thus, while it is true that TFL refuses to accord *predicate* status to relational expressions, it is not true that it does not recognize them as a special class of categoremata quite different from terms like 'man' or 'Socrates'. One can recognize the equivalence between 'Socrates sees Plato' and 'Plato is seen by Socrates' without parsing either sentence with a 'two-place predicate'. This is so because the rules that allow us to rewrite the first as the second are quite independent of what one takes as the logical predicates of the sentences.

There are a number of reasons for the failure of TFL to develop an adequate logic of relations, none due to any intrinsic advantage of the logical syntax of MPL over TFL. One main reason was its failure to achieve a formal notation for representing categorical propositions—relational and non-relational alike—that was felicitous for a logical calculus. I shall show in chapter 9 how to repair this characteristic defect of TFL. Another defect has to do with pronouns. Traditional logicians did not make explicit the logical form of pronouns in a manner that would have been consistent with their own view of the logical subject as a complex expression. Lacking this, they were unable to read a proposition like 'every man loves himself' as 'if someone is a man then he loves himself', an inability which places obstacles in the way of formalizing relational inferences involving pronouns. Because of the lack of an adequate notation for pronouns within the logical syntax of TFL, there was a tendency to rely very heavily on converse forms of a relation. Thus, where MPL could get by with 'loves' in representing both 'every boy loves some girl' and 'some girl is loved by every boy', TFL was forced to invoke rules governing transformations from the active to the passive form. In MPL, this is taken care of by a change in the order of quantifiers. For example, using quantifiers we may represent 'someone is seen by every one' as 'someone, y; everyone, x (x sees y)' thus getting by with 'sees' alone and not introducing 'is seen by'. In the translation, the 'x' in the matrix '(x sees y)' appears before the 'y' but the order of the antecedents is opposed to this. This tension between the order of the antecedents and the order of the variables that are bound by them produces the effect of a passive transformation. The practical advantage of this effect is especially evident in cases where no natural converse is available. Thus we can say 'Socrates has a disease' but 'a disease is had by Socrates' is unnatural. A formula such as 'some disease, y; everyone, x (x has y)' can represent 'there is a disease that everyone has' without requiring us to say something like 'some disease is had by everyone'. Another example: let 'Pxyz' represent 'x persuades y to do z'. Then '$(\exists z)(y)(\exists x)(Pxyz)$' would express what the traditional logician might express by 'something was effectively urged on everyone by someone' but the formula of the modern logician does not use anything but the original relation 'x persuades y to do z'.

Without the quantifier variable apparatus and without an adequate representation of pronouns to compensate for it, it is natural to use the converse passive forms. These, however, can always be defined from a single form of a relation. Indeed, given any n-place relation R_1 there will be other relations $R_2 \ldots R_n$, that are converses to R_1. Take for example the 3-place relation '. . . gives . . . to . . .' There are six (3!) permutations of the three places and these give us six equivalent forms: x gives y to z; x gives z, y; y is given by x to z; y is given to z by x; y gets from x, z; y gets z from x.

It is useful to have some systematic way of representing the relation that corresponds to a given permutation of the subjects.[1] Let G^{123}_{abc} represent the proposition 'a gives b to c'. Since we are here construing 'a', 'b' and 'c' as subjects with quantity, we stipulate that *all have the same quantity*. This stipulation is unnecessary in the case of singular subjects but we wish our discussion of relations to hold for *any* subjects, singular or general. Corresponding to G^{123} there will be other relations, G^{132}, G^{213}, . . . G^{321}, any two of which are converse to one another and any one of which is a converse to G^{123}. We then have six equivalent propositions:

$$G^{123}_{abc}, \ G^{132}_{acb}, \ G^{231}_{bca}, \ G^{213}_{bca}, \ G^{312}_{cab}, \ G^{321}_{cba},$$

any two of which are converse equivalents.

The set of relations corresponding to the permutation possibilities for subjects will be called a *converse* set. It is obvious that we can define converse sets for any relation. For example, we can, beginning with P^{123}_{abc} –for 'a persuades b to do c', define five more relations ending with P^{321}_{cba} any two of which are converse equivalents. For instance, P^{231}_{bca} and P^{312}_{cab} would represent the equivalent propositions 'b is persuaded to do c by a' and 'c is effectively urged by a on b'.

Generally then if ϕ is an n-place relation and $a_1 \ldots a_n$ are n subject expressions, all of which have the same quantity, there will be a set of n! propositions, $\phi^{1 \ldots n}_{a_1 \ldots a_n}, \ldots, \phi^{n \ldots 1}_{a_n \ldots a_1}$, any two of which are converse equivalent. The relation of converse equivalence is an analytic relation. Where the modern notation can get by with a single form of relation, traditional logic will often use the analytical converse form.

---

[1] The superscript numeration is due to David Bennett of the University of Utah.

This advantage of modern logic over traditional logic could only be a practical one and not a theoretical one. For the modern logician must still appeal to the definitions of converse equivalents at the atomic level if he is to explain such inferences as 'Plato sees Socrates hence Socrates is seen by Plato'. If the modern logician tried to 'get by' with just 'sees' here, he would represent the inference as

Plato sees Socrates hence Plato sees Socrates

leaving it up to us to read the conclusion as a form equivalent to 'Socrates is seen by Plato'. Of course, that is no explanation and the recourse to the definition

y is seen by x = x sees y

is here necessary. Although the definition is needed at this level, the use of converse forms is later dispensable, a considerable practical advantage, which however should not be conflated to a theoretical one.

2. Even the practical advantage is altogether dissipated in a fully expressive TFL language complete with ways of representing pronouns. In such a language we can map any MPL formula and avail ourselves of whatever economy the former may have by its avoidance of converse forms. For example, we can express 'some man is seen by every man' as (roughly) 'some one is a man and if anyone is a man then the latter sees the former'. Not that this is really the more economical way of representing 'some man is seen by every man'. Indeed, for most purposes of logical reckoning, the proposition may be left as it stands. But the possibility of mapping '$(\exists x)[Mx\&(y)(My \rightarrow Syx)]$' into a corresponding TFL equivalent that is free of quantifiers is theoretically important and it shows that TFL is not forced to use the converse forms. The possibility of mapping becomes available as soon as one allows for intersentential pronominalization. This breaks up the characteristic quantificational formula in which the pronoun figures as bound variable in the same sentence as its antecedent (quantifier).

The bridge between the quantifier and the bound variable in the matrix is supplied by the notion of 'such that'. The expression '($\exists$x)(Px)' is read as 'something is such that it is P'. Russell once said that 'such that' is *sui generis*, an unanalysable and indispensable logical notion. In TFL the pronoun can appear in a sentence that is independent of the sentence containing the antecedent. We may then conjoin two sentences to give us the effect of binding. '($\exists$x)(Px)' then becomes 'ˌsomething$_{\text{Jj}}$ exists and it (*J) is P'. We may similarly render '(x)Px' as 'if ˌa thing$_{\text{Jj}}$ exists, then it (*J) is P'. A more complicated formula like '(x)($\exists$y)(Bx → (Gy&Lxy))' (which translates 'every boy loves some girl') could be rendered as

if there is a boy then there is a girl and he loves her.

In a more formal rendering we should introduce proterms and give the pronouns wild quantity.

The discussion of the syntactical relation of TFL to MPL is best left to the later chapters when we shall have developed a formal notation for TFL and shown its usefulness for logical reckoning. For the present, we note the possibility of mapping formulas of MPL into equivalent formulas of TFL. We shall not take advantage of this possibility in the discussion of the present chapter but in section 4 we shall outline a procedure for mapping from TFL into MPL.

2.1 It is customary, in reciting the advantages of MPL over TFL, to point out that in the notation of modern logic we can distinguish clearly between two meanings that might be given to 'every man sees a man', one being that every man sees some man or other, the other being that there is some man such that every man sees him. The second would be represented by having a different order of antecedents than the order of variables in the matrix: 'some man y; every man x (x sees y)'. This advantage is closely related to the advantage in expressive power that MPL is reputed to enjoy over TFL which has just been discussed. But it is even less real. First it is recognized even by some disciples of Frege that there is no ambiguity in 'every man sees a man' since most of us would read this in the first way.[2] The traditional logician who wants 'there is a man such that everyone sees him' would use the converse form and say 'some man is seen by every man'. But even if the ambiguity is a

---

[2] See Dummett, *Frege*, p. 12.

social fact, there is nothing to prevent us from stipulating that 'some y' in 'R (every x, some y)' should always be read with confused *suppositio* as 'some y or other'. We will, in fact, adopt a convention that applies to any relational proposition with several subjects of mixed quantities:

> A subject expression of form 'some S' is to be understood as 'confused' (i.e., read as 'some S or other') when and only when it is preceded by but not followed by a universal subject expression.

It might be said that MPL has no need of any such convention. But this is not so. The convention corresponds to the one implicitly applied by the modern logician in interpreting the quantifiers that precede the matrix of a. formula. If an existential quantifier is preceded by but not followed by a universal quantifier, its effect is that of 'something or other'. Thus '(x)(∃y)(Lxy)' is a translation of 'everyone loves someone or other' whereas '∃x(y)(Lxy)' is read as 'someone loves everyone'. In the first formula, the existential quantifier is indefinite in its interpretation. In the second it is definite.

3. It is in any case not accurate to say that MPL enjoys an advantage of explicitness and clarity over TFL in respect to the confused and determinate interpretations of subject expressions of form 'some S'. The only serious problem facing TFL is that of logical reckoning. How could TFL justify the inference of 'every man sees some man' from 'some man is seen by every man'? How does he infer 'everyone who draws a circle, draws a figure' from 'every circle is a figure'. This is the logistic problem which must in the end be faced by TFL. The challenge of Frege is, in this respect, genuine. For Frege showed how to reckon logically with relational propositions and in this area TFL was decidedly a failure. An example of the kind of inference that is easily handled by MPL is

> (1) since every circle is a figure, everyone who draws a circle draws a figure.

Leibniz and Jungius before him, realized the importance of being able to explain the validity of (1) and they made repeated attempts to provide a syllogistic chain of reasoning which would have 'every circle is a figure' as one premiss and 'everyone who draws a circle, draws a figure' as the conclusion. In effect, they assumed that (1) and arguments similar to it were enthymenes and the problem was to formulate the platitudinous missing premisses which could show a clear derivation of the conclusion. One of Leibniz's attempts actually succeeded but it was never generalized, and not further developed by him or by his immediate successors—a fate typical of many of Leibniz's logical discoveries. In the case of the proof of (1) the situation was not helped by Leibniz's cumbersome formulation of several tacit premisses which could all have been reduced to a single tautological premiss. The proof is the second 'demonstration' in 'A specimen of a demonstrated inference from the direct to the oblique sent by Leibniz to Vagetius (January 1687)'. When its irrelevancies are cleared away, its general form is seen to be the following one:

every X is Y
every R to an X is R to an X
_____
(so) every R to an X is R to a Y

Here we have an application of the syllogistic principle according to which we may substitute in any proposition '. . . X . . .' containing a term 'X' that is undistributed, the predicate term 'Y' of a universal premiss 'every X is Y'. This substitution principle is the rule corresponding to the *Dictum de Omni*: what's true of every X is true of (what is) an(y) X.

The *Dictum de Omni* was originally formulated for non-relational categorical propositions but it is general enough to apply to relational propositions. As a general principle, the *Dictum* sanctions conclusions that are the result of replacing 'an M' in a premiss of form 'an M is an S' or 'an(y) S is an M' or 'an(y) S is R to an M' by any expression that applies to every M. For example, given a premiss of form 'every M is P' and another of form 'some S is R to an M' we can draw the conclusion 'some S is R to a P'. Other schemas are:

some B is R to every M
some M is an S
_____
some B is R to an S

every B gives every M to some C
every S is an M

every B gives every S to some C

some S is R to every M
some G is R to an M

(so) some G is R to (what) some S is R to

Note that in the third example, the first premiss claims that 'what some S is R to' applies to every M so this expression may supplant 'an M' in the second premiss. A more mechanical method for applying the *Dictum de Omni* is obviously desirable and one will be offered in chapter 9. For the present, the following formulation is general enough. Let 'H' represent the expression claimed to be applicable to every M and let 'H: every M' represent the proposition in which this claim is made. Then the schema of the *Dictum* can be represented thus:

H: every M
an M

H

This schema clearly shows that the *Dictum de Omni* is a substitutivity principle allowing for the replacement of 'an M' by the expression applicable to every M.[3] Specifically it governs the replacement of the undistributed occurrence of 'a circle' in the context 'draws a circle' thus explaining the inference:

every circle is a figure
(everyone who draws a circle draws a circle)

∴ everyone who draws a circle draws a figure

One often hears that TFL cannot handle arguments with multiply general propositions.[4] A favourite example is the inference 'some girl is loved by every boy so every boy loves a girl'. It is accurate to say that this and other inferences of the same kind were not systematically treated by traditional logicians. But the claim, made on behalf of Frege's systems, that for the first time it was possible to account for the boy-girl

---

[3] The distribution condition for substitutivity is always satisfied when the major premiss is an identity statement '(every) M is H'. See the discussion in chapter 6.

[4] See Dummett, *Frege*, chap. 2.

inference is quite baseless. For as we said it is open to TFL to represent the premiss as a (B-type) pronominalization in two sentences:

(1) ⌞some one⌟$_j$ is a girl
(2) every boy loves her (*J)

The proof proceeds:

(3) if ⌞some one⌟$_j$ is a girl then she (*J) is a girl
(4) *J is a girl
(5) every boy loves a girl

Premiss (3) is a platitude. (4) follows from (3) and (1) by *modus ponens*. (5) follows from (4) and (2) by the *Dictum de Omni* if we read (4) as 'every J' is a girl and (2) as 'every boy loves some J'. A similar attempt to derive 'some girl is loved by every boy' from 'every boy loves some girl' will fail. Geach calls the inference of 'some girl is loved by every boy' from 'every boy loves some girl' the 'boy–girl fallacy' and he says this of it:

We observe that the traditional formal logic is wholly incompetent to resolve it . . . . Since there are still Colleges of Unreason where traditional formal logic is taught as the only genuine logic, this is worth pointing out.[5]

Incidentally, I fully agree with Geach that modern logic should be taught in all colleges. But that is irrelevant to the claim that traditional formal logic is 'wholly incompetent' to handle inferences with multiply general sentences and mixed quantities.

For we have shown that traditional formal logic is not incompetent to deal with the circle–figure argument and generally with arguments of form 'every A is B therefore every R to an A is R to B'. And we have now shown the same thing for the boy–girl argument and generally for arguments of form 'some A is R to every B therefore every B is R'd by some A'. The boy–girl argument can be traditionally accounted for if we expand the premiss as a pronominalization: someone is a girl and she is loved by every boy. It must however be acknowledged that our method, which involved the use of pronouns in analysing the premiss of the boy–girl argument, is not likely to

[5] Geach, *LM*, p. 5.

impress Geach and the many other logicians who have persistently claimed that TFL is unable to handle it. It is after all a matter of historical fact that TFL had no systematic treatment of pronouns and indeed that such a treatment is a justly celebrated accomplishment of MPL (wherein pronouns are represented as bound variables). This reaction would not be unreasonable. In effect one who defends TFL from the charge of incompetence is challenged to provide an account of the boy–girl argument that is confined to the kind of techniques available to the pre–Fregean logicians. This challenge was met for the circle–figure argument. All that was needed there was the addition of a tautological premiss of form 'every R to an A is R to an A' which conjoins with the given premiss 'every A is B' to yield the desired conclusion by the *Dictum de Omni*. Can something similar be done for the boy–girl argument? Indeed it can. According to the *Dictum de Omni*, whatever is true of every M is true of whatever *is* M. For example, if Sam loves every M and Trudy is an M, then Sam loves Trudy. Accepting this rule of inference we take as valid any argument of form

. . . every M . . .
some S is M
_____
. . . some S . . .

Our premiss is 'Some girl is loved by every boy'. To this we add a tautological second premiss.

(1) some girl is loved by every boy
(2) everyone loved by every boy is loved by every boy.

In general 'every B is R'd by every A' is the converse equivalent of 'every A is R to every B'. So from (2) we derive a second tautology:

(3) every boy loves everyone loved by every boy

Taking 'loved by every boy' as M and applying the *Dictum* to (3) and (1) yields the desired conclusion:

every boy loves some girl.

Clearly the charge of incompetence is unwarrented in both the boy–girl type argument and the circle–figure type of argument.

Since both types of arguments are very often cited to show the superiority of MPL over TFL one may well wonder how this false charge has received such widespread and enduring acceptance by responsible logicians. That they were anxious to persuade the students that the older logic was superseded is not by itself a sufficient explanation. A minimal attention to the methods of proof available to pre-Fregean logic would have given them pause. One doubts it could happen that two generations of modern geometers could falsely claim that Euclidean geometry could not prove certain theorems that are easily provable in some non-Euclidean systems. But then mathematicians who do modern geometry are not as tendentious as philosophers who do modern logic.

4. TFL is sometimes pejoratively called a 'subject–predicate' logic. Geach's criticism of Chomsky alludes to this: he is chiding Chomsky for retaining the old subject–predicate framework in his 'noun-phrase/verb-phrase' approach to the syntax of natural language. And Russell's criticism of Leibniz and his own view of the fundamental importance of the difference between 'Socrates is a man' and 'every man is mortal' is grounded in the conviction that the logician must free himself from the subject-predicate analysis of TFL. This general view is also invoked in criticizing TFL for its failure to develop a logic of relational sentences, a failure attributed to treating them as having subject–predicate form.

To such animadversion, the best response is to subvert the thesis that MPL is *not* a subject–predicate logic. In this section I shall show how to give a subject–predicate (noun-phrase/verb-phrase) analysis of vernacular sentences that corresponds exactly to the structure, in MPL, of the sentences that translate them. We shall see that quantificational translations of relational sentences have a definite, albeit covert, subject–predicate structure. In showing this I shall incidentally indicate how one may teach students who have difficulty in translating the vernacular into the language of MPL a mechanical way of mapping the cannonical sentences of natural language into their canonical MPL translations. My purpose here is constructive as well as polemical. For those interested in the problem of translating from English into standard logical languages I provide an easy mapping method for translating a sentence like 'some Senator Knows someone who has Lobbied for every Major oil company' as

$$(\exists x)[\,Sx\,\&\,(\exists y)\,((z)(Mz \to Lyz))\,\&\,Kxy)]$$

The more important constructive side is to show how the original natural language sentence may be analysed as a subject–predicate expression that nests other subject–predicate expressions. We shall indeed see that a relational sentence of natural language is to be viewed as an expression of subject–predicate form whose relational terms must themselves be construed as having a subject–predicate structure.

We shall be concerned with sentences of the vernacular that have been regimented to exclude all logical words except 'every', 'some', 'not', 'and', if 'then', and 'or'. The form of the elementary sentences is categorical being an assertion or denial of 'every/some X is Y'. The terms 'X' and 'Y' may be compound (e.g. 'female engineer' regimented as 'female and engineer') or relational (e.g. 'taller than some Swede'). The order of the subjects in a relational sentence will indicate whether the form 'some S' is to be understood with confused suppositio. For example the sentence 'a sailor is giving a toy to each of the children' would be regimented as 'some Sailor is Giving every Child some Toy'. This would ensure the confused suppositio we want here, since presumably the sailor is not presenting some one toy to all of the children but giving to each of them some toy or other. We represent 'some S' as '$\lfloor S \rfloor$', 'every S' as '$[S]$' and 'is P' as '$\langle P \rangle$'. The sailor sentence would be initially represented as

$$\lfloor S \rfloor\,\langle G^3[C]\lfloor T \rfloor \,\rangle.$$

A sentence like 'no horse's tail is a reptile's tail' would be regimented as 'not: some tail of some Horse is a tail of some Reptile' and represented as

$$-(\,\lfloor t^2 \,\lfloor H \rfloor\rfloor \,\langle t^2 \,\lfloor R \rfloor \,\rangle).$$

(Numerical superscripts indicate whether a relational expression is dyadic, triadic, etc.)

Note that in 'some tail of some Horse is a tail of some Reptile', the subject term is 'tail of some Horse'. This expression may itself be treated as having a subject and a predicate. Putting the subject on the left and the predicate on the right we may represent this term as '$_\llcorner H_\lrcorner \langle t^2 \rangle$'. Any expression consisting of a subject followed by a predicate will be called a 'supred'. The subject and predicate terms of the sentence before us are supreds. Putting subject expressions to the left and predicate expressions to the right we rewrite our representation of 'no tail of some Horse is a tail of some Reptile' in a supred canonical form:

$$- (_{\llcorner\llcorner} H_\lrcorner \langle t^2 \rangle_\lrcorner \langle _\llcorner R_\lrcorner \langle t^2 \rangle \rangle).$$

This form will be called a *transcription* of the original regimented sentence in *subject–predicate normal form* (SNF). In putting a sentence into SNF we make sure to order the subjects and predicates so that each subject expression is followed by its own predicate expression. Applied to 'some Sailor is Giving every Child a Toy' we have the sequence

$$_\llcorner S_\lrcorner \langle G^3 [C]_\llcorner T_\lrcorner \rangle$$
$$_\llcorner S_\lrcorner \langle [C] \langle G^3 _\llcorner T_\lrcorner \rangle \rangle$$
$$_\llcorner S_\lrcorner \langle [C] \langle _\llcorner T_\lrcorner \langle G^3 \rangle \rangle \rangle.$$

The last transcribes the sentence in 'supred normal form'. The expression '$\langle [C] \langle _\llcorner T_\lrcorner \langle G \rangle \rangle \rangle$' is predicate to the subject '$_\llcorner S_\lrcorner$', the expression '$\langle _\llcorner T_\lrcorner \langle G^3 \rangle \rangle$' is predicate to '[C]', and '$\langle G^3 \rangle$' is predicate to '$_\llcorner T_\lrcorner$'. The example illustrates how a nested subject–predicate analysis can be given to relational sentences in accordance with the analytic technique of TFL which treats 'some X' and 'every X' as the basic subject expressions. Expressions of form '$_\llcorner X_\lrcorner \langle Y \rangle$' or '$[X]\langle Y \rangle$' are supreds. Although singular sentences are analysable as expressions of these forms, it is useful to give them a special representation. We shall use upper corners for singular subjects, representing a sentence such as 'Socrates is wise' as '$^\ulcorner Socrates^\urcorner \langle wise \rangle$'.

According to TFL every categorical sentence is a supred and every relational term is a supred. The supred form of 'R to Some A' is '$_\llcorner A_\lrcorner \langle R^2 \rangle$' that of 'R to every A' is '$[A]\langle R^2 \rangle$'. A sentence is in supred normal form (SNF) when each of its subjects has its predicate. The analysis can be applied to sentences containing relational products like 'acquainted with an author of'. For example 'some Senator is Acquainted with someone who has

Lobbied for every Major oil company' would first be represented as '$_{\llcorner}S_{\lrcorner}\langle A^2{}_{\llcorner}L^2[M]_{\lrcorner}\rangle$'. Its SNF is

$$_{\llcorner}S_{\lrcorner}\langle{}_{\llcorner}[M]\langle L^2\rangle_{\lrcorner}\langle A^2\rangle\rangle$$

We now show that supred analysis corresponds to quantificational translation. The basic mappings are given in three rules:

R1 $\ulcorner\alpha\urcorner\langle P\rangle = P\alpha$
R2 $_{\llcorner}S_{\lrcorner}\langle P\rangle = (\exists x)(Sx\,\&\,Px)$
R3 $[S]\langle P\rangle = (x)(Sx \rightarrow Px)$.

Two other rules are fairly obvious and useful in translation procedures. The first has to do with compound terms. A sentence such as 'Some Engineers were Female Pilots' would be represented as '$_{\llcorner}E_{\lrcorner}\langle F\,\&\,P\rangle$' and then transformed by R2 into '$(\exists x)(F\,\&\,P)x$'. We may obviously distribute the 'x' in '$(F\,\&\,P)x$' thereby permitting us to replace this expression in the formula. This gives us '$(\exists x)(Ex\,\&\,(Fx\,\&\,Px))$'. A second rule allows the importation of a singular term to the dominant predicate expression. For example 'α Loves a Girl' transcribes as '$\ulcorner\alpha\urcorner\langle{}_{\llcorner}G_{\lrcorner}\langle L^2\rangle\rangle$' which, by R1, becomes '$({}_{\llcorner}G_{\lrcorner}\langle L^2\rangle)\alpha$' and by 'importation' becomes '$_{\llcorner}G_{\lrcorner}\langle L^2\alpha\rangle$'. And, generally, any expression of the form '$(\ldots\langle R\rangle)x$' is equivalent by importation to an expression of form '$\ldots\langle Rx\rangle$'.

Given 'Zuleika was Cool to everyone who Admired her' we first represent it as '$\ulcorner Z\urcorner\langle C^2[A^2\ulcorner Z\urcorner]\rangle$' and then give its SNF as '$\ulcorner Z\urcorner\langle[\ulcorner Z\urcorner\langle A^2\rangle]\langle C^2\rangle\rangle$'. Applying the rules:

$([\ulcorner Z\urcorner\langle A^2\rangle]\langle C^2\rangle)z$	R1
$[\ulcorner Z\urcorner\langle A^2\rangle]\langle C^2 z\rangle$	Importation
$(x)((\ulcorner Z\urcorner A^2 x) \rightarrow C^2 zx)$	R3
$(x)(A^2 xz \rightarrow C^2 zx)$	R1

Applying the translation procedure to 'every tail of a Horse is a tail of an Animal' we have first '$[t^2{}_{\llcorner}H_{\lrcorner}]\langle t^2{}_{\llcorner}A_{\lrcorner}\rangle$' and then '$[{}_{\llcorner}H_{\lrcorner}\langle t^2\rangle]\langle{}_{\llcorner}A_{\lrcorner}\langle t^2\rangle\rangle$' which maps as follows:

$(x)(({}_{\llcorner}H_{\lrcorner}\langle t^2 x\rangle) \rightarrow ({}_{\llcorner}A_{\lrcorner}\langle t^2 x\rangle))$	R3
$(x)(\exists y)((Hy\,\&\,t^2 xy) \rightarrow (\exists z)(az\,\&\,t^2 xz)$	R2, R1

Applied to the transcription of 'some Senator is Acquainted with someone who has Lobbied for every Major oil company' we have

$$\llcorner S \lrcorner \langle \llcorner [M] \langle L^2 \rangle \lrcorner \langle A^2 \rangle \rangle \qquad \text{SNF}$$
$$(\exists x)(Sx \& (\llcorner [M] \langle L^2 \rangle \lrcorner \langle A^2 x \rangle)) \qquad \text{R2}$$
$$(\exists x)(Sx \& (\exists y)(\llcorner [M] \langle L^2 y \rangle \lrcorner) \& A^2 xy) \qquad \text{R2}$$
$$(\exists x)(Sx \& (\exists y)((z)(Mz \to L^2 yz) \& A^2 xy)) \qquad \text{R3}$$

And finally, when applied to the transcription of 'some Sailor is Giving every Child a Toy' we have

$$\llcorner S \lrcorner \langle [C] \langle \llcorner T \lrcorner \langle G^3 \rangle \rangle \rangle \qquad \text{SNF}$$
$$(\exists x)(Sx \& ([C] \langle \llcorner T \lrcorner \langle G^3 x \rangle \rangle)) \qquad \text{R2}$$
$$(\exists x)(Sx \& (y)(Cy \to (\llcorner T \lrcorner \langle G^3 xy \rangle))) \qquad \text{R3}$$
$$(\exists x)(Sx \& (y)(Cy \to (\exists z)(Tz \& Gxyz))) \qquad \text{R2}$$

The mapping procedures clearly show that the final translation has an underlying subject–predicate structure with '$(\exists x)(Sx \& \ldots$' playing the role of 'some S is ...' and '(x) $(Sx \to \ldots$' playing the role of 'every S is ...'.

The structure of the translations is a nesting of supreds. Viewed in this light the subject–predicate (noun-phrase/verb-phrase) forms of the vernacular sentences exposes the structure of the quantificational formulas that are their canonical equivalents. This strongly suggests that philosophers like Geach, Harman, and linguists such as McCawley and Lakoff, who have looked to the structure of quantificational formulas for insight into the structure of sentences in natural languages, are facing in the wrong direction. This applies also to the pro-gramme of Sir Peter Strawson whose recent book *Subject and Predicate in Logic and Grammer* is on the right track facing the other way. Strawson takes the atomic form as paradigm and then tries to fit 'derivative' and secondary forms like 'some S is P' into the picture. The inspiration comes from the fundamen-tal predicate tie found in the atomic sentences of a standard logical language. But this way of approaching the question of subject and predicate is literally wrong-headed. The place to start is natural syntax which treats 'some S' and 'Socrates' as noun phrase subjects. Here grammar has priority. Strawson's book should have been titled 'Subject and Predicate in Grammar and Logic'. But then it would not have been the Fregean work it is. Strawson is a good example of a philosopher who has carried the teachings of Fregean syntax to its logical and linguistic conclusions. But the correctness of a conclusion is no better than the correctness of the starting point. And any starting point that initially treats 'some S' as a non-subject is the poorest of guides to a general theory of subject and predicate in logic or language. If the formulas of MPL are themselves disguised supred formulas it should be possible to do logic without disguising this essential fact about logical structure. In chapter 9 we shall show that this is indeed the case and that an overt subject–predicate logic along classical lines is comparable in inference power to standard systems of modern predicate logic.

8

Propositions and States of Affairs

1. I have been saying that the historical failure of traditional logicians to develop an adequate term logic was not due to some inherent deficiency in the two-term theory of propositions. The failure is a historical fact but it was not inevitable. This is even less controversial when said of the logic of propositions. All the materials for the development of a logic of propostitions were present since the time of the Stoics but they were neglected and unappreciated by the best of the traditional logicians. One reason for the neglect was the tendency on the part of TFL to give priority to term logic by construing all propositions as saying something about something.[1] We find Keynes saying that 'if p then q' could be understood to say of every circumstance in which p that it is a circumstance in which q. Thus let '[p]' represent 'state of affairs in which p'. Then the following ways of reducing compound (truth functional) propositions to categorical propositions are available:

for '−p'	the [p] does not obtain
for 'p and q'	some [p] is a [q]
for 'if p then q'	every [p] is a [q]
for 'p or q'	every [−p] is a [q]

The actual extent of a serious programmatic effort to construe compound propositions as categorical in form is very hard to assess but even if the ideal of categoricalness is only an implicit one, it must have made the independent development

---

[1] The eighteenth-century Cambridge logician, John Wallis, made one of the early serious attempts to recast conditionals and conjunctions as categorical propositions. See W. Kneale and M. Kneale, *The Development of Logic* (Oxford, 1962), p. 306, and W. S. Howell *Eighteenth Century British Logic and Rhetoric* (Princeton, 1971), p. 29. For the nineteenth century, De Morgan is typical. See for example *Formal Logic* Augustus De Morgan (The Open Court Co., 1926), p. 2.

of a propositional logic unlikely. In Leibniz's case the ideal of reducing compound propositions to subject–predicate categorical form played a significant part:

If, as I hope, I can treat all propositions as terms and hypotheticals as categoricals, and if I can treat all propositions universally, this promises a wonderful ease in my symbolism and analysis of concepts and will be a discovery of the greatest importance.[2]

Later, after Leibniz has devised a way of treating propositions as terms, he says:

We have discovered how absolute and hypothetical truths have one and the same laws and are contained in the same general theorems so that all syllogisms become categorical.[3]

Leibniz has here in mind that fact that the so-called hypothetical syllogism becomes categorical when we map into terms:

| if p then q | every [p] is a [q] |
if q then r	every [q] is a [r]
if p then r	every [p] is a [r]

The categorical interpretation of conditional propositions tempted Frege himself. Speaking of the proposition 'if the sun has already risen the sky is very cloudy', Frege says:

Here it can be said that a relation between the truth values of the conditional and dependent clauses has been asserted, viz., such that the case does not occur in which the antecedent stands for True and the consequent False.[4]

In effect, a proposition 'if p then q' is viewed as the assertion that no case in which 'p' stands for the True is a case in which 'q' stands for the False, or what is the same thing, every case in which 'p' stands for the True is a case in which 'q' stands for the True. This occurrence in Frege of a categorical interpretation of the conditional is isolated and indeed one cannot take it seriously on pain of circularity since the Fregean analysis of

---

[2] Leibniz's *Logical Papers*, ed. G. H. R. Parkinson (Clarendon Press, Oxford), p. 66. Hereafter referred to as *LLP*.

[3] *LLP*, p. 78.

[4] Black & Geach, p. 74.

propositions of form 'every . . . is . . .' characteristically makes use of the conditional.

It is then more accurate to say that Frege 'reduced' the categorical form to a conditional form 'if x is S then x is P'. And here too we have the contrast with Leibniz, for Leibniz reduced the conditional to the categorical. This contrast between Frege and Leibniz is a consequence of their disagreement over atomicity. If with Frege we hold that a proposition is either atomic or constructed out of atomic materials, then since 'every S is P' is not atomic, we must find its analysis in terms of atomic propositions. This leads quite naturally to seeing it as a function of 'it is S' and 'it is P' and the function is of form 'if it is S then it is P'. Leibniz does not hold that 'a is P' is atomic in Frege's sense; there is therefore, no temptation to think of 'every S is P' as a compound of atomic propositions. On the other hand, since Leibniz saw 'every S is P' as an elementary form, not analysable into further propositional elements, it is quite natural for him to attempt the categorical construal of compound forms for success in this attempt would enable him to think of all propositions—elementary or compound—'universally'.

That we can go either way, treating 'if p then q' as a categorical proposition about states of affairs or 'every S is P' as a conditional proposition, suggests a theory in which neither type of proposition is viewed as analytically prior to the other but both are viewed as structurally isomorphic. I shall later argue for a position of this kind, between Leibniz and Frege, in which terms and propositions are the elements of abstract structures governed by laws that can be interpreted to hold indifferently for categorical propositions or for compound propositions. This sort of theory seems to have been an explicit ideal for Leibniz even though in practice he succumbed to the reductivist temptation to give categorical form to compound propositions.[5]

2. Whatever one thinks of the priorities or lack of priorities between categorical and compound propositions, there seems

[5] Leibniz's examples of the law of identity includes 'if p then p' along with 'every A is A', cf. Leibniz, *Philosophische Schriften*, ed. C. I. Gerhardt (Berlin, 1895–90), volume 7, p. 299.

little reason to deny that a proposition of the form 'if p then q' cannot be true unless—to use Frege's phraseology—every case of 'p' standing for the True is also a case of 'q' standing for the True. Let '[p]' be read either as 'case of "p" standing for the True' or—more neutrally—as 'state of affairs in which p'. A proposition whose terms are '[p]' and '[q]' will be called a state proposition; the terms of a state proposition will be called propositional terms.

The attempt to carry out the systematic transformation of compound propositions into categorical state propositions is of historical interest. Also it casts some light on the obscure but hardly dispensable idea of a state of affairs or a circumstance. (Recall Frege's definition of the truth value of a proposition as 'the circumstance that it is true or false'.) The idea of a state of affairs is somewhat better understood if we attend to those state propositions that are counterparts of theorems of propositional logic. Take for example the theorem which asserts that 'if p then q' follows from 'p and q'. The state correlate to this is that '*some* [p] is [q]' entails '*every* [p] is [q]'. Now this suggests that state propositions have singular subjects and that the term '[p]' or 'state of affairs in which p' applies to no more than one thing. This would account for our readiness to speak of *the* state of affairs in which p.

It appears, however, that we can also show that there is no more than one state of affairs and that the truth of 'p' and 'q' cannot mean that there are two different states, one specified by 'p' and the other by 'q'. Consider the following valid propositional inference and its state counterpart:

$$\frac{p}{\therefore q \to p} \qquad \frac{a\,[p]\ \text{obtains}}{\therefore\ \text{every}\ [q]\ \text{is a}\ [p]}$$

This tells us that if a state in which p obtains then *every* state is a state in which p. Now this result is sufficiently paradoxical to want resolving even though some recent philosophers are quite content to say that there *is* only one state of affairs, a thesis that fits well with Frege's doctrine that all true propositions have a single referent: the True.

We shall hold to the intuitively acceptable position that there are many and distinct states of affairs. Our problem is to reconcile this position with the results one gets when pursuing the correspondence of 'state' propositions with the truths of propositional logic. From the standpoint of traditional logic, we are interested in state propositions because they afford one way of understanding what compound propositions are asserting. There is, after all, something attractive in the idea that 'if p then q' can be construed as saying something categorically about states of affairs or about the world thought of as a totality of such states. But our way of transforming compound propositions into state propositions has led us to the intolerable conclusion that there is only one state of affairs, one case, one Fact. It may be, however, that our way of transforming compound propositions into propositions that contain propositional terms is faulty. So let us try another way.

Let T be a totality of distinct states of affairs—what Wittgenstein calls *a world*—and let 'p' and 'q' specify two states within the totality so that the T will have a [p] and a [q] as two of its components. T is composed of states but we need not think of T itself as a state; indeed, we shall assume that T is not itself a state. Even so, it is possible to say of T that it is *in part* a state of affairs in which p. Similarly, I can say that T is a [p] and a [q] if I mean by this to say that it is a [p]-in-part and a [q]-in-part.

An analogy may be helpful here. It is generally true that nothing can be red and blue. But it is also true that the American flag is red, white and blue. It is customary to explain this by distinguishing two meanings of red, a 'partly' meaning in which 'red' is synonymous with 'partly red' or with 'red-in-part' and an integral meaning in which it is synonymous with 'red-all-over'. There are other explanations; in saying that the flag is red and blue I might be said to have used 'is' to mean 'has parts that are'. We could call this the componential sense of 'is' and distinguish it by means of an asterisk. Thus 'A is* B and C' is the same as 'A has components that are B and C'. Still a third explanation might be that 'the flag is red and blue' is to be parsed as a conjunction: 'part of the flag is red and part of it is blue'. It seems to me the second and third explanations amount to the same thing: 'A is B and C' means the same as 'part of A is B and (another) part of it is B'. Note also that in these two explanations the terms 'red' and 'blue' do not have a 'partly' sense; in saying that part of the flag is red I say that that part is red-all-over.

If we think of a state proposition as a way of construing a compound proposition as a subject-predicate proposition, then we must recognize the use of an integral sense of '[p]' will not do. Beginning with 'p and q' we try 'some [p] is [q]'. Even if we ignore the fact that this way of reducing 'p and q' to a categorical form soon gets us the intolerable consequence of a single state, we see that this way of understanding what 'p and q' says about states of affairs is faulty. For example, the proposition 'Wittgenstein met Russell and Frege died in July 1925' is true but in what sense is it true that the state of affairs in which Wittgenstein met Russell is a state of affairs in which Frege died in 1925? As a systematic equivalent to 'Wittgenstein met Russell and Frege died in July 1925' this 'state proposition' is palpably implausible. Indeed there is little meaning to the formula 'a [p] is a [q]', for how are we to understand that a description that specifies one state is applicable to another state? Similar considerations apply to 'every [p] is a [q]'—the alleged state correlate to 'if p then q'. If the condition for saying that a state in which p is a state in which q is merely that both states obtain, then the sense of 'state' must be different from the sense in which we can say of two states that obtain that one is different from the other. It is clear that the assumption of a diversity of existent states prohibits the predication of 'is a state in which q' of a state in which p simply on the grounds of the truth of 'p and q'.

If we move on to the forms 'T is a [p] and a [q]' and 'T is a [q] or a [−p]' as ways of saying categorically what 'p and q' and 'if p then q', respectively, say, then we must again be careful. For it is false to say of the totality of states of affairs that it *is* a [p]. Or at least it is false if '[p]' is taken in an *intergral* sense. So the price of getting a categorical transformation of a compound proposition is the use of the 'partly' sense of the propositional terms. The price is not inconsiderable, for the partly use of a term requires great care. If—using the propositional terms in the partly sense—'some [p] is a [q]' is a state proposition corresponding to 'p & q', it cannot be taken to mean that 'it is a q' is true of a state of affairs in which p; instead it should be taken to mean that something (the 'totality') that is in part a [p] is in part a [q]. Now the partly use of a term can be quite misleading and ought perhaps to be avoided. (For example, it might allow one to say 'that flag is red and not-red'.) But if we avoid it for state terms, there seems to be no way of formulating a categorical transform of a compound proposition that allows for more than one state of affairs.

Respectable or not, the partly use of terms is familiar enough in such sentences as 'the flag is red, white and blue'. If we employ 'partly' state terms the Leibnizian programme of getting a categorical form for each compound seems to be a realizable one. It is interesting that the carrying out of the programme commits us to an ontology of states of affairs and, more particularly, to a Wittgensteinian world; for Wittgenstein thought of the world not as a domain of individuals but as a totality of states of affairs or cases of something being so and so. We saw above that the thesis of a single state was not unwelcome to the Fregean. The idea of a single totality of 'atomic' states of affairs is perhaps equally congenial to him; after all, the *Tractatus* Wittgenstein was a Fregean. The idea of a single state of affairs and the idea of a single referent for all true propositions are first cousins to Wittgenstein's 'World' as a totality of states of affairs. But only the latter idea allows us to carry on with the programme of giving compound propositions a categorical form while allowing for a diversity of states, cases or facts.

3. The discussion of the present chapter suggests that the policy of analysing 'if p then q' or 'p and q' as a categorical subject-predicate proposition, even if it is a possible one, is not a desirable one. And the discussion of the previous chapters suggests that the modern policy of analysing categorical propositions as functions of atomic propositions is also suspect. Our own standpoint is that 'p and q' and 'some A is B' (or, 'if p then q' and 'every A is B') share a common structure which makes one or the other style of analysis possible but that neither analysis is necessary or even desirable. If this is right, then 'p and q' and 'some A is B' are analytically autonomous and structurally isomorphic. In support of this, we must reveal the common structure of categorical and compound forms in a manner that does not analyse one in terms of the other as Leibniz and Frege—each in his own way—do. If our standpoint is correct, then the syncategoremata that are characteristic of categorical propositions and those that are characteristic of compound propositions will have a common representation. For example, the syncategorematic elements of 'some A is B' and the syncategorematic elements of 'p and q' have a logical affinity which makes it possible to use 'and' in analysing the former and 'some is' in analysing the latter. But if neither of these is logically prior to the other, they must both share a *common* structure and it should then be possible to represent 'and' and 'some is' in some common notation. Thus, let '#' be a functor that operates on a pair of elements. If the elements are terms, the functor '#' will have as its interpretation the sycategorematic expression 'some . . . is . . .' If the elements represent whole propositions, then the functor '#' will be interpreted as 'and'. A similar functor must be available for 'every is' and 'if then'. Paradoxically, the parity and mutual independence of term and propositional logic implies that the syncategoremata which seem respectively specific to terms and to propositions must have important formal affinities. That this is indeed the case will be borne out in the next chapter.[6]

4. The syntactic thesis that any sentence, elementary or compound, consists of two categorematic expressions (two terms or two sentences) and a syncategorematic expression that connects them is generally applicable to all of the logically canonical sentences of a natural language. Where the categorematic expressions are themselves not simple, they are analysable as binary expressions. We saw how this can be done for sentences with relationsal terms by embedding binary expressions in other binary expressions. Thus 'a boy gave a girl a flower' is analysable as: 'a boy (a girl (a flower (gave)))' in which each subject expression is followed by its own predicate expression. In this manner one can represent the structure of the most complicated sentence on a binary tree that exhibits the embedding of basic binary forms.

The syntactic thesis goes hand in hand with the semantic thesis that a sentence such as 'a boy gave a girl a flower' and more generally any sentence of form 'an A is a B' denotes a state

---

[6] For more on States of Affairs see Appendix B.

of affairs. It seems best to hold this thesis in a minimal way for we have no need of negative or compound states of affairs in accounting for the truth of negations and compound sentences. Thus let p be an elementary affirmative sentence. Then to say that p is true is just to say that the [p] obtains and to say the [p] is false is just to say that the [p] does not obtain. The absence of the [p] in the totality of states of affairs suffices to define a sense of 'true' for ' − p'; we do not in addition need to countenance anything like the existence of a negative state of affairs. Thus we do not talk of a [− p] or of a [that p is false]. Similarly where 'p and q' is true, this is to be accounted for by the presence of the [p] and of the [q] in the totality of actual states and not by the presence of a compound state of affairs. The semantic thesis appropriate to a neoclassical logic of terms and propositions thus limits the correspondence of true sentences to states of affairs denoted by elementary affirmative sentences. Negations and compound sentences are themselves non-denotative but are interpreted as affirming or denying the existence of the states denoted by their elementary component sentences; the truth or falsity of any non-elementary sentence is not to be accounted for by the existence of a negative or compound state denoted by it but by the existence or non-existence of the 'elementary states' denoted by the elementary components. The neoclassical thesis differs from Frege's view in not assuming that every true sentence denotes something actual (in Frege, this is the True). Where Frege economizes by maintaining that all true sentences have a single denotatum, the neoclassical approach recognizes distinct denotata but economizes by confining sentential denotation to elementary sentences.

One question left open is whether to count sentences of form 'every A is B' as negative and non-denotative or as positive and denotative. We shall argue below that 'every A is B' is defined by way of 'no A is non-B' and not the other way round. The priority of 'no' to 'every' has strong consequences, one of which may be that universal sentences do not denote states of affairs. In favor of including such states as the [every raindrop is colourless] within the actual totality of states is the consideration that the sentence 'every raindrop is colourless' though defined by the negation of 'some raindrop is coloured' is not itself about a state of affairs but about raindrops. Now it seems gratuitous to hold that a sentence asserting or denying the existence of states of affairs should itself denote a state of affairs. For example, a proposition to the effect that the [p] obtains (or fails to obtain) is equivalent to one that says of the totality of states that it contains (fails to contain) the [p] but *this* proposition does not itself denote a state of affairs in the totality of states. In contrast to propositions that affirm or deny the existence of states of affairs we have propositions like 'some raindrops are colourless' and 'every raindrop is colourless'. It seems then that we may harmlessly count both as state-denoting propositions. On the other hand we find what appear to be good reasons to deny denotability to universal sentences. Philosophers sometimes disagree on the priority of 'seeing that' to 'seeing'. I see a black cat and some philosophers hold that my seeing that it is black is epistemologically prior to seeing the black cat. Others hold to the reverse order of priority. But both parties to this disagreement agree that seeing the black cat and seeing that it is black are closely related. Note that the use of 'that is' is shared by both sorts of seeing. I see a cat that is black. Here 'that is' is like 'and'; what I see is a cat *and* black. I see that the cat is black. Here 'that is' is like 'some is' for what I see it the [some cat is black]. Let 'perceive' be used in an epistemically neutral way for objects and for states of affairs. And let # be the neutral functor representing 'and' or 'some is'. Then seeing a black cat is perceiving a (cat # black thing) and seeing that a cat is black is perceiving a [cat # black]. The structure of expressions denoting the state of affairs perceived and the thing perceived is the same and this comes to the syntactical surface in the use of 'that is' for seeing an A *that is* B and seeing *that* an A *is* B.

It is, I think, significant that the affinity between what is denoted by 'an A that is B' and 'that an A is B' can have no parallel in an affinity between what is denoted by 'a thing that is not A or B and a state denoted by 'every A is B'. We do not, I think, perceive that every A is B and even if we do, this is in no sense equivalent to perceiving something that is either not an A or a B in the way that perceiving that some A is B is equivalent to perceiving an A and B thing. This appears to me to be a good argument for denying that universal sentences are state-denotable. Other arguments can be given for confining denotability to particular sentences but none that I know of seems to me to be quire decisive. The reader will find some further discussion of this question at the end of Appendix B but there too the discussion is sketchy and the question whether to countenance states of affairs denoted by universal sentences is left open.

In conclusion, we have in this chapter examined the two reductionist trends in the history of logic. Classical term logic tends to view compound sentences as general categorical sentences about states of affairs. Modern predicate logic goes the other way by analysing general categorical sentences as functions of atomic sentences. The latter approach is responsible for giving the logic of propositions and truth functions primacy. (As if the Stoics should have logically preceded Aristotle since to understand categoricals of form 'every A is B' one must first understand 'if p then q'.) The categorical approach leads finally to thinking of propositional compounds as being not about states of affairs but about the totality of states of affairs, not a natural way of construing compound sentences. Avoiding either sort of reduction, we recognize categoricals and compounds as two kinds of sentences each with its own kind of material elements and its own kind of connectives that join them. Having paid our respects to the parity of propositional and term logic we note all the same that the connective expressions joining terms and sentences have important formal affinities. In the next chapter we shall be exploiting these affinities at the level of logical syntax by developing a notation suitable for transcribing the logically canonical sentences of natural language in a direct and natural way. That the direct transcriptions are suitable for logical reckoning will also be shown.

9
The Algebra of Traditional Formal Logic

1. Scholastic logicians distinguished two kinds of expressions which they called categorematic and syncategorematic. In 'every A is B and C' the terms A, B and C are categoremata. In 'if p then not q' the propositions p and q are categorematic 'material components'. Words like 'and', 'not' and 'every', expressions like 'if then' and 'except for' are syncategorematic 'formative components'. Categorematic expressions apply to things or states of affairs; syncategorematic expressions do not.

The scholastic characterization of syncategoremata is essentially negative; it tells us what these expressions are not and quite pointedly fails to tell us what they are. This is commendably modest but is immodest in its presumption that there are effective ways of determining the class of categorematic expressions. Contemporary logicians are equally modest and immodest but they tend to give a negative characterization to the categoremata: thus Quine calls categoremata 'extra-logical' expressions; the positive characterization is reserved for a finite list of syncategorematic expressions. Whether one favours the class of logical expressions (syncategoremata) or the class of categorematic expressions (extra-logical) does not much matter as long as we are given a principle of determining the members of the favoured class. But neither the medieval nor the modern logician tells us how to determine the class of categoremata or syncategoremata and we are no better off today than our predecessors of the fourteenth century were to distinguish the logical from the non-logical. Dummett believes we *are* better off and that Frege deserves the credit:

The suggestion is made that the term 'logical constant' cannot be defined save by listing the expressions to which it is to apply . . . But, in fact, ever since Frege inaugurated the era of modern logic there has been to hand a simple and precise principle of distinction. The basic idea of the step by step construction of sentences involves a distinction between two classes of sentences and correspondingly between two classes of expression. Sentences can be divided into atomic and complex ones: atomic sentences are formed out of basic constituents none of which are or have been formed from sentences, while complex sentences arise, through a step by step construction, from the application of certain sentence forming devices to other sentences . . . beginning with atomic sentences. The expressions which go to make up atomic sentences—proper names (individual constants), primitive predicates and relational expressions—form one type: sentence-forming operators such as sentential operators and quantifiers which induce reiterable transformations which lead from atomic to complex sentences form the other . . . Logic properly so called may be thought of as concerned only with words and expressions of the second type . . . [1]

Dummett is objecting to the scepticism of those philosophers (Tarski and Quine are among them) who suspect that the logical expressions are characterized only as belonging to a finite list of expressions whose membership answers well enough to the concerns of the logician. These philosophers are not convinced that the distinction between logical and extra-logical expressions can be more positively characterized. Dummett himself does not attempt a positive characterization of the class of logical expressions. Instead he is positively medieval in his reliance on an effective way of determining the class of categoremata. His appeal is to the division of sentences into atomic and complex. The class of atomic sentences determines the class of categorematic (extra-logical) expressions: all and only those expressions that enter as names or predicates in atomic sentences are categorematic and atomic sentences are themselves categorematic. Now this would be quite straightforward if only we knew how to distinguish the class of atomic sentences. Let us grant that the class of atomic sentences exists (not a small concession: what Leibniz and the traditional logician deny is here being set up as foundational) and turn to the question of recognizing its members. This is not at all an easy thing to do. Frege, for example, held 'the sun is

[1] Dummett, *Frege*, p. 21.

hot' to be an atomic sentence; Russell thought it was complex. And the mention of Russell in this connection reminds us that Quine showed how to parse out all proper names, introducing quantifiers and individual variables in complex sentences that say the same thing as the original atomic sentences. One must wonder how hard these atoms can be if it is possible to do this systematically. There is, in addition, the question of primitive predicates. The logical expression 'is identical with' will satisfy the test of belonging to the class of extra-logical expressions since (in the standard Fregean system) it is a relational predicate in atomic sentences. Dummett sees this and he struggles valiantly to get identity back into the class of logical expressions. I find his efforts unconvincing but even if he could succeed, it would only raise the question of other primitive predicates. If the relational expression 'identical with' is a logical sign, why not also 'greater than', 'as tall as', 'is a member of' and other relational expressions some of which denote relations with analytical properties like symmetry or transitivity. It should be obvious anyway that the class of atomic sentences cannot itself be fixed independently of the class of categoremata. Indeed, one way of saying what an atomic sentence is is to say that it is the kind of sentence that contains only categorematic expressions. There is, therefore, little reason to grant Dummett his class of atomic sentences from which to draw the distinction between logical and extra-logical expressions. More generally, it seems that any effort to positively characterize the class of categoremata must be futile. That class is potentially infinite and if its membership has not yet been specified by any universally accepted principle, it does not seem likely that it ever will be.

A more promising line is to concentrate on some equally adequate list of syncategorematic expressions. Here we deal with a finite and small number of expressions and it is quite possible we may yet find something more interesting to say of them than that they belong to a group of expressions that logicians find it convenient to keep fixed for purposes of inference.

2. We accept some traditional assumptions concerning the logical syntax of natural language. Among them: (1) that terms and not Fregean names or predicates are the categoremata of the elementary sentences; (2) that each elementary sentence has two terms; (3) that, in addition, each elementary sentence contains a syncategorematic expression that joins the terms—a 'term connective' such as 'some is' or 'every is'.

The contrast here is between the atomic sentences of a standard Fregean language that have no syncategorematic elements and the elementary categorical sentences of the termist language that have both categorematic and syncategorematic parts. The shift back to a traditional termist syntax immediately provides a simple and uniform conception of the well-formed formulas of propositional and term logic. Let '#' be a connective and let 'α' and 'β' be either two terms or two propositions. Then '$\alpha \# \beta$' is a well-formed formula. So conceived, any well-formed formula (proposition) consists of two material elements of the same kind joined by a (term or by a propositional) connective.

The next sections are devoted to the exposition of a notation for logical words and expressions like 'not', 'and', 'some', 'every', 'if then', 'or' and other logical particles that figure in systems of roughly first order strength. The purpose is twofold:

(1) To show that such seemingly disparate signs as 'not', 'every', 'and' and 'some' have a common character that distinguishes them sharply as syncategorematic signs.

(2) To exhibit the structural isomorphism of 'and' as a connective between propositions and 'some is' as a connection between terms and to do the same for 'if then' and 'every is'. To indicate how these isomorphisms are related to characteristic modes of sentence composition in modern predicate logic.

Our task is to characterize a canonical sub-set of the statement-sentences of natural language that satisfies the following conditions:

(1) The syntax of the sentences in the sub-set is easily specifiable.

(2) The elementary sentences have a noun-phrase/verb-phrase ('categorical', subject–predicate) structure.

(3) Any statement-sentence of natural language is either

  itself canonical or else is paraphrasable as a sentence in
  the subset.
(4) The syntactic structure of any sentence in the set fully
  determines its logical relations to other sentences in the
  set.

We shall initially be restricted to a primitive part of the
logically relevant sentences of natural language in which a
single commutative functor (represented by a dagger sign)
connects two terms (represented by Roman *upper case* 'term
letters') or two propositions (represented by Roman *lower case*
proposition letters). When the dagger sign joins two term letters
(as in 'A † B') the proposition formed is elementary (being read
as 'an A is a B' or as 'some A is B'). When the dagger sign joins
two propositions (as in 'p † q') the proposition formed is
compound (being read as 'p and q'). The use of a single sign for
the primitive connective brings out important formal affinities
between 'an A is a B' and 'p and q', for example both 'A † B' and
'p † q' obey the law of commutivity. The dagger sign is also used
to form compound terms. A compound term in the primitive
notation is always a conjunction. Thus 'A † B' is read as 'an A
and B thing' or as '(an)A that is (a)B'. To distinguish 'A and B'
from 'an A is a B' we shall always enclose the former in angular
brackets. For example 'an A that is B is a C' is represented as
'⟨A † B⟩ † C'. Finally it will be necessary to introduce another
style of brackets for conjoining two propositions when each
one has an explicit internal structure. We then enclose each
conjunct in square brackets. For example 'an A is a B and a C is
a D' is represented thus:

  [A † B] † [C † D]

Generally, any expression enclosed in square brackets will be
given a propositional reading (as opposed to being read as a
compound term).
  The following expressions illustrate the use of the notation:

A † B	some A is B
p † [q † r]	p and (q and r)
⟨A † B⟩ † C	Some A that is B is C
[A † ⟨B † C⟩] † [D † ⟨E † F⟩]	Some A is B and C and Some D is E and F

2.1 Not all syncategorematic expressions play a logical role in a given argument. For example the argument 'No senator is a non-citizen and some senators are very rich, therefore some senators are very rich and no senator is a non-citizen' has the form 'p and q ∴ q and p': the syncategorematic expressions internal to each of the conjuncts play no part. The form of the argument 'no senator is a non-citizen, therefore no non-citizen is a senator', is 'no X is Y ∴ no Y is X' in which 'no' plays a logical role but 'non' does not. When we speak of the logical and extra-logical parts of a given expression we usually understand it to have been analysed within some argument under consideration that contextually determines the distinction between its logical and extralogical parts. We can however view the parts of propositions more generally, distinguishing those that can play the role of syncategoremata contrasting them with those that cannot. In a general discussion of logical syntax, one takes the second approach in analysing propositions into logical and extra-logical parts.

3. The fundamental categoremata are *terms* (including relational expressions) and *propositions*. Both terms and propositions come in opposed pairs. Opposed terms are called logical contraries. Examples are *'citizen'*; *'non-citizen'*; *'coloured'*; *'colourless'*; *'wet'*; *'dry'*; *'lover of'*; *'non-lover of '*. Opposed propositions are called contradictories. Examples are 'a man spoke'; 'not a man spoke'; '(it is true that) the king is dead'; 'it is not true that the king is dead'.

3.1 *Contrary Terms*: Contrariety is primarily an opposition of terms and only derivatively of propositions. In a natural language like English we may form the logical contrary of a term, P, by prefixing it with or affixing to it a negative particle such as 'un-' or '-less' or by forming the term 'thing that fails-to-be P'. What fails to be P is un-P. What fails to be un-P is P. Terms like 'black' and 'white' are also called contraries but they are not *logical* contraries since what fails to be black is not necessarily white and what fails to be white is not necessarily black. A pair of logical contraries exhausts a range of predicability. Thus 'is either coloured or colourless' is true of whatever it makes sense to predicate colour terms. In our discussion 'contraries' will always mean 'logical contraries'. We drop the qualifying adjective for convenience.

If P and Q are contraries it is, more often than not, natural to consider one to be positive, the other negative. But from a logical point of view a positive-negative assignment is arbitrary. Given say 'pure' as the positive term, 'impure' will be considered negative. But we could define 'pure' to mean 'uncontaminated' in which case the positive term 'contaminated' would be its contrary. In characterizing the contrariety of P and Q, the relation of incompatibility between P and Q together with the fact that their union exhausts a range of predicability counts for more than the arbitrary assignment of positive and negative qualities to one or the other of the two terms. For just as Q fails to be P so does P fail to be Q and even where the contrary of P is given an overtly negative form (non-P) it is always possible to introduce a term Q with the denotation of non-P and then to understand P as equivalent to non-Q.

Contraries will be represented as positively or negatively charged expressions. Thus '$+P$' and '$-P$' are contraries, it being understood that we may introduce definitions like '$+Q = -P$' to reverse the assignment of positive and negative qualities to the contraries.

If p is a proposition, not p is its contradictory. We represent p as '$+p$' and not p as '$-p$'. There are different ways of forming the contradictory of a proposition but we are at present concerned with propositions whose connective functors are 'some is' or 'and' and for such propositions the formation of a contradictory involves the use of a negative particle of sentential scope. Thus two ways of contradicting 'a child of mine was unfed' are 'not a child of mine was unfed' and 'no child of mine was unfed'. These two ways are essentially the same; the word 'no' in the latter sentence is not—as Geach and Strawson, following Sir William Hamilton, hold—a sign of quantity but a negative sign of sentential denial qualifying '(a) child of mine was unfed'.

We just made the point that an assignment of positive or negative quality to each of a pair of contrary terms is arbitrary because we can always introduce a new term of opposite quality to denote what a given term denotes. The corresponding point does *not* hold for contradictories: given a proposition of negative quality, there is no positive proposition with the same truth conditions. This means that whenever S_1 and S_2 are contradictories there is an irreducible asymmetry of quality between them. We shall speak of a difference in *valence*, characterizing 'a child of mine was unfed' as *positive* in valence and 'no child of mine was unfed' as *negative* in valence. Later we shall extend our analysis to consider contradictories of form 'every X is Y' and 'some X is not Y'. Since 'every X is Y' will be defined by 'no X is non-Y' we shall say that universal categoricals have negative valence and particular categoricals have positive valence. For the present we are confined to propositions of forms '$(\pm X)\dagger(\pm Y)$' and '$-((\pm X)\dagger(\pm Y))$' and we note that *convalence is a necessary condition of equivalence*: there is no way to form a positive equivalent to any proposition of form '$-((\pm X)\dagger(\pm Y))$' and no way to define a negative equivalent to a proposition of form '$(\pm X)\dagger(\pm Y)$'. This principle of convalence figures as an important constraint on the allowable transformations of any formal term logic. The reader will find a discussion of the reasons for the asymmetry of propositional divalence in Appendix B.

4. The system of term logic in which 'some is' and 'and' are the sole connectives will be called a Primitive Term Logic (PTL). The general form of a proposition in PTL is

$$\pm((\pm\alpha)\dagger(\pm\beta))$$

where 'α' and 'β' are two term letters or two proposition letters and the plus and minus signs signify the positive or negative quality of a term or of the proposition itself. The connective functor '$\dagger$' is read as 'some is' when 'α' and 'β' are term letters. It is read as 'and' when 'α' and 'β' are proposition letters. Since we use lower and upper case Roman letters, respectively, for propositions and for terms the reading of the dagger sign will be unambiguous. The positive signs of quality in '$+((+\alpha)\dagger(+\beta))$' could be omitted. We shall usually follow the customary arithmetic practice of dropping plus signs of positive quality. Thus 'p and q' will be transcribed as '$p\dagger q$' and 'some non-P and Q is R' will be transcribed as '$\langle(-P)\dagger Q\rangle\dagger R$' and not as

'$+(\langle(-P)\dagger(+Q)\rangle\dagger(+R))$'.

4.1 A relational proposition is one that contains a relational term. A relational term consists of a relational expression followed by one or more subject expressions of the form 'some X'. Examples of relational propositions are 'a boy is admiring a girl', 'a sailor gave a child a toy', 'an owner of a cow was protesting'. It is clear that we can partially transcribe 'a boy is admiring a girl' as 'boy † admirer of a girl'; but how are we to transcribe the relational term 'admirer of a girl'? The discussion in chapter 7, section 5 is relevant to this question. We there argued that relational terms have a subject predicate structure so that we could understand 'a boy is admiring a girl' as

some boy is what some girl is being admired by

or, in the active voice, as

some boy some girl is admiring

which transcribes as 'boy † (girl † admiring^2)' or straight-forwardly as

boy † (admiring^2 † girl).

Similarly 'a sailor is giving a child a toy' transcribes as:

(2) Sailor † (giving^3 † child † toy).

This is justified by giving the original a nested subject–predicate form in which each subject phrase has its predicate: 'A sailor is what a child is what a toy is given to by' or, again in the active voice, as 'a sailor a child a toy is giving' whose 'SNF' transcription is:

sailor † (child † (toy † giving^3)).

The nested form is useful for mapping TFL forms into MPL. For our purposes here the direct linear transcription is appropriate. Generally, then, a relational term of form 'R^n some $A_1 \ldots$ Some A_{n-1}' transcribes as:

$R^n † A_1 † A_2 \ldots † A_{n-1}$

Examples of relational sentences and their PTL transcriptions are:

Some boy loved a girl who
owned a cow $B † (L^2 † \langle G † (O^2 † C) \rangle)$

An owner of a cow was
protesting $(O^2 \dagger C) \dagger P$
A senator was influenced by
a friend of a gangster $S \dagger (I^2 \dagger (f^2 \dagger G))$

4.2 *Singular Terms*: Terms of restricted denotation, including singular terms that denote no more than a single individual, are called U-terms.[2] A proposition with a U-term, ϕ, in subject position has the form 'Some ϕ is ψ'. When the U-term is singular 'Some ϕ is ψ' entails 'no ϕ is non ψ'. For example, 'Socrates' is a singular U-term and 'Socrates is wise', which transcribes as '$S \dagger W$', entails '$-(S \dagger (-W))$'.

4.21 The proterms of pronouns are U-terms. A pronominaliz-ation such as 'a woman is on the phone; she is asking for Harry' is a conjunction of the antecedent sentence 'a woman is P' and the pronominal sentence 'she is Q'. Conjunctive propositions have the form 'p $\dagger$ q'. But where the conjuncts have explicit internal structures, they are encased in square brackets. In our example the conjuncts are '$W_J \dagger P$' and '$J \dagger Q$' and the complete transcription is:

$[W_J \dagger P] \dagger [J \dagger Q]$.

Since 'J' is a proterm '$J \dagger Q$' entails '$-(J \dagger (-Q))$'. We intro-duce a convention to indicate this by writing '$J \dagger Q$' as '$*J \dagger Q$'. The entailment is also valid in the case where 'J' is plural. For example 'some women are P; they are Q' may be transcribed as

$[W_J \dagger P] \dagger [*J_s \dagger Q]$

A proposition such as 'some sailor is giving every child a toy' contains the word 'every' and cannot be transcribed in PTL but its PTL equivalent *can* be given if we use proterms:

Some person$_J$ is a sailor
and it is not the case that
some person$_K$ is a child and J fails-to (give K some toy)
$[P_J \dagger S] \dagger [-([P_K \dagger C] \dagger [-(J \dagger G^3 \dagger K \dagger T)])]$

4.3 The functor '$\dagger$' is additive in the sense that the terms or the propositions joined by it, obey the laws of commutation and

---

[2] See discussion in chapter 5, section 2.1.

association. Thus 'Some X is Y' and 'Some Y is X' are equivalent and so too are 'Some X is Y and Z' and 'Some X and Y is Z'. Generally, if α, β, and γ are three terms or three propositions the following laws hold:

i) $\alpha \dagger \beta = \beta \dagger \alpha$ ii) $\alpha \dagger (\beta \dagger \gamma) = (\alpha \dagger \beta) \dagger \gamma$

We shall presently exploit the additive character of the primitive connective '$\dagger$' in a system of term logic that uses '$+$' in place of '$\dagger$'. Here we note that a single additive functor for concatenating positively and negatively charged elements suffices for the basic logical language. Pronominalization needs no additional logical syntax since it is effected by the introduction of special terms (proterms). Identity is non-relational so no new logical sign is needed for representing identity sentences. In effect PTL can be developed as a system roughly equivalent to that of a standard first order logic whose logical particles consist of the existential quantifier and the signs for conjunction, negation and identity.

5. We now give a formal description of PTL and later proceed to extend it to a system called TFL capable of directly expressing propositions containing 'every', 'if ... then', 'or' and other syncategorematic expressions that PTL cannot transcribe.

FORMAL DESCRIPTION OF PTL

Vocabulary

The vocabulary of PTL consists of material elements and formative elements.

   I. Material Elements
      (i) a) Term letters.
         b) Singular term letters.
      (ii) Relation letters (n-place, n > 1).
      (iii) Proposition letters.
   II. Formative Elements
      (i) Signs of quality: '$+$', '$-$'.
      (ii) A sign of concatenation '$\dagger$'.
      (iii) Brackets: '$($, $)$'; '$\langle$, $\rangle$'; '$[$, $]$'.

Formation Rules

Terms

(1) If α is a term letter or a relation letter then $\pm \alpha$ are terms or relations, i.e. $+\alpha$ is a term (or relation) and so is $-\alpha$.
(A term is singular if it is of form $+\alpha$ where α is a singular term letter).

(2) If α and β are two terms (or relations of the same degree) then $\langle \alpha \dagger \beta \rangle$ is a (compound) term (or a compound relation).

(3) If R is an n place relation and $\alpha_2, \ldots \alpha_n$ are terms then $R \dagger \alpha_2 \ldots \dagger \alpha_n$ is a term.

(4) Nothing is a term unless by 1, 2, or 3.

Propositions

(5) If α is a proposition letter then $\pm \alpha$ are propositions.
(6) If α and β are terms then $\alpha \dagger \beta$ is a proposition.
(7) If α and β are propositions then $[\alpha] \dagger [\beta]$ is a proposition.
(8) Nothing is a proposition unless by 5, 6, or 7.

5.1 Exploiting the similarities of logic to arithmetic led nineteenth-century logicians, notably Boole and Schröder to common laws shared by propositional and term logic. Our investigation is in this tradition, which indeed goes at least as far back as the researches of Leibniz. The formation rules of PTL have obvious points of similarity to the familiar rules for constructing well-formed numerical expressions. According to the formation rules for arithmetic, if α is a number then $+\alpha$ is a positive number and $-\alpha$ is a negative number. Also if α and β are numbers so are $\alpha + \beta$ and $\alpha - \beta$. The plus and minus signs do double duty, functioning in a unary way in signifying the positive or negative quality of a number and in a binary way when connecting two numbers to form a third number. The dual use of the signs facilitates arithmetical calculation and it suggests that the functor which connects the material signs of our logical language may be usefully represented by the sign that signifies positive quality. Instead of '$\dagger$' we will now write '$+$' reading the plus sign as 'and' when it connects two propositions and as 'some is' when it connects two terms.

The idea that 'and' is like 'plus' is intuitively plausible; indeed these words are often used synonymously. And the idea that '$+$'

could serve as a term connective was suggested by Hobbes and enthusiastically endorsed by Leibniz. We carry out this suggestion by systematically replacing the dagger sign by the plus sign in the formal description of PTL.

5.2 Having remarked on the similarity of logical and arithmetical notations we take note of some fundamental differences. One difference concerns closure. In arithmetic but not in logic the addition of two elements always results in an element of the same kind. Thus if a and b are two numbers 'a + b' will also be a number. In logic, on the other hand, the addition (predication) of two *terms* A and B may result in a *proposition*. Here is one source of the disanalogies one finds between logical and ordinary arithmetical calculation. Certain operations permitted in arithmetic are not permitted in logic, while, on the other side, certain operations (for example the replacement of 'p' by 'p + p') permitted in logic are not permitted in arithmetic. We are about to extend PTL to the more general system of TFL. In presenting the set of transformation rules for TFL we make the customary stipulation that only operations explicitly licensed by the rules are allowable. All other operations, including some allowed by the rules for manipulating expressions in standard arithmetic, are prohibited. The caveat of constraint is of special significance here. For we are introducing an unfamiliar use of a very familiar notation whose manipulation for the standard arithmetical interpretation is second nature. On the other hand the logical constraints on standard operations are surprisingly few and very quickly mastered. Moreover the resulting ease of transcribing sentences of natural language into a notation that makes it possible to do logic in an arithmetical way makes it quite worthwhile to master them. Or so I trust the reader will find.

5.3 *Amplifying PTL*: It has been remarked that the expressive power of PTL is that of a standard language of modern predicate logic (MPL) whose syncategorematic elements are '∃x', '∼', '&', and '='. As is well known, such systems can be augmented to include the universal quantifier as well as signs for connectives such as '→' and '∨' by means of such definitions as

$$(x)(..x..) = df \quad \sim (\exists x)(\sim ..x..)$$
$$p \rightarrow q \quad = df \quad \sim (p\& \sim q)$$

In extending PTL to TFL we make use of parallel difinitions of this sort.

In transcribing 'some S is P' and 'p and q' into the notation of PTL we used only a single sign, '†' to connect the material elements. Our goal now is the transcription of such term and propositional connectives as 'every is', 'if then', 'some isn't', and 'or'. As a start, we shall find it useful to transcribe 'some S is P' and 'p and q' as of form '$+\alpha + \beta$'. With this modification the transcription of 'Some S is P' becomes linear since the first sign of '$+ S + P$' may be read as 'some' and the second as 'is'. Similarly one may read the first plus sign of '$+ p + q$' as 'both' and the second as 'and'.

The following examples illustrate the new style of transcription:

(1) Some A is R to some B
    $+ A + (R^2 + B)$
(2) An A loved a B and he married her
    $+ [+ A_j + L^2 + B_k] + [+ J + M^2 + K]$
(3) Some S is non P
    $+ S + (- P)$
(4) not both p and not q
    $- (+ p + (- q))$

5.31 '*Isn't*' *and* '*Andn't*': The English contraction of 'is not' to 'isn't' corresponds to the arithmetical contraction of '$+ -$' to '$-$' in $a + (- b) = a - b$. This suggests that we can extend the expressive power of PTL to allow for the transcription of sentences of form 'Some S isn't P'. The following definition accomplishes this:

(D1) Some S isn't P = df   Some S is nonP
    $+ S - P = df + S + (- P)$

The suggestion that the negative copula 'isn't' should be represented by a minus sign had been made by Hobbes and Leibniz. It is a natural suggestion and we shall adopt it.

In some languages there are contractive forms for 'and not'. If English had the word 'andn't' we could interpret '$+ p - q$' as 'both p andn't q' by way of the definition:

(D2) $+p - q = df + p + (-q)$
        p andn't q = df p and not q

In forming definitions we bear in mind that the definiens and the definiendum must be convalent as well as algebraically equal. Indeed it is a feature of the algebraic system that we are developing that logically equivalent categorical propositions are a) algebraically equal and b) convalent. These two conditions are sufficient as well as necessary for equivalence as the word 'equivalent' conveniently suggests.

5.32 *'Every'*, *'If then'*, *and 'Or'*: Denying 'Some S isn't P' results in a proposition equivalent to 'every S is P'. Now 'not some S isn't P' is expressible in PTL and this suggests that we can use it to define an algebraic expression for 'every S is P'.

(D3.1) $-S + P = df - (+S - P)$
           every S is P = df not: Some S isn't P

Similarly, using 'not both p and not q' we may define an algebraic expression for 'if p then q':

(D3.2) $-p + q = df - (+p + (-q))$
           if p then q = df not both p and not q

Finally we define an expression for 'p or q':

(D3.3) $-(-p) - (-q) = df - [+(-p) + (-q)]$
           p or q = df not both not p and not q

In using four minus signs to represent 'or' we abandon the policy of trying to match an English word to each logical sign. The fact that English hasn't got the words is responsible. If the word 'thenn't' were available as a contractive form for 'then not' we could read '$-(-p) - (-q)$' in a linear way as 'if not p thenn't not q'.[3]

---

[3] In some languages 'or' is repeated in disjunctions ('or fish or fowl'). If 'orn't' were available '$-p - q$' could be read as 'orn't p orn't q' and defined by '$-(+p +q)$'. In choosing a notation, I have tried to retain a linear correspondence to English. In a language where 'if' characteristically appeared between consequent and antecedent, 'q if p' could be represented as 'q $-$ p' with a single binary sign. Similarly where the verb phrase characteristically precedes the noun phrase we could represent 'every S is P' as 'P $-$ S' and 'some S is P' as 'P $+$ S'. Though impractical for transcription from English the use of a single connective sign is of theoretical interest.

5.4 *Singular Terms*: If 'α' is a singular term the proposition 'α is P', which transcribes as '$+\alpha + P$', entails '$-\alpha + P$'. For example, '$+$ Socrates $+$ wise' entails '$-$ Socrates $+$ wise'. Strictly speaking 'Socrates is wise' is an elementary particular proposition. But it has the logical power of a universal proposition. To indicate that it has this power we often transcribe 'Socrates is wise' as '*S + W' or even as '$\pm$ S + W'. The expression '$\pm$ Socrates' *may* be read as 'Some-or-every Socrates' provided that we do not make the mistake of thinking that 'Socrates is wise' is actually a conjunction of the particular and universal forms.

5.41 Having shown how to represent 'every' and such connectives as 'if . . . then' and 'or' we are able to transcribe directly from the regimented vernacular any sentence translatable in a standard language.

The following transcriptions illustrate the versatility of TFL in giving algebraic expression to canonical forms of English sentences:

(1) if some A is B then every C is D and E
    $-[+A+B]+[-C+\langle +D+E \rangle]$
(2) some A is R to every B
    $+A+R^2-B$
(3) Some A is B and it is C
    $[+A_J+B]+[+J+C]$
(4) every A is either B or R to every C
    $-A+\langle --B--(R^2-C) \rangle$

5.5 The general form of a proposition in the algebraic language of TFL is

$$\pm(\pm(\pm\alpha)\pm(\pm\beta)$$

Where α and δ are two terms the general form has the following interpretation:

yes	some	α	is	β
not	every	not α	isn't	not β

Where α and β are two propositions it will not always be possible to assign an English equivalent to each plus and minus sign. If English had contractive forms for 'and not' and 'then not' we could interpret the omnibus form thus:

$$\frac{\text{yes}}{\text{not}} \quad \frac{\text{both}}{\text{if}} \quad \frac{\alpha}{\text{not } \alpha} \quad \frac{\text{and}}{\text{andn't}} \bigg/ \frac{\text{then}}{\text{thenn't}} \quad \frac{\beta}{\text{not } \beta}$$

5.51 Counting denials of particular propositions as universal and denials of universal propositions as particular we can consider the valence of a proposition to be its logical quantity, or, since valence is the more general characteristic (applying as it does to conjunctions and disjunctions of propositions as well as to categorical propositions), we may say that *a particular proposition is a proposition of positive valence and a universal proposition is a proposition of negative valence*. Similarly if we count negations of conjunctions as disjunctions and negations of disjunctions as conjunctions then *a conjunction is a proposition of positive valence and a disjunction is a proposition of negative valence*. Conditionals count as disjunctions.

The valence of a proposition may be mechanically read from the *first two signs of its explicit algebraic form*: '$\pm (\pm \ldots)$'. If these are the *same* the valence of the proposition is positive. If these *differ* the valence is negative. Note now that the so-called affirmative proposition 'every S is P' has negative valence as is clear from its transcription: $+ (-S + P)$. Similarly the so-called negative proposition 'not every S is P' is positive in valence because the first two signs of its transcription '$-(-S + P)$' are the same. In what follows we continue our policy of suppressing signs of positive quality. A traditional schedule of the four standard categorical propositions then looks like this:

A	every S is P	$- S + P$
E	no S is P	$-(S + P)$
I	some S is P	$+ S + P$
O	some S isn't P	$+ S - P$

I have transcribed 'no S is P' as '$-(S + P)$' instead of as '$-(+S + P)$' to make its algebraic form correspond to the original vernacular which has 'no' as a contraction of 'not:some'. A more elegant schedule from a formal standpoint would have two propositions beginning with 'every', or else with 'no', and two beginning with 'some':

A	$-S + P$	$-(S - P)$
	every S is P	no S isn't P
E	$-S - P$	$-(S + P)$
	every S isn't P	no S is P
I	$+S + P$	$+S + P$
	Some S is P	Some S is P
O	$+S - P$	$+S - P$
	Some S isn't P	Some S isn't P

According to the much maligned doctrine of distribution, the predicate terms of E and O propositions and the subject terms of E and A propositions are distributed while the predicate terms of I and A propositions and the subject terms of I and O propositions are undistributed. The distribution value of a material element in a proposition is perspicuous in its algebraic representation: in TFL the question whether a given term is distributed or undistributed in a proposition is the question whether its algebraic value in that proposition is negative or not. If we extend the idea of valence to the internal categorematic parts of the proposition we may consider the distribution value of an element in a proposition as the valence of that element. In determining the distribution value (or valence) of the elements of an expression we simplify its algebraic representation by driving the minus signs in as far as possible. The result will be an algebraic expression in which each element is either negative or positive. Negative elements are distributed, positive elements are undistributed. For example to determine the distribution values of A, B, C, and D in

if no A is B then no C is D

we first transcribe it algebraically as:

$$-[-(A + B)] + [-(C + D)]$$

and then simplify:

$$A + B - C - D$$

The simplified expression has no interpretation but it serves to show that in the original proposition, A and B are undistributed and C and D are distributed.

Similarly the valences or distribution values of 'p', 'q' and 'r' in 'if p and q then r' can be found by giving this formula its algebraic representation '$-(+p+q)-r$' and simplifying to '$-p-q+r$' which shows that 'p' and 'q' are distributed and 'r' is undistributed. The valence of a proposition and the valence of its elements determine its logical powers. In particular, convalent propositions whose elements are convalent are logically equivalent. For example, 'every A is B' and 'no non-B is non-A' are convalent (both being universal). In both propositions A has negative valence (being distributed) and B has positive valence (being undistributed). The propositions are therefore equivalent.

6. We are now ready to give a more formal account of the algebraic system of term logic.

FORMAL DESCRIPTION OF TFL

Material Elements

The material elements of TFL are the same as for PTL, namely terms, relational expressions, and propositions. The formative elements lack the dagger sign but are otherwise the same, consisting of brackets and plus and minus signs. (But in TFL the minus sign is not only used for negative quality but also for 'every' and 'if' in the binary functors 'every is' and 'if then'.)

Formation Rules

Terms

(1F) If α is a term or relation letter then $(\pm\alpha)$ are terms or relations. That is to say $(+\alpha)$ is a term (or a relation) and so is $(-\alpha)$.

A term is singular if it is of form $(+\alpha)$ where α is a singular term letter.

(2F) If α and β are two terms (or two n-place relations) then $\pm\langle\pm\alpha\pm\beta\rangle$ are terms (or n-place relations).

(3F) If R is an n-place relation and $\alpha_2 \ldots \alpha_n$ are n-1 terms then $R\pm\alpha_2 \ldots \alpha_n$ are terms.

(4F) Nothing is a term unless by 1, 2, or 3.

Propositions

(5F) If α is a proposition letter then $(\pm\alpha)$ are propositions.

(6F) If α and β are terms then $\pm(\pm\alpha\pm\beta)$ are propositions.

(7F) If α and β are propositions then $\pm (\pm[\alpha] \pm [\beta])$ are propositions.

(8F) Nothing is a proposition unless by 5, 6, or 7.

Rules of Transformation and Derivation

(1) *Laws of Commutation*
   (i) $+\alpha + \beta = +\beta + \alpha$
   (ii) $--\alpha --\beta = ---\beta --\alpha$

For example where α and β are two terms we read (ii) thus: every non α isn't non β = every non β isn't non α. Where α and β are propositions (ii) is read: α or $\beta = \beta$ or α

(2) *Laws of Association*
   (i) $+\alpha + (+\beta + \gamma) = +(+\alpha + \beta) = \gamma$
   (ii) $--\alpha --(--\beta --\gamma) = --(--\alpha --\beta) --\gamma$
The term interpretation of (ii) is:
   every non α isn't neither β nor γ = everything that is neither α nor β isn't non γ.

(3) *Laws of External 'not' Distribution (DeMorgan's Laws)*
   $-(\pm\alpha \pm \beta) = \mp\alpha \mp \beta$
For example $-(-\alpha + \beta) = +\alpha - \beta$
which, propositionally interpreted, is
   not: if α then $\beta = \alpha$ andn't β

(4) *Laws of Internal 'not' Distribution*
   (i) $\pm\alpha - (\pm\beta) = \pm\alpha + (\mp\beta)$
   (ii) $\pm\alpha_1 - (R \pm \alpha_2 \ldots \pm\alpha_n) = \pm\alpha_1 + (-R) \mp \alpha_2 \ldots \mp \alpha_n$
For example, the propositional reading of $+\alpha - (-\beta) = +\alpha + \beta$ is:
   α andn't not $\beta = \alpha$ and β
The term reading is:
   some α isn't non β = some α is β

(4ii) is exclusively a term law. An example is
   $-\alpha_1 - (R - \alpha_2) = -\alpha_1 + (-R) + \alpha_2$
i.e. every α_1 isn't R to every α_2 = every α_1 is non-R to some α_2

(5) *Law of Double Negation*
   $--\alpha = \alpha$
   not not $\alpha = \alpha$

(6) *Laws of Iteration*

  (i) $+\alpha + \alpha = \alpha$

    α and $\alpha = \alpha$

  (ii) $--\alpha--\alpha = \alpha$

    α or $\alpha = \alpha$

(7) *Laws of and/or Distribution*

  (i) $+(--\alpha--\alpha)+(--\beta--\gamma) = --(+\alpha+\beta)$
$$--(+\alpha+\gamma)$$
$$\alpha \text{ and } (\beta \text{ or } \gamma) = (\alpha \text{ and } \beta) \text{ or}$$
$$(\alpha \text{ and } \gamma)$$

  (ii) $--(+\alpha+\alpha)--(+\beta+\gamma) = +(--\alpha--\beta)$
$$+(--\alpha--\gamma)$$
$$\alpha \text{ or } (\beta \text{ and } \gamma) = (\alpha \text{ or } \beta) \text{ and}$$
$$(\alpha \text{ or } \gamma)$$

Laws of Derivation

(8) *Dictum de Omni* (DDO)

  (i) $-\alpha \pm \beta$ (ii) $\pm \beta + \alpha$

    $\underline{\quad .. \alpha .. \quad}$ $\underline{\quad .. -\alpha .. \quad}$

    $.. \pm \beta ..$ $.. \pm \beta ..$

where '$-\alpha$' has the meaning 'every α' or 'if α' and the conclusion is equal to the sum of the two premisses. The DDO is a general rule of inference comprehending as instances such laws as *BARBARA*, *modus ponens*, and the Substitutivity of Identity.

(9) *Conjunction*

  p

  $\underline{\quad q \quad}$

  $+p+q$

(10) *Disjunction*

  $\underline{\quad p \quad}$

  $--p--q$

(11) *Simplification*

  $\underline{+p+q}$

    p

(12) *The Law of Wild Quantity*

$$\frac{+\alpha_i + \beta}{-\alpha_i + \beta}$$

where α_i is a singular term. Because of its wild quality, $+\alpha_i$ is often written as $*\alpha_i$ or as $\pm\alpha_i$.

(13) *Laws of Predicative Distribution*

   (i) $+\alpha + \langle --\beta --\gamma\rangle = --[+\alpha+\beta] --[+\alpha+\gamma]$
      some α is β or γ = some α is β or some α is γ

  (ii) $-\alpha + \langle +\beta+\gamma\rangle = +[-\alpha+\beta]+[-\alpha+\gamma]$
      every α is β and γ = every α is β and every α is γ

Note where α is a *singular* term the distribution works for *both* 'and' and 'or'.

(14) *T-Laws*

   (i) $-A+T$
     every A is a thing

  (ii) $\pm A + B = \pm T + \langle \pm A + B\rangle$
     a) Some A is B = Something is A and B
     b) every A is B = every thing is if A then B

 (iii) $\pm A + B = \pm [+Tx + E] + [\pm [\pm x + A] + [\pm x + B]]$
     a) Some A is B = Some thing exists and it is A and it is B
     b) every A is B = if some thing exists then if it is A then it is B.

(15) *The Law of Converse Relations*

$$\frac{\pm\alpha_1 + R^{\cdots i \cdots j \cdots} \ldots \pm\alpha_i \ldots \pm\alpha_j \ldots \pm\alpha_n}{\pm\alpha_1 + R^{\cdots j \cdots i \cdots} \ldots \pm\alpha_j \ldots \pm\alpha_i \ldots \pm\alpha_n}$$

where $R^{\cdots i \cdots j \cdots}$ is an n place relation and $R^{\cdots j \cdots i \cdots}$ is one of its $n!-1$ converses and provided that no particular subject, $+\alpha_j$ moves left across or into a position occupied by a universal subject.

For example

$$+\alpha_1 + R^{123} + \alpha_2 - \alpha_3$$

entails

$$+\alpha_1 + R^{132} - \alpha_3 + \alpha_2$$

as in

$$\therefore \frac{\text{Some sailor read a(certain) poem to every girl}}{\text{Some sailor read every girl a poem}}$$

The reverse entailment would be illegitimate because it would violate the prohibition of the leftward movement of 'a poem' into the position occupied by 'every girl'.

Laws (12), (13), (14) and (15) are semantic laws whose validity depends on the special properties of certain categorematic elements. Thus (12) and (13) hold because singular terms have unique denotation. (14i) holds because T has universal denotation and (15) holds because relational converses (e.g. the active form and the passive form of binary relations) bear certain analytic relations to one another (e.g. a loves b = b is loved by a).

Tautological Forms in TFL

(1) $-\alpha + \alpha$ is a tautology
(2) if H is a tautology, so is $-\alpha + H$
(3) if H_1 and H_2 are tautologies so is $+H_1 + H_2$
(4) Any proposition entails a tautology.
(5) Any proposition is a contradiction if its negation is a tautology.

Definitions of Inconsistency and Validity

(1) A set of propositions is inconsistent if and only if a contradiction is derivable from the conjunction of its members
(2) An argument whose premisses are consistent is valid if and only if the set formed by its premisses and the denial of its conclusion is inconsistent.

7. In illustrating how the algebraic system of traditional formal logic applies in proofs of validity, I shall first consider the sort of argument that was the focus of attention in antiquity and the scholastic period. The arguments to which I refer have the following formal features.

a) each argument has as many terms as sentences
b) each term occurs twice in different sentences

Any argument with these features will be called a classical term argument (CTA). Thus a CTA is an argument of n categorical sentences and n recurrent terms. When n = 3 the CTA is a standard syllogism. The counter-set of a given CTA is the set of sentences consisting of the premisses of the CTA and the *denial* of its conclusion. For example the counter-set of 'every M is P, every S is M, therefore every S is P' is 'every M is P, every S is M, not every S is P'. Any CTA is valid if and only if the conjunction of sentences in its counter-set is inconsistent. We can therefore prove validity or invalidity by showing whether the counter-set is inconsistent or consistent. It is in fact easy to test any counter-set for inconsistency. The following principle which will be stated without proof tells how:

The P-Zero Rule

A set of n categorical propositions with n recurrent terms is inconsistent if and only if

    a) The set contains exactly one particular proposition.
    b) The algebraic sum of the propositions in the set is zero.

Consider a CTA for the case n = 2:

$$\therefore \quad \frac{\text{Some A isn't B}}{\text{Some B isn't A}} \qquad \frac{+A-B}{+B-A}$$

Its counter-set is

$$+A-B$$
$$-(+B-A)$$

This contains exactly one particular proposition but it doesn't sum to zero. The counter-set is consistent so the argument is invalid.

The reader can quickly satisfy himself of the ease with which he can deal with any syllogism or sorites in algebraic transcription. One first checks to see whether the counter-set contains exactly one particular proposition (counting denials of universal/particular propositions as particular/universal). If this first condition is satisfied, add up the propositions to see whether all terms of the counter-set cancel out. One may, for example, wish to determine whether the following form of sorites is valid:

Some C is D	$+C+D$
every non-B is non-D	$-(-B)+(-D)$
no C is non-M	$-(C+(-M))$
$\therefore$ Some B is M	$\therefore \ +B+M$

The counter-set is:

$$+ C + D, \ -(-B)+(-D), \ -(C+(-M)), \ -(+B+M)$$

Here both conditions of the P-Zero Rule are satisfied. The sorites is valid.

For contrast consider:

Some A isn't B	$+A - B$
Some B isn't C	$+B - C$
∴ Some A isn't C	∴ $+A - C$

Counter-set:

$$+A - B, \ +B - C, \ -(+A - C)$$

which violates the P-Zero Rule by having two particular propositions. The syllogism is invalid.

7.1 The reader will find a discussion of proof and model theory for a version of TFL in Appendix F by Clifton McIntosh. A discussion of the relation of TFL to the term-theoretic mapping of MPL that Quine has developed is given in Appendix E by Aris Noah. Here we may indicate that TFL has the sort of inference power one associates with MPL. The following examples illustrate the manner that one may apply the rules in proofs for arguments that were not satisfactorily dealt with by the pre-Fregeans. The first is a textbook example adapted from one devised by Quine:

A. (1) all who entered unaccompanied by a member were searched
   (2) none of the Frenchmen were searched
   (3) some of the Frenchmen entered unaccompanied by anyone else
   ∴ some of the Frenchmen are members

The conclusion transcribes as '$+ F + M$'. We deny it and conjoin it with the others:

(1) $- \langle + E + (-(A + M)) \rangle + S$
(2) $- (F + S)$
(3) $+ F + \langle + E + (-(A + (-F))) \rangle$
(4) $- (+ F + M)$

By immediate inference (4) is equivalent to

(5) $-M + (-F)$

and (2) is equivalent to

(6) $-F + (-S)$

Adding (6) to (3) we get

(7) $+(-S) + \langle + E + (-(A + (-F))) \rangle$

Adding (5) to (1) we get

(8) $- \langle + E + (-(A + (-F))) \rangle + S$

Adding (8) to (7) gives

(9) $+(-S) + S$

a contradiction.

The second is a well-known example.

B. $\therefore$ $\dfrac{\text{every horse is an animal}}{\text{every owner of a horse is an owner of an animal}}$

Here too we may deny the conclusion and derive a contradiction.

(1) $-H + A$
(2) $-(-(O^2 + H) + (O^2 + A))$
(3) $-(-(O^2 + A) + (O^2 + A))$ (1) (2) DDO
(4) $+(O^2 + A) - (O^2 + A)$ DM

The third and fourth examples illustrate how TFL deals with statements containing singular terms. The fourth and final example involves an identity statement, i.e., one with singular terms in both subject and predicate position.

C.   Sartre is a famous philosopher
        Sartre is a novelist
    $\therefore$ Some novelist is a famous philosopher

We use a direct proof:

(1) $+S + P$ premiss
(2) $+S + N$ premiss

| (3) $-S+N$ | (2) wild quantity |
| (4) $+N+P$ | (3) (1) DDO |

D.   Tully envies everyone else
         He doesn't envy Cicero
_____
   ∴ Tully is Cicero

We shall use an indirect proof

(1) $+T+e-(-T)$	premiss
(2) $+T+(-e)+C$	premiss
(3) $-(+T+C)$	denial of conclusion
(4) $-T+(-C)$	(3) DM
(5) $+T+e-C$	(4) (1) DDO
(6) $-T+e-C$	(5) WQ (Wild Quantity)
(7) $-(-T-(-e)+C)$	(2) DM
(8) $-(-T+(e-C))$	(7) Not Distribution

(8) contradicts (6)

8. Monadic term logic is decidable but for inferences involving relational propositions the Dictum de Omni is still the basic rule in proof procedures of TFL—including methods of proof analogous to those used in MPL. In one such method the validity of an inference is shown by exhibiting the inconsistency of the conjunction of the premise with the denial of the conclusion. For example, one may show that (B), 'every owner of a horse is an owner of an animal', follows from (A), 'every horse is an animal', by exhibiting the joint inconsistency of (A) with (B)'s denial, (C) 'some owner of a horse is not an owner of an animal'. The method consists of instantiating to atomic propositions and finding a contradiction. Here one first gives (C) a canonical form and instantiates its existentially bound variables. The canonical translation of (C) is:

$$(\exists x)(\exists y)(Hy \,\&\, Oxy \,\&\, (z)(A_z \to -O_{xz}))$$

Putting 'a' for 'x' and 'b' for 'y' we get

(1) $Hb \,\&\, Oab$
(2) $(z)(Az \to -Oaz)$

Instantiating the universally bound variable in (2) and using 'b' gives

(3) $Ab \to -Oab$

Instantiating again in '(x) (Hx → Ax)'—the canonical translation of (A)—we get

(4) Hb → Ab

(3) and (4) yield

(5) Hb → − Oab

which is equivalent to

(6) − (Hb & Oab)

contradicting (1).

The TFL proof procedure for this example is more direct. The transcriptions of (A) and (C) are

(A)   − H + A
(C)   + (O² + H) − (O² + A)

from which the contradiction

+ (O² + A) − (O² + A)

follows by the DDO.

8.1 The MPL method is longer because MPL construes every general sentence as a pronominalization whose antecedent is a quantifier and whose pronouns are the variables it binds. TFL sees no pronouns in (C) but MPL sees no less than three. In its proof procedure MPL must de-pronominalize by dequantification and instantiation before it can derive the desired contradiction.

It is open to TFL to construe any categorical sentence as a pronominalization in the manner of TFL. Thus 'something is A' which transcribes as '+ T + A' can be expanded as a pronominalization, '+ [+ Tx + E] + [+ X + A]', 'something exists and it is A'. One may even think of '+ T + A' as an expression that uses the functor '+ +' to depronominalize 'something is such that it is A'. To my mind this is the wrong way round but to a Fregean it might look like that.[4]

Quine, for whom MPL formulas are canonical, has shown how one may deploy a finite set of functors operating on terms and on relational expressions to render any quantificational

---

[4] The Fregean may balk at this way of de-pronominalizing because it treats 'thing' as a (categorematic) term.

formula as a pronoun-free expression. We have seen how the binary functors 'some is' and 'every is' suffice to do this for simple categoricals. These natural functors are represented algebraically in TFL. But the plus-minus notation does not suffice for a full program of de-pronominalization. There is, for example, no natural way to give a pronoun-free equivalent for 'every cat cleans itself'. (Quine introduces a special 'self' functor which here would operate on 'cleans' to eliminate the pronoun). And while one may introduce a permutation functor operating on 'has' to change 'there is a social disease that is harmless but every man has it' to 'some harmless social disease is had by every man', the latter, pronoun-free sentence, is deviant. More generally the *systematic* application of the permutation functor to any n-place expression to generate its n! − 1 converses is suitable for a formal system of predicate functor logic but not for a system that adheres to the logical syntax of natural language.

8.2 That the possibilities for pronoun-free expression are limited in a logical system that seeks to adhere to the syntactic resources of natural language is no reflection on its inference power. From a logical point of view there is no more reason to eliminate pronouns where they naturally occur than there is reason to proliferate them in the manner of MPL by treating every general sentence as a pronominalization. The natural resources for pronoun-free expression coincide with the arithmetical functors comprehended by the plus-minus notation for the basic logical particles. Other natural resources, such as passive permutation and self-functors do exist in the natural languages but have only an occasional application to certain expressions. Where pronouns are not naturally avoidable the syntactic resources of TFL are adequate for their overt expression. A pronominalization in TFL is, after all, syntactically unremarkable, consisting simply in the introduction of a proterm in a pronominal sentence alethically joined to an antecedent sentence. Corresponding to MPL's '$(\exists x)(. . x . .)$', we have 'something exists and . . . it . . .'. Corresponding to '(x) $(. . x . .)$', we have 'if anything exists then . . . it . . .'. The form '$+[+Tx+E]+[\pm X+A]$' is syntactically on all fours with '$+[+T+E]+[+T+A]$'. Admittedly the proterm introduced in the pronominal sentence has special semantic properties but any questions concerning its semantic role do not affect its syntax: the rules governing the formulation of 'something exists and it is A' are the same as those governing the formation of 'something is A and some B is C'. From a naturalist standpoint, therefore, the quantifier-construed as an operator binding the variables in a matrix is a superfluous bit of logical syntax. Where pronominalization is naturally unavoidable—as in 'every cat cleans itself'—quantification is not needed to effect it: we may for example express it as a conditional 'if something is a cat, then it cleans it(self)' which is syntactically unremarkable. Here, once again, we encounter the question whether to think of a pronoun as a bound variable whose antecedent is the quantifier that binds it, or whether to allow that it may be a proterm with semantic ties to a syntactically independent antecedent sentence.

9. It is obviously important to be clear about the relationship between the well-formed quantificational sentences of MPL in which pronominalization is a primitive affair of binding and corresponding Boolean forms of quantification that take place between an antecedent sentence of the form 'something exists' and a pronominal sentence '. . . it . . .' connected to the antecedent sentence by 'and' 'if . . then'. I shall presently argue that the intersentential Boolean form may be properly understood as an analysis and interpretation of the quantifier matrix relation. Here I present without comment some correspondences of MPL and TFL.

MPL			TFL	
Ax	$\Leftarrow$	x is A	$\Rightarrow$	$\pm x + A$
p & q	$\Leftarrow$	p and q	$\Rightarrow$	$+ p + q$
p → q	$\Leftarrow$	if p then q	$\Rightarrow$	$- p + q$

Two correspondences of particular prominence for quantified formulas are

R1 $(\exists x)(Ax \& (.. x ..)) \Leftarrow (.. \text{some A} ..)$ $\Rightarrow + [+ Tx + E]$
$+ [+ [\pm x + A] + [.. x ..]]$

R2 $(x)(Ax \rightarrow (.. x ..)) \Leftarrow (.. \text{every A} ..)$ $\Rightarrow - [+ Tx + E]$
$+ [- [\pm x + A] + [.. x ..]]$

The following equivalences that hold within TFL are called rules of expansion. These are important for expressing sentences in the form of pronominalizations that correspond to the quantificational formulas of MPL.

(E1) $+A+B$ $= +T+\langle +A+B\rangle$

some A is B $=$ something is A and B

(E2) $-A+B$ $= -T+\langle -A+B\rangle$

every A is B $=$ everything is if A then B

(E3) $\pm x+\langle +A+B\rangle = +[\pm x+A]+[\pm x+B]$

(E4) $\pm x+\langle -A+B\rangle = -[\pm x+A]+[\pm x+B]$

(E5) $+A+B$ $= +[Tx+E]+[+[\pm x+A]$
                         $+[\pm x+B]]$

(E6) $-A+B$ $= -[+Tx+E]+[-[\pm x+A]$
                         $+[\pm x+B]]$

Two basic rules of correspondence derivable from the earlier correspondence rules are

R1* $(\exists x)(Ax \& Bx) \Leftrightarrow +A+B$
R2* $(x)(Ax \rightarrow Bx) \Leftrightarrow -A+B$

9.1 Another set of rules correspond to Laws of *Instantiation* and *Generalization* in MPL:

(I1) $+[Tx+E]+[.. \pm x ..] \Leftrightarrow .. \pm \dot{J} ..$
(I2) $-[+Tx+E]+[.. \pm x ..] \Leftrightarrow .. \pm J ...$

A formula '$\pm [+Tx+E]+[.. \pm x ..]$' is called a pronominal expansion of its pronoun-free equivalent. The expansion of a particular or universal sentence is a B-type pronominalization. Particular sentences expand as conjunctions, universal sentences expand as conditionals. For example the expansion of 'some horses are grey' is 'something exists and it (*x) is a horse and it is grey'; the expansion of 'every horse is an animal' is 'if a(ny) thing exists, then if it (*x) is a horse then it (*x) is an animal'. In the conjunction the B-type pronoun has mock reference to some individual that would verify the sentence and the whole instantiates as '*$\dot{K}$ is a horse and *$\dot{K}$ is grey', the dotted letter being introduced as an instantial name denoting 'the thing in question'. In the conditional there is no pretense of reference to a particular individual under consideration; there the proterm of the pronominal sentences is analogous to a universally bound variable and the conditional instantiates as a potentially infinite conjunction of sentences of form 'if $*\dot{K}_i$ is a horse then $*\dot{K}_i$ is an animal' each of which is said to be an instance of the original universal sentence.

Replacing a proterm by a dotted letter corresponds to the introduction of a name for an existentially bound variable. Replacing a proterm by an undotted letter corresponds to 'universal instantiation'. One may understand the formula '. . J . .' to represent a conjunction of dotted formulas '. . $\dot{J}_i$ . .'. Equivalently, one may think of the undotted formula as being analogous to an open sentence that may be conjoined with any sentence of form 'some J is $\dot{J}_i$' to yield '. . J_i . .' by the DDO. Sentences of form 'Some J is $\dot{J}_i$' are analogous to the stipulation we make when we instantiate universally saying 'let x be a' thereby replacing the universally bound variable by an arbitrary name. In the universal case we can choose whatever name we please as often as we please. In TFL this amounts to the standing license to introduce at will any premiss of form 'some J is $\dot{J}_i$'. For example, given 'if anything exists it is created' we form the open sentence 'J is created'. We are then free to introduce the premiss 'some J is Jimmy Carter' and to conclude that Jimmy Carter is created. Universal instantiation is then understood as the application of the *Dictum de Omni* to sentences of form '. . . J . . .' and 'some J is $\dot{J}_i$' yielding '. . . $\dot{J}_i$ . . .'.

9.2 The method of instantiation characteristically used in MPL is available to TFL. I will sketch such a procedure to show that TFL is able to deal wth inferences in the manner of MPL and to show that the semantics that underlie the proof technique by instantiation are not essentially different for termist logic, or at any rate that interpretation models for MPL need not be significantly different for TFL. As our first example we show that 'every *man* has a *disease*' follows from 'there is a *disease* that every *man* has'. The premiss transcribes as

(1) $+[+Tx+E]+[+[\pm x+D]+[-M+h^2 \pm x]]$
(2) $\pm \dot{J}+D$
(3) $-M+h^2 \pm \dot{J}$ ⎫
(4) $-M+h^2+D$ (2) (3) DDO

    I.1

Our next example shows that 'some man loves himself' follows from 'some man loves every man'.

$$
\begin{array}{ll}
(1) & + M + L^2 - M \\
(2) & + Tx + E \\
(3) & \pm x + M \\
(4) & - [+ Ty + E] + [- [\pm y + M] \\
& \quad + [\pm x + L^2 \pm y]] \\
(5) & \pm \dot{J} + M \\
(6) & - [\pm K + M] + [\pm \dot{J} + L^2 \pm K] \\
(7) & + K + \dot{J} \\
(8) & - [+ \dot{J} + M] + [+ \dot{J} + L^2 \pm \dot{J}] \\
(9) & \pm \dot{J} + L^2 \pm \dot{J} \\
(10) & + [+ Tx + E] [+ [\pm x + M] \\
& \quad + [\pm x + L^2 \pm x]]
\end{array}
$$

pronominal
expansion of (1)

(3) (4)
I.1, I.2
letting K be $\dot{J}$
(6), (7) DDO
(5), (8) DDO
(5), (9), I.1

(10) represents 'someone exists and he is a man and he loves himself'. We may apply a rule to this expression that allows us to reduce it to ' $+ Mx + L + x$ ', 'some man loves himself'. The general rule which licenses the condensation of external pronominalizations to internal ones is

$$\pm [+ [+ Tx + E] + [\pm x + S]] + [\pm x + P] \Rightarrow \pm Sx + P.$$

The examples indicate that TFL can apply the method of instantiation in proofs. They also cast light on the relation of MPL to TFL at the level of singular sentences.

9.3 The relationship of TFL to MPL is further illuminated by translation or mapping procedures that enable us to find the MPL formula for any formula of TFL and vice versa. By applying the mapping rules we can take a vernacular sentence such as 'some sailor gave every child a toy', transcribe it as ' $+ S + G^3 - C + T$ ' and by a series of steps arrive at the canonical MPL formula $(\exists x)(Sx \& (y)((y \to (\exists z)(Tz \& Gxyz)))$. The reverse is also feasible. The reader will find an account of translation procedures between MPL and TFL in Appendix A. The basic mapping rules that apply are ' $(\exists x)(. . x . .) = Ex \& (. . x . .)$ ' and ' $(x)(. . x . .) = Ex \to (. . . x . .)$ ' where 'Ex' represents the sentence 'something exists' or 'there is a thing'. The forms 'Ex & $(. . x . .)$ ' and 'Ex $\to (. . x . .)$ ' are the Boolean counterparts to the standard quantificational forms. I shall speak here of Boolean quantification. Quine has said that bound variables are pronouns. Boolean quantification takes this seriously adding that pronominalization can be from sentence to sentence; if quantification is pronominalization then quantification can be construed in the Boolean way. We may therefore take 'Ex & (. . x . .)' as an *analysis* of '($\exists$x)(. . x . .)'.

Here the Fregean may object that 'something exists' cannot even be expressed in a standard language of MPL. But this only means that the formation rules of MPL are, in that respect, deficient. In any case one could add a rule for forming a sentence 'Ex' whose intended interpretation is 'something exists' or 'there is a thing'. After all, as matters now stand, '($\exists$x)' is introduced as primitive expression in MPL. If MPL were enriched by 'Ex', '($\exists$x)' could be contextually defined. We could then understand 'there is a thing such that it is P' as 'there is a thing *and* it is P'. In Boolean form, existential quantification is conjunctive; universal quantification is conditional. That a Boolean analysis of the quantifier is desirable and right is borne out by the fact that we can now dispense with the so-called law of quantifier interchange. For we can show that $(x)(Ax) = -(\exists x) - Ax$ by putting them both in Boolean form:

$$Ex \to Ax = -[Ex \& - Ax]$$

Another equivalence—called by Quine a 'law of passage'—is perspicuous in Boolean form:

$$(\exists x)Ax \to p = (x)(Ax \to p)$$
$$(Ex \& Ax) \to p = Ex \to (Ax \to p)$$

That such laws become mere instances of propositional laws counts in favour of the Boolean interpretation. It is worth remarking that the Boolean analysis of the quantifier-matrix relation supports Quine's view that the correct interpretation of the quantifier is objectual and not substitutional. Indeed if the Boolean analysis of the quantifier is adopted, the substitutional interpretation of quantificational formulas is incoherent.

Finally we note that the Boolean interpretation (in which the pronominal variables are semantically bound by the antecedent quantifiers but syntactically free) is not subject to the criticisms we made in chapter 4 of the view that 'pronouns of the vernacular' should be construed as syntactically bound by antecedent quantifiers. On the Boolean account of quantification the binding of the variable is intersentential; semantic binding can even occur into sentences used as questions, commands or other kinds of speech acts.

10.   Though termist logic takes strong exception to the doctrine that 'B-type pronominalization' is essentially intrasentential, it is not committed to the opposite thesis that pronominalization is always from sentence to sentence. Termist logic is in a position to respect the fact that in some pronominalization the antecedent and pronoun are in a single sentential unit, as for example in 'Some man loves himself'. One could of course view this sentence as the result of a transformation from 'Some man exists and he loves he' but this move is not forced.

The reader will recall that in our general account of pronominalization we distinguished between referential (A and D-type) pronouns whose antecedents focus on a particular individual taken for an S and non-referential B or E-type pronominalizations where the move from 'an S' to 'it' or 'that S' is made without epistemic focus on a particular thing being taken for an S. In the case of referential pronouns 'an S' is construed as 'a certain S' with the word 'certain' playing the role of a U-term indicator. Using the notation of the present chapter a referential pronominalization 'an S . . that S' may be represented as

$$+\hat{S}\ldots\ldots \pm\hat{S}\ldots$$

in which '$\hat{S}$' is a U-term denoting the individual under consideration. When I say that some man loves himself I *may* have a particular (self-loving) man in mind. I am then to be understood as saying

A *certain* man loves himself
$$+\hat{M}+L\pm\hat{M}$$

In chapter 5 section 5 we suggested that B-type pronominalizations also have U-terms in their antecedents but that their U-terms are instantial. If I say 'some man is P' and go *on* to say 'and he is Q' we may understand 'some man' to be of the form '$+\hat{M}_i$' where '$\hat{M}_i$' is an instantial U-term introduced to denote an unspecified but specifiable individual. (The circumflex in '$\hat{M}_i$' signifies U-term status; the subscript 'i' signifies that the U-term is here instantial.) It is as if I had said 'a *certain* man is P and he is Q'. And generally whenever 'some S is P' is followed by '... it ...' we retrospectively read the antecedent with a U-term. I may be convinced that some man loves himself without being able to answer the question 'who?' All the same 'some man' should be construed as 'some $\hat{m}an_i$'—'a certain man'. This 'instantial' use of 'a certain S' to focus on an unspecified but (in principle) specifiable individual occurs when I infer 'a certain S is P' from the purely existential claim that there is an S that is P. Clearly 'some S is P' entails 'a certain S is P'. And generally ' + S + P' entails $+ \hat{S}_i + P$' even where there is no epistemic focus on an identifiable individual taken for an S. Instantial U-terms, like variables, do not have rigid denotations. But from a syntactic standpoint they behave like referential U-terms and if we adopt the view that the antecedents of B-type pronouns also contain U-terms, then all pronominalizations will be characterized by recurrent U-terms. 'Some man (somewhere) loves himself' will then be transcribed as ' $+ \hat{M}_i + L \pm \hat{M}_i$'. Construed with recurrent U-terms any pronominalization 'a thing ... that thing' has the form ' $+ U ... \pm U ...$' in which antecedent and pronoun differ only sty-listically since both have particular quantity. Wild quantity is the mark of definiteness in the symbolic language of TFL. In actual language, a definite subject may have no quantity at all or it may be marked by a definite article which also serves as a U-term indicator. In pronominalization both 'an $\hat{S}$ ...' and 'it ...' entail universal propositions but only the pronoun is definite; its U-term has been previously introduced; in moving from 'a (certain) S' to '.. it ..' the speaker focuses on what was antecedently referred to in an indefinite manner (a certain S → that very S).

We have all along represented 'an S ... that S' as '$_{\iota}$some $S_{jj} ... *J ..$' thereby remaining neutral about adopting the recurrent U-term interpretation for B-type pronominaliz-ations. According to that interpretation the indexing of 'an S' amounts to according U-term status to the subject term represented later as 'J'. In effect a recurrent U-term reading does away with the need for indexing. Despite this important formal virtue I have chosen to retain the indexical style of representing the antecedent-pronoun relation because it captures the cross reference of the vernacular in a semantically uncommitted way. Reservations about the recurrent U-term reading arise because of its departure from the surface appearance of a G-term in the antecedent. When I say 'Some man will reach Mars in the nineties; he will become very famous' I do not appear to be referring to a certain man—perhaps not even in the mock focusing way that comes with the use of an instantial U-term. A more serious objection to the recurrent U-term reading concerns pronominalizations of form 'if an(y) S . . then that S . . . '. For when we read 'an(y) S' as 'an(y) certain S' we have if an(y) certain S . . then that S . . ' which looks and sounds deviant. I believe that these objections to the recurrent U-term interpretation can be overcome and that its virtues are considerable enough to warrant the effort and adjustments that may be needed to overcome them. Meantime it has seemed advisable to use the indexical style of representing the antecedent-pronoun relation of reference leaving open the question whether the two U-term interpretation is the proper analysis of this relation in the case of B-type pronominalizations.

11.   We have seen how inferences proved valid in MPL can by analogous procedures be proved valid in TFL. Are any inferences valid in TFL that are not valid in MPL? The question brings to mind the so-called weakened inferences from universal premisses to particular conclusions. Strictly speaking, nothing in the rules of TFL sanctions the entailment of 'Some S is P' by 'Every S is P'. On the other hand 'Some S is P' does follow syllogistically from 'Every S is P' in conjunction with 'Some S is S'. The question of the validity of 'Every S is P, hence some S is P' thus turns on the status of 'Some S is S'. If propositions of this form are acceptable we could treat the inference as an enthymeme with 'Some S is S' as a tacit minor premiss. It is tempting to regard 'Some S is S' as a logical truism since we need not assume that it imports the existence of an S. Nevertheless it is not hard to see that 'Some X is X' cannot be the form of a logical truth. If it were then any propositions of form 'Some X that is Y is an X that is Y' would be logically true.

But this has the intolerable consequence that any proposition of form 'some X is Y' would be logically true since such propositions follow from propositions of form 'Some X that is Y is an X that is Y'.

Although 'Some S is S' is not a logical truism a good case for the traditional thesis that weakened inferences are valid may still be made. In assessing the validity of 'every S is P, therefore some S is P' we bear in mind that 'every' propositions cannot be expressed in the primitive system of term logic (PTL) which has 'some is' as the sole term connective. In TFL 'every S is P' is defined as 'no S is non-P' provided that 'no S is P' is not also true. Where both of the contrary propositions 'no S is P' and 'no S is non-P' are true 'every S is non-P' is undefined. Here we come upon the nutritious grain of truth in the traditional thesis that of the two subcontrary propositions 'some S is P' and 'some S is not P' one must be true. This cannot be unqualifiedly sound logical doctrine, if only because 'some S is P or some S is not P' entails 'some S is S', and the view that 'some S is S' is logically valid has just been shown untenable. What *can* be said is that *whenever* 'every S is P' *has a truth value*, then 'some S is S' and 'some S is P or some S is not P' are true. The thesis that one of the two subcontraries must be true is stated in the context of the traditional square of opposition in which 'every S is P' occupies the top left position. And in that context the thesis is tenable and correct. (See below pp. 289 ff.)

12. Only a fragment of the sentences of a natural language are used in deductive reasoning. Among these we find 'Socrates is wise' and 'some editor is reading every novel written by an author of a trilogy', but not 'please try harder' or 'honour thy father'. The syntactic characterization of the cognitive fragment is a fundamental aim of logical theory. Sentences of this fragment that are not compounded from other sentences by conjunction or disjunction are variously called 'elementary', 'simple' or 'basic'. We have argued for the thesis that any basic sentence of the fragment either is, or is paraphrasable as, an assertion or denial of a sentence of form

Some/every X is Y

in which 'X' and 'Y' are grammatically interchangeable. Thus our thesis is that the sentences of the logical fragment (for our purposes restricted to the regimented paraphrases) are distinguished by having noun phrases of form 'some X' or 'every X'.

Traditionally such sentences are called categoricals. The label is vague but is made more precise when we specify them as sentences amenable to transcription into the algebraic notation of TFL. That the logical fragment consists of sentences whose noun phrases are of form 'some/every S' is not a thesis necessarily confined to traditional logic. It is true that orthodox Fregeans (among them Russell, Strawson, Geach, Dummett) reject it. But Quine accepts it when he suggests that singular as well as general categoricals can be parsed and regimented with the noun phrases that traditionally distinguish the class of sentences in the logical fragment.

Categorical sentences, albeit regimented, are sentences of natural language with the characteristic Noun-Phrase/Verb-Phrase (NP/VP) structure. This applies also to relational sentences like 'every boy loves some girl'. The idea that relational expressions like 'loves' are two place *predicates* has no place in classical linguistics or classical logic. In TFL the predicate or VP of 'every boy loves some girl' is 'loves some girl'—a phrase that itself has a noun and verb phrase. As we saw in chapter 7, a sentence like 'every boy loves some girl' has an iterated binary (NP/VP) structure: 'every boy some girl (doth) love' in which the predicate or dominant VP, 'some girl doth love', is itself an embedded sentence. Here we encounter one of the ways that MPL has affected contemporary linguistics. For some linguists are tempted by modern analysis to give 'every boy loves some girl' a ternary representation—a line of thought that threatens the classical NV/VP framework for constituent analysis of relational sentences. Chomsky himself has resisted the blandishments of Fregean syntax and remains committed to the classical binary analysis. In effect he gives each subject its very own predicate, treating 'loves some girl' much as one treats an embedded sentence. More generally, for any sentence of form '$\pm A_1 + R^n \ldots \pm A_n$' one can get what may be called its subject predicate normal form (SNF) by giving each subject phrase '$\pm A_i$ *its* predicate:

SNF $A_1 + R^n \ldots \pm A_n \Rightarrow A_1$
$+ (\pm A_2 + (\ldots + (\pm A_n + R^n)) \ldots).$

For example 'some sailor is giving every child a toy', whose *direct* transcription is

$+ S + G^3 - C + T$

has as its SNF:

$+ S + (-C + (+ T + G^3))$

Similarly the SNF of

$+ E + R^2 - (W^2 + (A^2 + T))$

—some editor is reading everything written by an author of a trilogy—is

$+ E + (-(+(+T + A^2) + W^2) + R^2)$

We saw also that the NP/VP or subject-predicate analysis represented by the SNF of a sentence maps directly into its canonical translation. For '$(\exists x)(Sx \,\&\, Px)$' corresponds to '$+ S + P$', and '$(x)(Sx \rightarrow Px)$' corresponds to '$- S + P$'. Applying these correspondence rules to the SNF of 'every boy loves some girl' we have

$- B + (+ G + L^2)$
$(x)(Bx \rightarrow (+ G + L^2 x))$
$(x)(Bx \rightarrow (\exists y)(Gy \,\&\, Lxy)).$

Applied to the SNF form

$+ S + (-C + (+ T + G^3))$

we have

$(\exists x)(Sx \,\&\, (-C + (+ T + G^3 x)))$
$(\exists x)(Sx \,\&\, (y)(Cy \rightarrow (+ T + G^3 xy)))$
$(\exists x)(Sx \,\&\, (y)(Cy \rightarrow (\exists z)(Tz \,\&\, G^3 xyz))).$

The last formula is the canonical translation of 'some sailor is giving every child a toy'.

12.1 It is instructive to see how a sentence in SNF corresponds to its linguistic constituent analysis on the one hand and to its canonical MPL form on the other. We take 'every boy loves some girl' for an example:

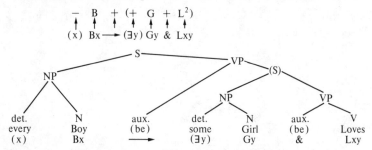

Note that the MPL translation is in exact correspondence to the SNF tree in which the classical subject–predicate structure of 'every boy loves some girl' is explicit and perspicuous. There is in this a historical irony that not everyone is in a comfortable position to appreciate. I have in mind philosophers like Geach and Dummett who continue to this day to hail Frege for the service he is alleged to have rendered in putting paid to the traditional 'subject-predicate logic'.

13. The Fregeans have supplemented their criticisms of traditional syntax with a confident attack on the traditional strategy of inference. There the claim was that pre-Fregean logic gave too central a place to syllogistic as the paradigm of inference. Implicit in this claim is that the *Dictum de Omni* gives way to principles like *modus ponens* since the primacy of propositional logic means that the basic rules of inference are propositional. We have seen however that *modus ponens* is simply a special application of the general rule of inference (the DDO in its abstract algebraic form) which comprehends syllogistic, propositional logic and even identity theory. According to that rule, inference with two or more premisses proceeds in algebraic fashion by cancellation of middle elements. That the DDO can ground identity arguments, propositional arguments and syllogisms, all of which are differently treated in modern predicate logic is made possible by the use of a uniform notation that represents propositional compounds, categorical propositions and identity propositions as a joining of two elements by a term or propositional connective. In representing the syncategorematic elements of a system roughly equivalent to standard first-order logic with identity, we take the first step in removing the stigma attached to traditional formal logic. For TFL has been considered incapable of doing what any logic must do in the way of formalizing inference. One immediate advantage in adopting a neoclassical system that conforms to the logical syntax of TFL is the solution to the problem we have encountered at the beginning of this chapter. The algebraic notation suggests the solution to the problem of defining a common nature for the syncategorematic elements of a standard deductive logic: the logical vocabulary of basic logic consists of signs of opposition. And it suggests that inference proceeds by cancellation and substitution according to the Dictum that traditional logicians have always considered to be fundamental and at the basis of deductive reasoning. The ability of TFL to handle inferences considered to be diverse in MPL is also in its favor. As we have seen the following inference forms are comprehended under the rule licensing substitution:

(i)   if p then q
$$\frac{\ldots p \ldots}{\ldots q \ldots}$$

(ii) a = b
$$\frac{\ldots a \ldots}{\ldots b \ldots}$$

(iii) every S is M
$$\frac{\ldots S \ldots}{\ldots M \ldots}$$

Each of these is an instance of the generic inference pattern '$-x+y, \ldots x \ldots; \ldots y \ldots$'. The algebraic notation teaches that *modus ponens*, Leibniz's law, and classical syllogistic are instances of the same generic pattern. One may therefore pointedly ask whether inferences involving identity and inferences involving propositions are indeed as diverse as they are made out to be in MPL. This question is not to be dismissed by an appeal to logical taste. In logic, the achievement of generality is always a mark of progress and the influence of logicians who adhere to unneeded distinctions is to be counted as retrograde.

There is also the psychological question of how we reason. Since Frege, logicians have been wary of viewing logic as the laws of thought. For all that, the question is legitimate, and alternative logistical systems with different logical syntaxes will one day receive confirmation or disconfirmation as models for the deductive processes actually taking place as we move from premisses to conclusions. It may be that neither MPL nor TFL will be confirmed. But the implausibility of MPL seems far greater. Consider again the fact that MPL translates 'some sailor gave every child a present' as

$$(\exists x)(Sx \,\&\, (y)(Cy \rightarrow (\exists z)(Tz \,\&\, Gxyz)))$$

where TFL transcribes it as '$+ S + G^3 - C + T$', and consider the processes that are required if we are to justify the inference to 'some sailor gave some athletes something expensive' ('$+ S + G^3 + A + E$') by the addition of the premisses 'some children are athletes' ($+ C + A$) and 'all the presents were expensive' ('$- P + E$'). It is far more likely that the actual procedures we use in getting from the premisses to the conclusion are closer to the model of cancellation than to the model of instantiation and generalization familiar to the practitioner of MPL.

And finally we consider once more the question of how the linguist would like to represent the structure of sentences that enter into deductive reasoning. Is he to accept Russell's claim that 'Socrates is wise' is altogether different in form from 'some human is wise', and further claim that 'Tully is Cicero' is different from both of these? Or is it simpler for him to remain logically naive and to accept the view of TFL that all these propositions have a structure that is basically the same? Why, after all, should the linguist complicate his life with the quantificationalist analysis of propositions when he has to hand the traditional system of logic that is in agreement with him in his classification of 'Socrates' and 'some man' as expressions of the same substitution class for grammatical purposes? Here we have a consideration that is not in the distant future. For a Fregean like Geach and a traditionalist like Chomsky have contemporary matters at stake and contemporary reasons for their divergent positions. Here, too, I venture to say that the linguist will opt for the logical syntax of TFL as the one that does least violence to his fundamental institutions concerning the structure of the basic sentences that enter into the cognitive process of deductive inference.

10

Truth and Logical Grammar

1. The sentence 'there is someone x, such that x is an American and x has walked on the moon' is modern logic's canonical way of saying 'an American has walked on the moon'. In giving canonical MPL expression to a statement of natural language, we put our syntax where our semantics is. The original, 'untranslated' sentence has no part that signifies existence. But it cannot be true unless there exists or has existed someone who is an American and who has walked on the moon and the canonical translation says as much. The translation is an expression whose truth conditions are existentially explicit.

When Russell maintained that 'the S is P' has the logical form of a compound existential sentence, he too applied the principle that the truth conditions of a statement determine its logical syntax. The idea that they do is very attractive but I shall argue for rejecting it and for replacing it with a more subtle account of the way that truth conditions bear on the analysis of a sentence. Briefly, my objections to determining syntax by way of truth conditions comes to this: two statements of form 'the S is P' may have different existential truth conditions and the canonical analysis will present intolerable alternatives of saying either (a) that they differ in their logical syntax or else (b) of reinterpreting them to give them both the same truth conditions. In practice, logicians, being logicians, adopt the second course but neither is acceptable. As an example, consider 'the horse that Bellerophon captured was white' and 'the horse that won the triple crown was grey'. Pre-analytically both are true but only the latter has an existential condition of its truth, namely the truth of 'a horse that won the triple crown exists'. Logicians impose a parallel truth condition on the former sentence but since this is done to save the thesis that truth conditions determine logical syntax, we may reasonably subject the thesis itself to the kind of scrutiny available to anyone who tentatively adopts the standpoint of traditional formal logic. TFL has no apparatus for regimenting sentences in a manner that makes truth conditions perspicuous. This may be thought of as a disadvantage; nevertheless, for that very reason, TFL does not find itself forcing standardized truth conditions on sentences of the same logical form. Of course, TFL must still show how its interpretation of 'the S is P' can tolerate different truth conditions. In satisfying this demand, TFL will not insist on uniform truth conditions because theory requires it.

Since Russell's theory of descriptions is the paradigm application of the thesis that I shall be criticizing, I will begin with it and with Strawson's objections to it.

In their dispute about how to interpret

(1) the present king of France is bald,

Russell and Strawson shared the assumption that its truth was conditional on the truth of

(2) the present king of France exists.

Russell held that (2) is entailed by (1); Strawson held that (2) is presupposed by (1). But both agreed that (1) could not be true unless (2) was true. I shall refer to this as the existential truth condition on (1), and I shall say of any statement subject to an existential condition similar to this one that it has existential import. Generally then, a statement of the form 'the S is P' has existential import if it could not be true unless 'the S exists' is true. Russell and Strawson interpret (1) with existential import but they account for it in different ways. Russell's idea that (1) entails (2) requires—so it seems—an interpretation of (1) that, roughly speaking, analyses (1) as containing an existential part; in effect, (1) contains (2) as a part of itself. (There exists a king of France, and only one, and he is bald). For how else could (1) entail (2)? Here again, Strawson agreed with Russell: (2) could not be entailed by (1) unless (1) asserts the existence of the present king of France. But Strawson denied that (1) could be correctly interpreted to assert this and so he denied that (1) entails (2). Instead we have Strawson's doctrine that (1) is neither true nor false unless (2) is true.

Strawson's objections to any reading of (1) that treats it as 'saying' there is a present king of France (one and only one) is plausible. For in saying that the present king of France is bald I do not appear to be saying that the present king of France exists even if what I say is subject to the existential condition. On the other side, Strawson's idea of a truth-value gap for (1) when (2) is false has struck many as an implausible way of accounting for the existential import of (1). There are many examples of false statements whose presupposition is false. Thus 'my car broke down' in excuse of lateness is false and not merely 'misleading'if I have no car. If Russell's account of the existential import of (1) appears weak because he interprets (1) as an overt existential assertion, Strawson's presupposition theory appears weak because it opens too wide a truth-value gap.

This brief survey of one important facet of the well-known controversy between Russell and Strawson suggests that an adequate explanation of the existential import of (1), and similar statements, will reject the second assumption shared by Russell and Strawson that (2) could not be entailed by (1) unless (1) is overtly existential. The rejection of this assumption seems to be required by a correct account of the existential import of (1) if such an account is to do justice to the fact (a) that (1) is a false statement and is so because there is no present king of France, and (b) that (1) does not overtly assert that the present king of France exists.

We hold then that (1) entails (2) and so we must explain the validity of the following argument:

(A1)   the present king of France is bald
_____

(hence) the present king of France exists

Since we are agreed that the premiss of (A1) is not existential, we must immediately grant that (A1) is not valid in the form we have presented it. Nevertheless A1 may be an enthymeme whose validity becomes evident after we make explicit a suppressed premiss whose truistic character has rendered it inconspicuous and unstated. It is easy to see that the tacit premiss we need for validity is 'every bald (person) exists'. The addition of this premiss to (A1) confers formal validity:

the present king of France is (a) bald (person)
every bald (person) exists
_____

(hence) the present king of France exists

Our standpoint is that of TFL and we need not attend to the syntactical scruples of modern logicians concerning the appropriateness of 'exists' as a predicate. The reader will already have noted that TFL allows for terms like 'thing' and 'existent' and that these terms can appear in subject or predicate position. The advantage of the tacit premiss explanation is clear. Our reading of (1) is sensitive to Strawson's objection to interpreting it as 'saying' there is a present king of France. At the same time, it avoids the truth-value gap explanation of why (1) is not true when (2) is false. For suppose (what is in fact the case) that the present king of France does not exist. Making the tacit premiss explicit, we have the valid and sound argument:

(A2)   it is not the case that the present king of France
        exists
        every bald person exists

        it is not the case that the present king of France
        is (a) bald (person)

The conclusion of (A2) is incompatible with (1). Since both of its premisses are true, (1) must be false. Thus the enthymemic explanation of the existential import of (1) does not require us to read (1) as an existential statement. Nor does it threaten a truth value gap.

Our account of (1) does not construe its logical form existentially. So one who says that the present king of France is bald has not said that the present king of France exists. But anyone who thus agrees that Strawson was right in objecting to interpreting 'the S is P' as a statement that asserts the existence of the S ought to be equally concerned about the existential interpretation commonly accorded to statements of form 'some S is P'. A reading of 'some Spaniards are proud' that construes it to 'say' that some Spaniards exist is surely as objectionable as a reading of 'the king of Spain is proud' that has it saying that the king of Spain exists. In his *Introduction to Logical Theory*, Strawson accepted the consequences of this.

He there offers an account of the square of opposition that treats 'some S is P' as a form of statement that presupposes but does not assert the truth of 'some S exist'. Unfortunately, the doctrine of presupposition fares no better for particular statements than it does for definite singular statements. Surely (3) 'some blue swans are omnivores' is not neither true nor false. It is false, and false because there are no blue swans. So even if one sympathizes with Strawson's position in *Introduction to Logical Theory*, that 'some S is P' does not assert existence, one cannot agree with his explanation of why it has existential import. Here too the tacit premiss theory resolves that difficulty. To explain why (3) is false even though it does not assert the existence of blue swans, we call on the additional premiss 'every omnivore exists' and add it to the true premiss 'no blue swan exists'. Together these yield the conclusion 'no blue swan is an omnivore' which contradicts (3). Since the premisses are true, (3) is false.

We have now seen how to account for the existential import of propositions of form 'the S is P' and 'some S is P'. Since the view of TFL is that singular propositions have wild quantity, we can simply say that any proposition of form 'some S is P' has existential import whenever it is appropriate to add to it the premiss 'every P exists'. This explanation of existential import will include singular statements of form 'the S is P' since these are equivalent to propositions with particular quantity. Once again we emphasize that a statement can have existential import without being an existential statement. The difference between 'some S is P' and 'some S that is P exists' is preserved by this account. In TFL, I can assert the existence of an S that is P by means of the latter form. But the ordinary form 'some S is P' is non-existential.

2. A non-existential reading of singular and particular statements has certain other advantages. For one thing, it allows us to count as true such statements as

    (4) some frictionless motion on an inclined plane is accelerated
    (5) a flying horse was captured by Bellerophon
    (6) the beast that Bellerophon captured was a flying horse
    (7) Pegasus is a flying horse.

(4) is a truth of physics even if there is no such thing as frictionless motion on an inclined surface anywhere in nature. And the judgement that (5), (6) and (7) are true is required of any student taking a True-False examination in classical mythology. The truth conditions of these and similar statements do not involve actual things to which these predicates apply or fail to apply. Whether any flying horses actually exist is irrelevant to whether (6) or (7) is true. And the predicate of (4) is also not here being claimed to apply to something actual; the truth of (4) is therefore not dependent on there being any constant motion in the actual physical world. Clearly, all these statements lack existential import. And the non-existential reading we are giving to 'the/some S is P' leaves room for this. But we must now explain how these statements differ from (1) and (3) in not being subject to the existential condition by way of the tacit premiss route. Put another way, if a statement like (5) is true and without existential import, then 'every P exists' cannot, in general, be true; if it were, we could not avoid the conclusion 'a flying horse exists'. But if 'every P exists' is not a logical truism, then the account we have given of the existential import of (3) and (1) would appear to be badly defective. For that account makes use of statements of the form 'every P exists' to explain the existential import of 'the/some S is P'.

Consider the two statements:

(8) Pegasus is a horse
(9) Secretariat is a horse.

I shall assume that both of these statements are made in a normal context and that both are true. If this is so, the term 'horse' will have been understood to be used with respect to different domains of application. In (8), 'horse' is not used to apply to things in the actual world; in determining the truth of (8), one would ignore the fauna of Greece, etc., and restrict oneself to a conventional non-actual state of affairs whose members or participants constitute a non-actual domain or 'world'—the world of Greek mythology. On the other hand, it is a condition of the truth of (9) that 'horse' applies to some member of the actual world and anyone who understands (9) will be aware of this condition for its truth. The use of a term with respect to a given domain of application will be called the amplitude of the term. The amplitude of 'horse' in (9) is *standard* since the domain in question is the actual world. In (8) 'horse' is used with *non-standard* amplitude since (8) could be true even if nothing in the actual world were a horse.

The amplitude of a term in a statement is determined by my knowledge of the meaning of that statement and this in turn is a matter of my knowing the existential conditions for the truth of the statement. If I have some understanding of 'the/some S is P', I must know some of the conditions that will have to obtain if the statement is to count as true. This pre-analytic knowledge is my basis for assigning to the predicate term 'P' a specific amplitude. In the case of (8) and (9), the truth conditions (whose knowledge is a condition of my understanding the statements in a normal context of utterance) determine different amplitudes for the term 'horse'.

This is not to say that 'horse' has different meanings in (8) and (9). In any domain of application a thing to which the term 'horse' correctly applies must be a mammal, hooved, a quadruped, and so forth. So, if the meaning or sense of 'horse' may be specified by the criteria for applying it in *any* given domain, we are at liberty to say that 'horse' is univocal in (7) and (8). I believe it is acceptable to speak of univocal terms with different amplitudes, even though, as we shall see, a difference of amplitude can have the same effect on the validity of inference as the equivocation of a term.

It will be useful to indicate the amplitude of a term by some notational device. Let 'horse (G)' indicate that 'horse' is being used to apply to members of a world Wg—the world of Greek mythology. And let 'horse (A)' indicate that 'horse' is being used with standard amplitude to apply to members of the actual world, Wa. Then (8) and (9) would be respectively represented as

(8) Pegasus is a horse (G)
(9) Secretariat is a horse (A).

To see why (9) has existential import, while (8) lacks it, we contrast the following arguments:

(A3) Pegasus is a horse (G)   (A4) Secretariat is a horse (A)
     Every horse (A) exists   Every horse (A) exists
     ———————————   ———————————
     Pegasus exists   Secretariat exists

The second premiss is equivalent to the truism that every horse (A) is a member of the actual world Wa. The argument (A4) is formally valid and sound. But (A3) is invalid because of the shift in the amplitude of the middle term 'horse'.[1]

We have said that statements of form 'the/some S is P' do not assert existence but that they sometimes 'import' existence. It is now clear why (4), (5), (6), (7) and (8) neither assert *nor* import existence. In each of these statements, the amplitude of the predicate term is non-standard and the addition to them of a tacit premiss of form 'every P(A) exists' will not gain us existential import because we will run afoul of the requirement of uniform amplitude for the middle term 'P'. On the other hand, whenever 'P' has standard amplitude in 'the/some S is P', we have existential import. Both Russell and Strawson agree that (1) cannot be true unless there exists some person who is bald. In other words, both agree that 'bald' in (1) has standard amplitude. This pre-analytical agreement should have been enough to account for the existential import of (1) since we now can add the truism 'every bald person exists' and conclude that 'the present king of France exists'. In this manner, we have shown that we need not go so far as to translate (1) as an existential statement nor need we place truth-value conditions on (1) in the manner of Strawson.

Our account of the difference between (8) and (9) shows that 'every P exists' is not a logical truth. On the other hand, 'every P(I) is a member of Wi' *is* a logical truth where Wi is some domain actual or non-actual. The following form of argument is generally valid:

the/some S is P(I)
every P(I) is a member of Wi

---

the/some S is a member of Wi.

Thus every statement of form 'the/some S is P(I)' is subject to the range condition 'the/some S is a member of Wi'. This condition is sometimes not satisfied in the case of non-standard amplitude. For example, one does not need to know anything

---

[1] We might try to add 'every horse (g) exists' to the first premiss of (A3). But this new statement is not a truism and is in fact false since it is equivalent to 'no horse (G) is non-actual'.

about the progeny of Medusa to know that 'the most famous progeny of Medusa was a flying kangaroo' is false. For implicitly we argue thus:

> the most famous of Medusa's offspring is a member of Wg
> no member of Wg is a flying kangaroo
>
> ---
>
> (hence) the most famous of Medusa's offspring is not a flying kangaroo

We have characterized the predicate terms of singular and particular statements as having an amplitude: a term P has amplitude 'I' in 'the/some S is P' if and only if this statement could not be true unless some member of the domain Wi is P. We have also assigned amplitude to terms in subject position and indeed there is good reason to speak of the amplitude of any term in a categorical statement including the subject and predicate terms of universal as well as particular statements and including proper names. It is easy to see that the subject terms of particular statements must have the same amplitude as the predicate terms. For 'some S is P' is equivalent to 'some P is S'; if the former cannot be true unless some member of Wi is P, neither can the latter be true unless some member of Wi is S. Since the existential truth conditions for both predicates is the same, they both have the same amplitude. To the terms of a universal statement, we assign the amplitude of terms in the contradictory particular statements. For example, if in 'some horse was unfed' the terms 'horse' and 'fed' have amplitude I, the same amplitude will be assigned to the terms of 'no horse was fed' and the terms of contrary and contradictory statements will all have the same amplitudes. That subject terms have the same amplitude as predicate terms applies also to subjects whose terms are proper names or definite descriptions. Thus 'Secretariat' has standard amplitude in (9) and Pegasus has non-standard amplitude in (8). It will be remembered that proper names have full status as terms and that they implicitly follow 'some' or 'every' in subject positions.

The amplitude of terms does not change under operations like contradition or contrariety. More specifically, the terms 'P' and 'un-P' will have the same amplitude in 'some S is P' and 'some S is un-P'. It is reasonable to make this a condition for assigning an amplitude to a term and we may note that some terms cannot satisfy this condition. Thus the term 'member of Wa' in 'some S is a member of Wa' will not satisfy this condition since it is an analytical condition of truth that 'member of Wa' must apply to something in the actual world if 'some S is a member of Wa' is to be true. But it clearly cannot be a condition that 'non-member of Wa' must apply to something in the actual world for 'some S is a non-member of Wa' to be true. For this reason, we shall say that the predicate term of an overtly existential statement like (10) 'some black swans exist' has no amplitude. The temptation to assign a standard amplitude wanes when we observe that the contrary term 'non-existent' or 'non-actual' cannot possibly have standard amplitude. In general then, any term of form 'member of Wi' will not be assigned an amplitude. Because terms of form 'member of Wi' have no amplitude, it is sometimes said of them that they are not really predicate terms. Thus 'existence' is sometimes said not to be a predicate term since its contrary 'non-existent' cannot apply to anything in the domain of application of 'existent'. This popular position is excessive and misleading. Although 'actual' 'existent' and other terms that apply to all and only members of the actual world lack applicable contraries they have applicable complements. Thus 'non-actual' applies to Pegasus and the like. The denial of term status to 'existent' because it has no contrary has given credence to the modern doctrine that 'exists' is a syncategorematic expression, a logical particle, and more specifically, a quantifier. The use of existence in the quantifier position gives the language of MPL a pervasive ontological cast: every proposition in the language either affirms or denies that a 'real' predicate like 'horse' or 'unicorn' is satisfied by some actual thing. As for sentences of form 'some S is P' they are invariably interpreted with existential import since the syncategorematic part 'some . . . is . . .' is rendered with 'exists'. As we have seen this places unnatural constraints on interpreting sentences from different domains of discourse; it is in any case to be avoided by a theory of logical signs that is based on some idea of what logical signs have in common. When expressions as different as 'or' and 'there exists' are both included in the list of the formative elements of a logical language, the philosopher has practically given up trying for a unified understanding of the logical formatives. In this fundamental area of logical theory the more traditional idea that logical signs are what confer distribution values on the terms of the proposition is much to be preferred.

3. Our account of singular statements whose terms have standard amplitude is in agreement with the Russell–Strawson thesis that 'the present king of France is bald' (and generally, 'the S is P') has existential import (where 'P' has standard amplitude). In a recent paper, Keith Donnellan has argued against this.[2] Since his objection applies to assertions in which 'P' has standard amplitude we shall consider it here. Donnellan observes that

(11) Smith's murderer is insane

may be a true statement even if no one has murdered Smith provided only that the speaker has used 'Smith's murderer' to identify someone who is in fact insane. In that case, (11) will be true even though

(12) Smith's murderer exists

is false. Similarly, one would have made a true statement if, referring to De Gaulle in 1965, one had said 'the present king of France is bald'.

In objecting to the Russell–Strawson thesis of existential import for (1) and (11), Donnellan is exploiting the difference between two ways of using 'the S' which Donnellan characterizes as 'attributive' and 'referential' respectively. Donnellan's point is that the truth of 'the S exists' is not a condition of the truth of 'the S is P' where the latter assertion embodies a purely referential or identificatory use of 'the S' and that Russell and Strawson have failed to take this referential use into account.

Donnellan is right in saying that Russell and Strawson have not considered the referential use of 'the S'. But their neglect is wholly benign since the case where 'the S' is purely referential in Donnellan's sense is irrelevant to the thesis of existential

[2] Keith Donnellan, 'Reference and Definite Descriptions', in *Naming, Necessity, and Natural Kinds*, ed. S. P. Schwartz (Cornell University Press, 1977), pp. 46–7.

import for (1) and (11). That thesis is formulated as a relation between 'the S is P' and 'the S exists' for the attributive use of 'the S', provided that this is its use in *both* statements. This is clearly seen if we adopt the tacit premiss account of the existential import of 'the S is P' (where 'P' is used with standard amplitude). Taking (11) as our example, we have

> Smith's murderer is insane (A)
> every insane person (A) exists
> _____
> (So) Smith's murderer exists.

Donnellan's objection gets what plausibility it has from the fact that in 'Smith's murderer exists', we have an attributive use of 'Smith's murderer'. It is arguable that the referential use would here be meaningless. On the other hand, in saying that Smith's murderer is insane, I may sometimes use 'Smith's murderer' referentially. All the same, it is misleading to suggest that neglect of the possibility of referential use vitiates either the entailment or the presupposition of 'the S exists' by 'the S is P'; all we need assume is the same use of 'the S' in both statements. Of *course*, we cannot argue for 'Smith's murderer exists' (attributive use) from 'Smith's murderer is insane' (referential use of 'Smith's murderer'). But why should we assume that anyone would commit this simple-minded fallacy of equivocation? On the other hand, if we assume – as we have a right to – that 'Smith's murderer' is univocal in the syllogism, or the presupposition or the Russell entailment, then Donnellan's point has no force.

Although Donnellan's distinction does not tend to undermine the Russell–Strawson position regarding the existential import of 'the S is P', it is valid and important within the Fregean framework which accords to 'the S' and other definite singular subject forms the role of identifying an individual object. Donnellan has rightly seen that an identification can be achieved by using 'the S' in two ways. Used as a name or conventional label, 'the S' identifies the individual by directly designating it. It may be that a group of people who are quite puzzled about the cause of Smith's death decide perversely to call Jones 'Smith's murderer'. This 'referential use' of 'Smith's murderer' is different from the attributive way of identifying an individual by unique description. The latter way was already noted by Frege when he said that we may identify an object by presenting it in a certain way, the mode of presentation being determined by the sense of the object word. Donnellan follows Frege in viewing the primary role of the definite singular subject to be that of identifying the individual object. We identify by using a conventional mode of designation or by using a unique description—but in either case, we identify. We have been contrasting this modern view of the role of the logical subject with the view of TFL. (1) TFL does not hold that only definite singular subjects refer and reference itself is not identification even when we do manage to pick out a single object for attention. (2) Recall that TFL analyses 'the S' as a referring expression of form 'some X'. It is true that in this case 'X' denotes uniquely but this is not essential to the reference of 'the S'. (3) For TFL, identification is no more than a fortuitous by-product of reference. To compare distinctions made within two quite different theoretical frameworks is hazardous even where it may be illuminating. Nevertheless we may say that the distinction made by Donnellan between the referential and attributive modes of definite singular reference is parallel to the distinction, to which we have called attention, between the two modes of indefinite reference—epistemic and non-epistemic—of subjects of form 'some S'.

4. We said a while back that the subject term and the predicate term of a statement have the same amplitude. This applies also to singular statements whose subjects are proper names or definite descriptions. Thus 'Secretariat' has standard amplitude in 'Secretariat is a horse' and 'Pegasus' has non-standard amplitude in 'Pegasus is a horse'. The idea of assigning amplitude to proper names in subject positions presents no difficulties for TFL since proper names have full status as terms capable of following 'some' or 'every' and accessible to predicate position. But when we move to MPL, we confront special difficulties. MPL distinguishes between predicate terms and names on semantic as well as syntactical grounds: a name identifies the object to which it applies, a predicate characterizes the objects to which it applies. The idea of different domains for the application of characterizing expressions is not problematic. But what are we to make of different domains of application for an expression whose primary function is to identify an individual? The problem becomes acute when a proper name is used as subject in two different statements whose predicate terms have different amplitudes. Consider for example

  (i) Socrates is snub-nosed
  (ii) Socrates is hook-nosed.

Let us suppose that the predicate term of (ii) has amplitude 'b' where Wb is some imagined world in which Socrates is not snub-nosed but hook-nosed. Some philosophers then take (ii) as a way of saying 'Socrates could (well) have been hook-nosed'. This way of understanding (ii) seems harmless but we now confront the problem of 'crossworld identity' of what is named or designated by 'Socrates' in (i) and (ii). I do not say there is no plausible solution; one may, for example, maintain that different domains can have objects in common and that 'Socrates' designates Socrates in Wb as well as in the actual world. In the next chapter, I shall offer a TFL version of this solution. But, for the present, I observe that a theory in which a problem arises is at a *prima facie* disadvantage when compared to one in which that problem does not arise; the point may be made even after we become aware of one or more acceptable solutions to the problem as it arises in the first theory. TFL, as augmented by the doctrine of amplitude, would parse (i) and (ii) in the following way:

  (i*) some/every Socrates (A) is snub-nosed (A)
  (ii*) some/every Socrates (B) is hook-nosed (B).

In (i) and (ii), the subject expression 'Socrates' refers in different domains. As a *term* 'Socrates' denotes an individual. Taken either way, 'Socrates' is not a 'designator'. If the meaning of a term is bound to its denotation, there is no reason to deny that 'Socrates'—whatever it means—means the same thing in (i) and (ii). Analogously, there is little temptation to say that 'horse' means different things in the following two statements:

  (iii) a horse is on the White House lawn
  (iv) a horse was captured by Bellerophon.

We should say that 'horse' means the same thing in both statements even though the domains of its application differ. Similarly, we ought to say that 'Socrates' means the same thing in both statements even though the domains of its application differ in (i*) and (ii*).

Although the term 'Socrates' can be said to have the same meaning when its amplitude differs, we may still wonder whether the subjects of (i) and (ii) refer to the same thing or whether (like 'a horse' in (iii) and (iv)) the subjects refer to different things. For TFL this is not so much a problem as it is a question; it is not a problem because neither subject has the primary function of identifying or designating an individual; nevertheless, both subjects are referring expressions and the question is legitimate. One may ask the question with respect to the singular term 'Socrates': does it denote the same thing in different domains or does it denote different things in different domains (the criteria for its application being the same in either case). In the latter case, despite the fact that 'Socrates' is singular, it will be like the general term 'horse' whose extension may differ with different amplitudes.

The question of the reference or denotation of 'Socrates' is of interest because of the obvious analogy to the controversy that has arisen in connection with the MPL theory of 'Socrates' as a designator. According to David Lewis, 'Socrates' designates different individuals in different domains; according to Saul Kripke, it designates Socrates in every domain of its application. In the next chapter, I shall argue that the correct theory of the reference of 'Socrates' is analogous to Kripke's idea of 'Socrates' as a rigid designator. However, my argument will not attribute this to the special characteristics of proper names but to general characteristics of cross-reference over different domains of application. For the present, it will suffice to say that we shall be offering reasons to hold that 'Socrates' as used in (ii) refers to the same person as it does in (i) and that what is referred to in (ii) is not a mere counterpart of what is referred to in (i).

5. In assigning amplitude, we rely on our pre-analytical knowledge of existential truth conditions. These, however, are not always determinate. There are statements for which we may reasonably accept diverse truth conditions. This is typically the case with statements made by sentences that embed other sentences in clauses of 'propositional attitudes'. An example is

> (A) George the Fourth wanted to know whether Walter Scott was the author of *Waverley*

in which 'George the Fourth' has standard amplitude and 'Walter Scott' has an amplitude that may or may not be standard depending on how we are prepared to verify (A). On one interpretation, we may count (A) true even if there were no such person as Walter Scott.
Analogously in

> (B) Ponce de Leon wanted to find the Fountain of Youth

the term 'Fountain of Youth' does not have standard amplitude; (B) is true even though there is no Fountain of Youth. It is, however, also reasonable to interpret (A) in a manner that determines standard amplitude for 'Walter Scott' and 'the author of *Waverley*'. So interpreted, the middle term 'Walter Scott' will have standard amplitude in both of the premisses of the following syllogism:

> George the Fourth wanted to know whether Walter Scott was the author of *Waverley*
> Walter Scott was the author of *Waverley*
> _____
> George the Fourth wanted to know whether the author of *Waverley* was the author of *Waverley*.

If we read (A) and (B) with non-standard amplitude for the terms of the embedded sentences, the syllogism will be invalid and there will be other conditions of truth. For (A) cannot be true unless George the Fourth occasionally thinks of Walter Scott and believes him to exist. And (B) cannot be true unless Ponce de Leon thinks about the Fountain of Youth and believes it to exist. So Scott and the Fountain of Youth must figure in the respective 'belief worlds' of George the Fourth and Ponce de Leon. It is easy to devise an example where this kind of condition will not be met. Consider for example

> (C) George the Fourth wanted to know whether the palace phones were tapped.

(C) must be false even if we do not give standard amplitude to 'palace phones' and 'tapped' since things like palace phones and tapped wires are not in the ken of George the Fourth, and their being in the ken of George the Fourth is a condition of the truth of (C).

The foregoing examples illustrate that a sentence like 'K believes that (some/every) A is B' may have a different amplitude for A and B than the amplitude of the terms of the embedding sentence. Consider for example

(D) Tom believed that some survivors reached the island.

The terms of the embedding sentence are 'that some survivors reached the island' and '(was) believed by Tom'. The terms of the embedded sentence are 'survivors' and '(those who) reached the island'. Clearly, (D) cannot be true unless there is something that Tom believed and just as clearly (D) could be true if there are no survivors. So the terms of the embedding sentence are standard while those of the embedded sentence are non-standard.

From the standpoint of the doctrine of amplitudes, the so-called opaque contexts of propositional attitudes are contexts that may reasonably involve a shift of amplitude for the terms of the embedded sentence (the latter expresses a belief held, a state of affairs hoped for and so forth). The assignment of a different amplitude for the terms of the embedded context is sometimes more reasonable than other times. It is reasonable to assign a non-standard amplitude for 'the Fountain of Youth' in (B) but not so reasonable to assign non-standard amplitude for 'the thirty-seventh president of the United States' in 'I believe that the thirty-seventh president of the United States was a tragic figure'. The reasons for finding this more reasonable in some cases than in others cannot be explored here.

It is unfortunate that Leibniz's Law is so often brought into discussions of embedded contexts. For that Law is commonly interpreted to apply exclusively to the definite singular terms of an identity proposition sanctioning their substitution 'salva veritate'. From the standpoint of TFL, definite singular terms in subject position are simply a species of expressions of form 'some X' or 'every X'. As for Leibniz's Law, that is a special application of a more general principle of substitutivity which permits the substitution of 'Y' for 'X' in a statement of form '. . . X . . .' in which 'X' has undistributed (positive) occurrence whenever we are given another premiss of form 'every X is Y'. A failure of substitutivity is inevitable whenever the middle term has an amplitude that differs from the amplitude of 'X' in the major premiss. This happens routinely with embedded middle terms in the minor premiss. And it makes no difference whether the middle term is singular or general. For example, suppose that Tom believes that some survivors reached the island and that Tom has never heard of logical positivists but that in fact all those who survived were logical positivists. We should then have two true premisses:

> all survivors were logical positivists
> Tom believes that some survivors reached the island.

It would be wrong to apply the general syllogistic substitution principle to derive the conclusion 'Tom believed that some logical positivists reached the island' because of the difference in amplitude of the middle term. The failure of substitutivity in this kind of inference is in principle no different from the failure in the commonly discussed cases where identity propositions are used for the major premiss. That discussion has centered on the failure of substitutivity of identity and is only one more manifestation of the bias for the singular case that is characteristic of modern post-Fregean analysis.

Finally, the following example, familiar in the literature on opaque contexts, illustrates amplitude disparity in the middle term of an invalid inference with a modal premiss:

(1) the number of planets is nine
(2) nine is necessarily greater than seven

(3) the number of planets is necessarily greater than seven

The amplitude of 'nine' in (1) is standard: (1) could not be true unless there were nine membered sets of things in the actual world. In (2), however, 'nine' occurs with non-standard amplitude; the truth of (2) is independent of what exists in the actual world.

6. In this chapter, I have argued for a doctrine of existential import that is intermediate between Russell and Strawson. I have assumed with Strawson that (1) 'the present king of France is bald' does not assert the existence of a present king of France and I have assumed with Russell that (2) 'the present king of France exists' is entailed by (1). To explain the entailment in the absence of an overtly existential interpretation of (1), I have proposed that the argument from (1) to (2) is enthymemic and that the missing premiss is 'every bald (person) exists'. This tacit premiss may be legitimately appended because 'bald' occurs in (1) with standard amplitude. The amplitude of a statement is determined by the existential conditions of its truth; since both Russell and Strawson agree that (1) cannot be true unless 'bald' applies to something actual, we have a determination of standard amplitude for 'bald' and we are justified in adding the premiss 'every bald (person) exists'.

I have assumed throughout that it is the *analysis* of (1) that is in question but that its 'pre-analytic meaning' as given by its existential truth conditions is known and agreed upon. That the truth conditions are not in question is shown in the fact that Russell and Strawson agree on the existential import of the statement. When Russell analyses (1) as an existential statement, he is following the Fregean policy of making one's logical syntax semantically explicit (putting one's syntax where one's semantics is). (1) cannot be true unless 'the present king of France exists' is true; it therefore seemed to Russell that we should construe the logical form of (1) in a way that makes this perspicuous. The policy of determining logical form by means of the truth conditions was judged to be mistaken. Once we get a logical form for 'the S is P', we are stuck with it and if we have given existential import to (1) on the basis of logical form, we find ourselves embarrassed by (6) 'the beast captured by Bellerophon was a flying horse', which is a true statement but which Russell's and Quine's analysis must treat as false. The doctrine of amplitudes is subtler and less impetuous. It does not impose existential form on 'the S is P', and its account of the way truth conditions are related to 'the S is P', by giving a semantic range to 'S' and 'P', seems altogether more reasonable. In addition, the doctrine of amplitudes allows also for a treatment of 'some S is P' which does not impose existential import on all statements of this form.

The effort to accommodate truths about Pegasus and other non-actual things has inspired more conservative attempts to revise standard interpretations of quantificational formulations. One suggestion is that the existential quantifier be interpreted 'substitutionally'. Another suggestion is to introduce distinctions in the meaning of the quantifier corresponding to different ranges of application for the predicates of the quantificational formulas. This latter device is similar to our own device of assigning amplitudes to the terms of a statement. Interpreted substitutionally a sentence like 'Ex (x is an American and has walked on the moon)' does not necessarily make an existence claim. And generally, a substitutional interpretation is in no danger of sinning by existential overstatement. Nevertheless, one of the most attractive virtues of the classical objectual interpretation has been lost: if translation of 'an American has walked on the moon' into canonical notation does not make a straightforward existence claim, then such a translation is not the semantically perspicuous thing it was vaunted to be and the point of the translation is badly blunted. The semantical perspicuity of quantification formulas as 'objectually' interpreted has always seemed to be their best claim to canonical status; if that is removed in favour of some more 'reasonable' interpretation of the canonical forms, then the classical tie between logical syntax and existential truth conditions is weakened and the idea of logical form as embodied in a semantically explicit formulation is undermined. It therefore seems to me that the philosophically interesting interpretation of quantificational formulas is the standard objectual one. But I have also argued that quantification formulas objectually interpreted are poor contenders for the logical forms of the sentences they purport to translate.

11

Proper Names and Other Pronouns

1. Frege's view of the elementary logical subject as a syntactically simple expression did not require him to distinguish between proper names and expressions of form 'the so and so'. But in recent years, and especially since Kripke's theories have become popular, no doctrine that fuses proper names and 'definite descriptions' can be uncontroversial. A difference between these two kinds of expressions had already been made important by Russell, but Quine's development of Russell's theory of descriptions had the effect of making light of it. For Quine 'parsed' proper names as descriptions treating 'Socrates' as (roughly) the definite description 'the Socratizer'. Where Frege had assimilated definite descriptions to proper names, Quine's expansion of Russell's theory assimilated proper names to definite descriptions. Kripke's views stand in firm opposition to both of these simplifications.

For Kripke, a proper name is a rigid designator; a definite description is a non-rigid designator. In Kripke's words, an expression is a rigid designator

. . . if in any possible world it designates the same object and it is a non-rigid or accidental designator if that is not the case. Of course we don't require that the objects exist in all possible worlds . . . When we think of a property as essential to an object we usually mean it is true of that object in any case where it would have existed.[1]

Kripke has an informal test for rigidity. If it makes sense to say 'D might not have been D' (where D is a designator expression), then D is non-rigid; otherwise, D is rigid. Applying this test, Kripke finds that 'Nixon' is a rigid

---

[1] Saul Kripke, 'Naming and Necessity' in *Semantics of Natural Language*, ed. D. Davidson and G. Harman (D. Reidel, 1972), p. 269. Hereafter referred to as *NN*.

designator and 'the president of the United States in 1970' is not:

Although someone other than the president might have been the president in 1970 (e.g., Humphrey might have been), no other than Nixon might have been Nixon . . . 'The president of the United States in 1970' designates a certain man, Nixon; but someone else might have been president of the United States in 1970, and Nixon might not have; so this designator is not rigid.[2]

Although Kripke says little or nothing about pronouns, they too satisfy the informal test for rigidity. Consider

   (i) A new president is in office. From what I can tell from his TV appearances, he seems to be an honest man.
  (ii) He could have easily lost the election, but he squeaked through.
 (iii) I think he will be a wise leader.

The pronoun in (ii) is rigid. We could understand (ii) to claim that in certain specifiable but non-actual circumstances he loses the election; and the person then designated by 'he' is still the person non-identifyingly referred to in (i) and (iii) where the context is not modal. The rigidity of 'he' is conventionally guaranteed by its special role which is that of referring to the very thing that was referred to in the antecedent proposition. We move from 'a new president' to 'he' and 'he' refers to the person in question. And, of course, it makes no good sense to say 'he might not have been he'.

    Kripke's account of the rigidity of proper names is part of his 'causal chain' theory.

The object may be named by ostension or the reference of the same may be fixed by description . . . An initial baptism takes place. When the name is 'passed from link to link' the receiver of the name must, I think, intend when he learns to use it with the same reference as the man from whom he heard it.[3]

This explanation (as Kripke acknowledges) 'takes the notion of intending to use the same reference as a given'. The success of the intention guarantees rigid designation passed from one

---

[2] *NN*. p. 270
[3] *NN*. p. 302.

user to another back to the object designated at the initial baptism.

A moment's reflection convinces one that the account Kripke has given cannot easily or even possibly be applied to pronouns. Construed as bound variables, pronouns are not passed from link to link since every bound variable must be contained in the sentence of the expression that binds it; and the connection between a bound expression and the expression that binds it is unmediated. I take it that the bound-variable theory is one that Kripke subscribes to. If we accept some form of the 'proterm theory' outlined in chapter 4, the causal account is not needed although the latter has interesting points of analogy with the proterm theory. It will be recalled that according to the proterm theory, a pronoun is a complex expression containing a sign of quantity and a term that is specifically designed to denote what the antecedent subject had referred to. The proterm theory thus allows for external pronominalization so we may have a series of pronominal references outside of the sentences that may serve as the antecedent background for the pronouns. Here we have something like a passing from link to link. Moreover, in the move from 'an S' to 'it', we even have something like a baptism with 'it' as the analogue of a name whose reference is fixed by the antecedent description. It would, however, be a mistake to take Kripke's causal account as primary. To speak of analogy here obscures what happens in pronominalization: the introduction of a term contextually defined to denote the thing or those things that antecedently have been indefinitely referred to. The proterm theory accounts for the rigidity of pronouns by pointing to the fact that the proterm of a pronoun is specifically designed to denote 'the thing in question'; a fact that explains why new tokens of the pronoun continue to designate that thing or those things in every context of use, including modal contexts.

2. I believe with Kripke in the importance of distinguishing rigid from non-rigid referring expressions. But where Kripke takes proper names to be the paradigm rigid expressions, I should point to pronouns. If I am right the phenomenon of rigidity whether in a pronoun or a proper name is entirely an effect produced by the introduction of a proterm to do a particular job of denoting an individual under consideration. The right way of understanding rigidity in proper names is to understand it in pronouns. And this is an easy thing to do as soon as one recognizes that *proper names are pronouns.* Consider

(i) a child has been born to the Nixons
(ii) it is a male
(iii) he weighs eight pounds
(iv) let's call him Richard Milhouse Nixon

Note that pronominalization *precedes* baptism. I shall argue later that one cannot think of a baptism in which this does *not* happen. We can thus view the official act of baptism as an act that introduces a *special duty* pronoun that may henceforth be used in place of the highly equivocal pronouns 'it', 'he' and 'him' that have hitherto been used to refer to the thing in question. In general, the baptismal formula 'let it be known as NN' may be understood to say:

Let 'it' be replaceable by 'NN'.

This thesis, that a proper name is an 'anaphoric' pronominal expression with implicit or explicit cross reference to some antecedent context of indefinite reference is what one might expect from a theory that considers all logical subjects to be syntactically complex expressions of form 'some X' or 'every X'.[4] Since this applies as much to proper-name subjects as to pronouns, it immediately confronts the question of the denotation of the terms of these subjects. In the case of pronouns, our answer was that the term of the pronoun (the proterm) denotes the thing(s) referred to by some antecedent subject. And our answer for proper names is the same: they too are anaphoric and they too have proterms that denote the references of antecedent expressions. These antecedent expressions need not have been actually uttered. I may, on discovering an island, immediately say 'Let it be called Tamler Island'

---

[4] The thesis that proper names are special duty pronouns has its MPL version in Quine's dictum: 'what distinguishes a name is that it can stand coherently in place of a variable in predication'. For Quine, the bound variable in '$(\exists x) Px$' is a pronoun; the instantiating move from '$(\exists x) Px$' to 'Pa' is an exemplary application of the dictum.

and then go on to use the name. But my use of 'it' in the baptismal formula may be understood to have anaphoric cross reference to some antecedently unexpressed proposition such as 'I've just discovered an island'. The descriptive expression 'an island I've discovered' here implicitly serves as antecedent background for 'the island I've just discovered' or 'it' and for 'Tamler Island'. One might say that the unexpressed proposition serves to fix the references of 'it' and 'Tamler Island'. For these new expressions have U-terms that denote the thing in question, in this case, the island I discovered.

Kripke thinks of a baptism as the *initial* ceremony in which the reference of a rigid designator is determined. But this ignores the fact that the thing in question about to be baptized must have already been introduced by pronominalization of the descriptive antecedent subject. Pronominalization always precedes nominalization. Once the pronominalization is at hand, the proper name we subsequently introduce in an act of baptism is nothing more than a new and convenient pronoun which may henceforth replace the original. As for the fixing of the reference, that must have already taken place in the pronominalization that preceded the naming ceremony. Viewed in this light the causal-chain account of proper names is no better than a confused attempt to do justice to the pronominal chain whose first link is an indefinite referring expression used in an epistemic context.

2.1 One of the controversies surrounding proper names concerns their 'connotativeness'. For reasons that will be clear later, I prefer not to ask whether proper names are connotative but to ask whether they are descriptive or not. If proper names are special duty pronouns, then we may expect that they are descriptive or non-descriptive in the way that pronouns are. Consider

(A) a child is on the roof
(B) it is not a child
(C) the child is not a child.

Note that while the denial 'it is not a child' is acceptable, 'the child is not a child' is not acceptable. This shows that 'it' is here not equivalent to the descriptive phrase 'the child in question' but to something like 'the individual in question'. The occurrence of 'it' in B is non-descriptive. Consider also

(1) a star is shining to the East
(2) call it Phosphorus
(3) Phosphorus is not a star (but a planet)
(4) it is not a star (but a planet)
(5) the star is not a star (but a planet).

(3) and (4) are acceptable but (5) is not. So here the proper name is introduced in place of a non-descriptive pronoun; its reference is fixed by the description 'a star' which serves as the common antecedent to both 'it' and 'Phosphorus'.

In these examples, the anaphoric expressions 'it' and 'Phosphorus' are both non-descriptive. We shall presently argue that the pronominal theory of proper names construes them non-descriptively, thus supporting the Mill-Russell-Kripke doctrine. On the other hand, and contrary to what Kripke suggests, most rigid designators are descriptive. In the next sections we explore the interplay of rigidity and non-rigidity and of descriptiveness and non-descriptiveness in expressions of form 'the S' as well as in proper names and standard pronouns like 'it'.

3. In *Word and Object*, Quine calls attention to the anaphoric or pronominal use of expressions of form 'the S'. I use 'the S' anaphorically in a context like 'we have a new president . . . the president is a Democrat'. This contrasts with the non-anaphoric use of the same expression in a context like 'the President of the United States is the Commander in Chief of the Armed Forces'. When 'the S' occurs anaphorically, there is implicit or explicit back reference to some antecedent context in which reference is made to an S: when there is no such cross reference, the use of 'the S' is non-anaphoric.

We said above that pronominal anaphors are rigid. This is true also of 'the S' when it occurs anaphorically. For then 'the S' is equivalent to rigid pronominal expressions like 'the S in question', 'he', or 'that S'. (One cannot say 'that S might not have been that S'.) Consider

(i) we have a new president
(ii) the president in question is a Republican

(iii) the president in question could have denied a pardon to his predecessor.

In (ii) and (iii), there is reference to the same person. And this is so even if one understands (iii) to claim that 'denied a pardon to his predecessor' applies to the president in some non-actual situation that we are entertaining. If so, the descriptive phrase 'the president' is a rigid designator. And generally, whenever 'the S' has anaphoric occurrence, it will designate the same thing in every situation where what it applied to is stipulated to exist. Kripke's observation that we can give a reading 'the S might not have been the S' is not a good general argument for the non-rigidity of 'the S'. For such a reading would require us to interpret 'the S' non-anaphorically—at least in the predicate. But where both occurrences of 'the S' are anaphoric, the reading makes no sense. It makes no more sense to say 'the president in question might not have been the president in question' than to say 'he might not have been he' or 'that man might not have been that man'.

4. In chapter 5 we analysed pronominal occurrences of 'the S' as expressions containing U-terms denoting the S antecedently referred to. Where something has been taken for an S, the later pronoun will contain a U-term 'S' denoting that S. The pronominal expression 'the S' is thus analysed with wild quantity and a U-term. The denotation of the U-term is fixed; it always denotes the same thing and our arguments here show that anaphoric occurrences of 'the S' are occurrences of rigid descriptions. The familiar Russellian accounts of 'the S' apply to non-anaphoric occurrences. When 'the S' is non-anaphoric, its categorematic parts are G-terms that may apply to different individuals in different contexts. Assuming that 'the inventor of bifocals' can occur as a non-anaphoric description, it will be possible to say that the inventor of bifocals might not have been the inventor of bifocals. For we may suppose that in the actual situation Ben Franklin invented bifocals and in some non-actual situation Tom Jefferson did. In that case the inventor of bifocals in situation A is not the inventor of bifocals in situation B. In this way we allow for the possibility that the S might not have been the S—for univocal non-anaphoric uses of 'the S'. It is however a mistake to think that the non-anaphoric use is somehow primary. On the contrary one could argue that all occurrences of 'the S' have implicit back reference to an S. As for 'the S might not have been the S' one could explain that by giving the two occurrences different background propositions in the different situations to which they apply. I shall not take a position on the question whether to construe *all* definite descriptions anaphorically except to say that often this seems to me to be not merely tempting but right.

4.1 A proper name may be explicitly introduced by an anaphoric description. A stipulation like 'let the first dog to be born on the moon be called "Leslie" 'should be understood in the context of an antecedent background and a mediating pronominalization that figures in the baptismal formula. Perhaps something like this:

> A dog who will have the distinction of being the first canine native of the moon will become famous in the next century. Let us now decide to call it Leslie.

Since all names are pronouns and since pronouns are rigid it will not be possible to form a non-rigid name. This is not to deny that one might *use* the word 'Leslie' as a direct substitute for a non-anaphoric description. But I shall argue later that 'Leslie' would then not be a proper name but a mere abbreviation for the description. That no proper name can be the direct equivalent of a definite description is in accord with Mill's view, recently revived by Kripke, that proper names are non-descriptive referring expressions. My disagreement with Kripke concerns the virtual neglect in his theory of reference of the anaphoric use of 'the S' and his implicit assumption that 'the S' is generally non-rigid and non-anaphoric. It is probable that most if not all uses of 'the S' are antecedently grounded in 'an S . . .'. If that is right, then most so-called definite descriptions are rigid referring expressions whose subject-terms are U-terms.

4.2 Before leaving the topic of descriptive and rigid referring expressions, I wish to comment on an argument of Kripke against the rigidity of 'the S'. Kripke's example is 'the length of this stick at time t'. There is, says Kripke, an intuitive difference between a name of a length like 'a metre' and a description of a length like 'the length of this stick at time t' (where the latter happens to apply to the length of a stick one metre long). We can say of the length of this stick that it might have been some other length, but we cannot say of a metre that it might have been another length. Kripke says that this intuitive difference indicates that 'one metre' is rigid and analogous to a proper name while 'the length of this stick at time t' is not rigid since it is a definite description. It is however a mistake to allow that we can say of the length of the stick that it might have been some other length. I can no more say of a given length, e.g. the length of this stick, that it might have been some other length than I can say of a metre that it might not have been a metre. It is of course true that the *stick* might have been of another length or that we can imagine it—in some non-actual situation—to have another length than the one it actually has. But if we are talking of its length, the alleged difference between 'a metre' and 'the length of this stick' is illusory—since it makes no literal sense to imagine the length of the stick to be, some other length in some non-actual situation. That we may be concerned with the length and not with the stick is evident from the fact that we can say that the length of this stick is the same as the length of that stick—same length, different sticks. When I speak of the length of this stick and then speak of the length of that stick (which, say, is one metre), then I am speaking of one metre and not of the sticks, although, as Wittgenstein recognized, the stick may serve in fixing the reference of what I *am* speaking about. It appears that Kripke does not see that 'the length of this stick' could be a descriptive designator for the length it has, and that we cannot literally say that the length of this stick might have been other than it is. He generally tends to read expressions of form 'the S' in a Russellian way; this allows him also to treat 'the length of this stick at time t might not have been the length it is' as saying of the *stick* (where 'the stick' is analysed à la Russell) that it might have been some other length. The shift from length to the object is converse to the one we make in interpreting 'I thought your yacht is longer than it is', ·a sentence devised by Russell to show that statements are often not about what they appear to be. One interpretation is given by the paraphrase 'the length I thought your yacht to be is greater than the length it is' which is clearly about lengths and not about yachts.

The more general error is the tendency to ignore the

anaphoric use of 'the S' as a descriptive anaphoric name. In the present example 'the length of S at t' rigidly designates a certain length and we may properly insist that it makes no sense to say that this length might have been some other length (which is not to say that we deny that the stick might not have been as long as it is).

5. We turn now to Mill's doctrine that proper names—the standard rigid kind—are always non-descriptive. Kripke's argument for this directs us to the open question. If a proper name 'NN' were equivalent to a definite description 'D' then it should not be possible to wonder whether NN is D or at least the question whether NN is D could not then make good sense. But it is always open for us to ask whether the NN is in fact D which shows that 'NN' is not descriptive.

The open question is appropriate only if we could be wrong in thinking that NN is D. The possibility that we could be wrong is epistemic and is to be distinguished from the metaphysical possibility that—granted NN is in fact D—this might well not have been the case. The latter sort of possibility allows that one may consistently conceive of counterfactual circumstances in which NN is not D, and this kind of possibility is consistent with 'NN' being equivalent to 'D' for unless being D is essential to the bearer of NN, we can conceive of NN not being D. Epistemic possiblity is another matter; if NN is equivalent to D, the question whether we could be wrong in thinking that NN is D is like the question whether we could be wrong in thinking that what is D is D. For example even if 'Aristotle' were equivalent in meaning to 'the most famous student of Plato' it would still be metaphysically possible that he who was in fact the most famous student of Plato could well not have been that. But we could not wonder whether Aristotle was indeed the most famous student of Plato.

The force of the open-question argument for the 'no-sense' doctrine of proper names is undiminished within the framework of the theory that proper names are special duty pronouns. The classification of pronouns as strongly or weakly referential and as descriptive and non-descriptive is relevant here. In the pronominal account, the thesis that proper names are non-descriptive expressions is the thesis that proper names are expressions that replace strongly referential non-descriptive pronouns. The reader will recall that strongly referential pronouns have antecedents that are originally asserted in contexts where something has been taken for a so and so. An example of pronominalization followed by nominalization where the antecedent is strongly referential is 'there appears to be a raccoon in the garden but whatever it is, I'm going to call it Leslie'. Here the name 'Leslie' is introduced for the strongly referential pronoun 'it' which refers to what appears to be a raccoon. Ordinary baptisms also fit this picture. Following the birth of a child we have 'it is a boy . . . he weighs seven pounds . . . let's call him Roger'. The context of pronominalization is epistemic—something has been taken for a child—but there is the epistemic possibility of a mistake: Roger may turn out to be non-human. And if it should turn out that Roger is really an otherwordly monster invading our planet, the name 'Roger' will have had this monster as its bearer from the moment of the naming.

It seems plausible that proper names should be strongly referential. But might it not be the case that a proper name can be introduced for a strongly referential *descriptive* pronoun (a 'D-type' pronoun)? Suppose that in fact there is a raccoon in the garden and that we decide to call it Willie. It may appear that we now replace 'the raccoon in the garden' by 'Willie'. And if that is what we do, then 'Willie' is a rigid referring expression equivalent to 'the raccoon we found in the garden'. I believe however that even then we would not introduce 'Willie' as the equivalent to the description. It is after all still possible that we have made a mistake and that Willie is not a raccoon. The force of the open question argument for denying descriptiveness to 'Willie' is that we can always wonder whether Willie is really what we take him to be. This argues that the pronouns that 'Willie' is doing duty for are not descriptive pronouns; we may think that 'Willie' is replacing 'the raccoon' but it is more accurate to say that 'Willie' is being introduced to replace the ascription 'what was taken to be a raccoon'. And generally, the open-question argument rules out the theory that a proper name may replace a referential descriptive pronoun.

5.1 Can we replace a weakly referring expression by a proper name? It may seem that we do this when we name a thing that is not yet in existence. Contrast the naming of Willie with the naming of the first dog to be born on the moon. We have for background, propositions like 'some day a dog will be born on the moon—it will be able to leap over a barn with ease—no dog before it will have been a native of the moon . . .'. We then say 'let's decide to call it "Leslie" '. Nothing as yet has been taken for the first dog to be born on the moon and the open question 'will Leslie really be the first dog to be born on the moon?' appears to be inappropriate.

It does seem that here we have a proper name acting as a descriptive B-type pronoun equivalent to the anaphoric definite description 'the first dog to be born on the moon'. Nevertheless appearance here is deceptive. What is it that we commit ourselves to do when we decide to call the first dog to be born on the moon Leslie? Clearly we cannot have committed ourselves to do more than confer the name on what we shall one day believe to be the first dog to be born on the moon. More than that we cannot have committed ourselves to. So the name we now confer has as its bearer what we shall later on, in good faith and with reasonable evidence, *take* to be the first dog native to the moon. Prior to the advent of Leslie one could speculate whether Leslie will in fact satisfy the description being used to fix the reference of its name. For even now, at the moment of baptizing Leslie, we cannot but be aware that things may go awry or be awry. It may for example be that Neil Armstrong and his crew had brought along a pregnant dog who had her puppies on the moon back in 1969. In that case what we shall later believe to be the first dog to be born on the moon will through no fault of ours, not really be that. This possibility is consistent with the decision to confer the name 'Leslie' on the creature we shall take to be the first native dog on the moon. All these variants of the open question show that 'Leslie' even now replaces an ascriptive pronominal like 'what we shall take to be the first dog . . .' and that it is not equivalent to a raw description. If so, 'Leslie' is a strongly referential name—a special duty A-type pronoun.

5.2 Let us call a name 'Millian' if it is introduced to replace an A-type (strongly referential and nondescriptive) pronoun.

A non-Millian proper name would be one introduced to do duty for an identifying definite description that refers to an individual in such a way as to make it possible for anyone to wonder whether the individual satisfies the description that identifies it and which gives the meaning of the proper name. Our arguments tend to show that a non-Millian name cannot be strongly referential. Frege placed a name like 'Louis' as an expression in the same category with 'the king of France'. He held that proper names have senses and his examples indicate that the sense of a proper name is equivalent to the sense of a definite description. Contemporary Fregeans who feel the force of the open-question argument (especially as it has been deployed by Kripke) have begun to realize that the thesis that all proper names are equivalent to definite descriptions is untenable. One begins to see interpretations of Frege that avoid equating a proper name with the meaning of a definite description. But this move has its dangers. Unless some proper names are equivalent in meaning to definite descriptions, the position that proper names belong in the same category with definite descriptions would be tacitly abandoned to Kripke and other Millians who hold that proper names and definite descriptions are radically distinct kinds of referring expressions in just this way: that proper names are never equivalent to definite descriptions. To avoid a Kripkean face, the Fregean position must be defended by distinguishing proper names from definite descriptions in some other way. In practice this means that the orthodox Fregean is forced to allow and to argue for the descriptiveness of some proper names. Dummett sees the necessity for this. We shall presently discuss his example of a descriptive proper name not subject to the open question.

As the controversy between the Fregeans and the Millians attests, there is no well defined class of proper names to which all can appeal to adjudicate the question whether proper names are descriptive or not. 'Louis' is a proper name but is 'The Sun King'? Answers to questions like this one cannot be given apart from some theory which specifies the kind of expression a proper name is. On the whole it does violence to linguistic practice and intuition to classify 'the king of France' along with 'Louis' as proper names. But if a distinction between proper names (properly so called) and definite descriptions is to be made, it should be supported by more than intuitions concerning what belongs inside the class of proper names. And in this respect the pronominal theory has the advantage of affording an independent way of distinguishing between classes of referring expressions. Taking into account that the requirement that anything referred to by a proper name is subject to the open question concerning any description associated with the name, one sees that proper names, as Mill and Kripke conceive of them, are stylistic variants of referential non-descriptive pronouns (A-type pronouns). Kripke has suggested that the explanation for the referential rigidity and non-descriptiveness of proper names is to be sought in their causal histories. From the pronominal standpoint the causal account misses the point: proper names are anaphoric pronominal expressions and any explanation of their special characteristics is to be found in the theory of anaphoric reference.

5.3 In the remainder of this chapter I shall take care to disambiguate the common and convenient ambiguity attaching to the term 'proper name' and to instances of it. The term 'proper name', as we have had occasion to remark, is sometimes used to denote a special kind of term and other times used to denote a special kind of subject expression in which that special kind of term plays the role of subject term. The ambiguity attaches to a proper name like 'Caruso' which itself may be understood as a subject expression (elliptical for '*Caruso') or as the term *within* this subject expression. We have usually read 'NN' as elliptical for '*NN' but we shall no longer indulge this practice. Thus 'St. Anne' will be construed as the subject *term* and contrasted with '*St. Anne'; the subject will always be represented with its sign of quantity explicit.

So far we have seen that a no-sense theory of proper names assigns them to the class of A-type pronouns. This accords with the observations that proper names appear to be expressions whose referents are subject to the open question. But we have not yet ruled out the possibility that some proper names are not subject to the open question. In the framework of the pronominal theory there is the possibility that proper names may be introduced for weakly referring (B-type) pronouns

whose antecedents are uttered in contexts where a so and so is
weakly referred to and where no individual has been taken for a
so and so. Dummett's example of a proper name not subject to
the open question is 'St. Anne' which may be thought of as
having a background like the following one:

> the mother of Jesus had a Galilean mother
> she is not known to us
> we shall refer to her as Anne.

Dummett believes that the reference of 'St. Anne' is fixed by a
single description:

> The reference of the name 'St. Anne' can be taken as fixed in
> essentially one way, namely by means of the description 'the mother
> of the Blessed Virgin Mary' . . . we can claim to know nothing
> whatever about its referent, save for the obvious facts that she was a
> married Jewish woman living at the end of the first century BC,etc. [5]

Given this sort of history, Dummett claims that we cannot ask
whether St. Anne was indeed the mother of Mary. In terms of
the pronominal theory, the example suggests that a proper
name may be introduced to do duty for a non-referential
pronoun. For when one speaks of a Galilean mother of Mary
one is not taking anyone to be that, and the pronoun 'she' only
weakly refers to the mother of Mary even though no more than
one person could satisfy the description 'the mother of Mary'.
    The case of 'St. Anne' is not dissimilar to the following one:

> a masked man has just robbed Tiffanys
> he got away with some very precious jewels
> we shall refer to him as 'Mr X'.

Is 'Mr X' a proper name? The only difference I can see between
'Mr X' and 'St. Anne' is that 'Anne', unlike 'Mr X' appears in
the lists of proper names one finds at the end of unabridged
dictionaries. On the other hand there may be no good reason to
withold the honorific label 'proper name' from any expression
that is introduced for a proterm, and the fact that 'St. Anne'
and 'Mr X' are instantial terms should not be considered
prejudicial. The question whether such names are genuinely
proper names cannot be unbeggingly answered in the negative

---

[5] Dummett, *Frege*, p. 112.

by merely pointing to the fact that they are instantial, and by remarking that their bearers, if any, are not subject to open questions concerning the applicability to them of the descriptions that fix their references.

Without prejudging the status of 'St. Anne' as a proper name we may insist that no name can be considered proper unless it refers to an individual that could in principle be identified by a description other than the one that has been used to fix the reference of the name. And in fact Dummett overstates the case when he says that only one definite description is available as a way of fixing the reference of '*St. Anne'. It is not only that we could in principle find some other identifying descriptions that hold good of St. Anne; even now it isn't true that we could not have used other descriptions purportedly characterizing the same individual. Thus the cult of 'St. Anne' might have used 'the maternal grandmother of Jesus' or even 'the mother-in-law of Joseph'. And it may happen that we find the remains of some women in a grave near Tiberius and have good reason to believe that these are the remains of the maternal grandmother of Jesus. In that case it would be true that St. Anne was *the* woman whose remains are in that grave.

The actual multiplicity of identifying descriptions of St. Anne casts doubt on the assumption that 'St. Anne' means 'the mother of Mary'. If the two are equivalent it would not be possible for St. Anne to turn out not to be the mother of Mary. Suppose however that a new scroll is found which confirms the traditional Jesus story except in the one detail that the wife of Joseph and the mother of Jesus was a woman called Hannah who died within a few days of having given birth to Jesus. The scroll relates that before she died Hannah charged her best friend Mary to take care of the infant Jesus and to see to it that he became a Nazarene. According to this new account Mary was indeed a virgin but she was not the mother of Jesus. Let us assume that the scrolls themselves are well authenticated and internally consistent so that after much debate this version of the story is accepted by the Church and by the cult of St. Anne. How is it reasonable to react to the new information? It is I think reasonable for a celebrant of the cult to say that St. Anne is still in most respects what we thought her to be: she is the woman whose remains we have discovered, and whose grave remains sacred as the maternal grandmother of Jesus, she is the mother-in-law of Joseph but she is not the mother of Mary.

We may also expect that some members of the cult, perhaps a minority, react by saying that the scrolls have shown that St. Anne, the mother of Mary, is not the mother of Jesus' mother, not the mother-in-law of Joseph and not the woman whose grave had been thought of as the grave of St. Anne. This minority view steadfastly holds that 'St. Anne cannot but be the mother of Mary'; she is so 'by definition'. There is nothing inconsistent in this position but it should be clear that '*St. Anne' is now being deployed as an expression introduced in place of an instantial pronoun. An instantial term denotes an individual in the comprehension of the sentence that serves as the antecedent in a pronominalization sequence of form 'an S is P; it is Q' where no one is taking a particular thing for an S. The term denotes something in the comprehension of 'an S is P', namely it denotes the S that is P indefinitely referred to. Instantial terms are descriptive proterms and if '*St. Anne' is indeed given as the replacement for 'the mother of Mary' then its subject term is descriptive and what it denotes is not subject to the open question.

If on the other hand the bearer of 'St. Anne' is subject to the open question, then 'St. Anne', despite its history of association with 'the mother of Mary', is not a descriptive term. In deciding to name the mother of Mary 'St. Anne', we recognize from the outset the possibility that we could some day make discoveries that could require us to withdraw the description 'the mother of Mary' from St. Anne. And this means that at the moment of naming what we are naming is not necessarily the mother of Mary though trivially it necessarily is what we take to be the mother of Mary.

It comes down then to the question whether we are to recognize names that replace instantial terms as proper names. *This* question is verbal though not for that reason entirely trivial. Proper names are pronouns. We have the choice of thinking of them as a unitary type of expression that replace A-type pronouns or as a hybrid type of expression that replace both A and B-type pronouns. The *standard* proper name is A-type; we have little reason to complicate the category of proper names by treating expressions that have been introduced to replace instantial terms in a B-type pronoun as belonging to the category of proper names. The pronominal perspective on proper names provides an independent distinction (between two types of pronouns) which adjudicates the controversy concerning descriptive names by suggesting that the standard and hence genuine proper name is an expression that replaces an A-type pronoun. This accords with the Millian position. It is on the whole to be preferred to any position that invites us to view proper names in a non-unitary way. The reader who is acquainted with the writings of Kripke is aware that our discussion owes much to Kripke. It owes this much: whenever I have been tempted to allow for descriptive proper names, Kripke's critical way with descriptivism has led me to look deeper into the possibility that the bearer of the descriptive name is after all subject to the open question. I have not found a proper name whose bearer is not subject to the open question and which seems to be nonetheless deserving of being characterized as a proper name.

To sum up: proper names properly so called are expressions standing in for the proterms of A-type pronouns. Although this means they are non-descriptive, it does not entirely accord with the Mill-Kripke theory that names have no sense. Here the proterm theory diverges from the theory that names are rigid designators whose causal history confers on them what meaning they have. A proper name has its reference fixed by the antecedent in some epistemic context. Something is taken for an S said to be P and to denote this something we form a term later replaced by a proper name. The term itself has this much meaning: it stands for whatever satisfies the ascription 'taken for an S and said to be P' and that much is not subject to the open question. For while we can discover that the thing in question was neither an S nor a P we cannot discover that the thing in question was not so taken to be or said to be. In section 7 we shall discuss the question of connotativeness of proper names somewhat further. Here we simply note that a proper name does have sense in the sense of being equivalent to some definite ascription associated with the antecedent that fixes its reference in the original epistemic context.

6. A termist account of definite subjects will reject Frege's category of proper names which includes definite descriptions like 'the deaf composer of nine famous symphonies' along with 'Beethoven' in the one category of proper names. It is helpful to locate the termist account of definite descriptions with reference to the position generally associated with Strawson. Strawson has long stressed the importance of what he sometimes calls descriptive names. With Frege, and in opposition to Russell (and now Kripke), Strawson classifies 'the S' as a logical subject in 'the S is P' rejecting Russell's treatment of it as a predicative description. Strawson also follows Frege in holding that a logical subject must designate an object; one that fails to do so cannot be the logical subject of a proposition: when reference fails 'no proposition is asserted'. In the case of descriptive names of form 'the S' the name must designate an object that satisfies the description 'is an S' and the existence of such an object is a condition of reference. The existential proposition that expresses this condition is in no way a constituent part of the proposition whose logical subject is the descriptive name. It is, instead, presupposed by the latter proposition.

In the theory I have been proposing, 'the S' is usually treated as a pronominal anaphoric expression related to some propositional background (which may be implicit rather than explicit) in the way that a pronoun refers back to an antecedent. If I mistakenly believe that the table at which I am sitting has a waiter assigned to it, I may say 'the Waiter assigned to this table is neglecting me' and what I say is false (and not neither true nor false). As for the implicit antecedent, 'this table has been assigned a waiter', it too is false. In general, while 'the S . . .' cannot be true unless 'an S . . .' is true, both can be false. The situation with vacuous subjects of form 'the S' is like that of 'it' in 'Socrates owned a kangaroo and it bit him'. Here 'it' is a descriptive anaphoric subject—a B-type pronoun—equivalent to 'the kangaroo' or 'the kangaroo that Socrates owned.' The subject of 'it bit him' is vacuous and the proposition is false.

The anaphoric theory does not treat singular propositions as being without quantity. And the difference with Strawson turns on just this point. For he thinks of 'the S' as a descriptive Fregean name, an 'object word' whose use presupposes the existence of the object named or described (and so the truth of an existential proposition) where the anaphoric theory treats the descriptive name as it treats any name in the position of logical subject: as an expression with a sign of quantity and a (descriptive) term. From the standpoint of the pronominal theory, Strawson errs in having accepted the Fregean dogma of the simplicity of the logical subject whose relation to its designation is that of name to bearer.

The Frege–Strawson view ignores the pronominal character of 'the S'. As Quine has observed: when 'the S' is anaphorically used, it behaves like the pronoun in 'an S is P and it is Q'. If 'the S' is pronominal, there is no need for the heavy apparatus of existential presupposition to support its use as a logical subject—pronominalization is familiar enough and it can do the job. Finally, if 'the S' is pronominal and if pronominals too have the form of traditional logical subjects ('every X', 'some X'), then even where reference fails cross reference will have succeeded in conferring a denotation on the proterm. The failure to refer will therefore not have the consequences it has in Strawson's theory of descriptive names where the lack of S's is fatal to the use of 'the S' in a proposition.

7. Proper names are non-descriptive. But being ascriptive they 'connote' their descriptions. To one who had learned the name 'Aristotle' as the name of the man who taught Alexander the Great, the name connotes the teacher of Alexander. Now this does not mean that 'Aristotle' is equivalent in meaning to 'the teacher of Alexander', or even to a cluster of descriptions of this kind. (For the open question may still be asked: Did Aristotle teach Alexander the Great?). Nevertheless, part of what 'Aristotle' means for that person is given by 'the teacher of Alexander' in the sense that 'Aristotle' has been defined as the man said to have taught Alexander. The expression 'the man said to have been the teacher of Alexander the Great' is one of a cluster of expressions that define 'Aristotle'. Expressions of form 'the thing said to be S' are descriptions only by courtesy. We are referring to them as ascriptions. Strictly speaking, 'Aristotle' is a non-descriptive name in the sense that we can always ask whether the man who was said to have taught Alexander the Great did in fact teach Alexander the

Great. We here distinguish between descriptions (expressions of form 'the S') and ascriptions (of form 'the thing said to be S') and correspondingly between expressions that—to use Kripke's phrase—'fix the referent' of a name and those that are its meaning. The name 'Aristotle' connotes 'the teacher of Alexander the Great' to one who has learned 'Aristotle' by way of that description. Also, that description fixes the referent of 'Aristotle' and the corresponding ascription is part of the meaning of this name to one who has learned it by way of this description. And generally, if I have learned the name NN by way of the description 'the S' then, among other things, NN will mean 'the thing said to be S' and in this sense the name NN connotes 'the S'.

It might be objected that 'Aristotle' cannot mean 'the person said to have taught Alexander' (or any cluster of similar ascriptions) for we can easily and without contradiction imagine or stipulate a situation in which no one had ever said of Aristotle that he was the teacher of Alexander the Great. Anyone who asks whether Aristotle was said to have taught Alexander would be asking whether the man who is said to have taught Alexander was ever said to have taught Alexander. That is the only meaning we can give to the question he asks. Indeed, since our postulated personage is ignorant of the fact that Aristotle was ever said to have taught Alexander, it is not likely that the question would arise for him. But if it did, the question must be understood by us to be referring to a person who was said to have taught Alexander. We need not talk here of possible worlds. If my neighbour comes in to ask me whether Aristotle had ever been said to have taught Alexander, I will understand him to have asked about the man who *was* said to have done this, *whether* he was said to have done it. Obviously, this is not how *he* would understand the question, but this is explained by the fact that he has learned his 'Aristotle' by way of ascriptions that do not coincide with mine. (He may be asking whether the author of the *Nichomachean Ethics* was ever said to have taught Alexander the Great.) So to him, 'Aristotle' does not connote 'the teacher of Alexander' although there will be a core of some common ascriptions that enable us to discuss Aristotle and to refer to the same man in our discussions.

8. I have tried to show how the anaphoric approach to definite subjects fares on some contemporary issues in the theory of reference. As against Frege, I believe with Kripke that the paradigm proper names are without sense—in the sense of being non-descriptive. That Fregean senses of proper names are equivalent to descriptions is clear enough although some apologetic writers have sought to de-emphasize it.[6] It is well to remember that Frege did not even bother to separate proper names and definite descriptions when it came to specifying the class of logical subjects; both sorts of expressions were called proper names. It is, therefore, plausible to attribute to Frege the doctrine that the sense of a proper name can be expressed by some definite description or perhaps by some cluster of definite descriptions. On this matter, I think that Frege was wrong. And by now, the reader knows that the grounds of my objections are similar to Kripke's.

I hold with Frege and Strawson (as against Russell and Kripke) that definite descriptions belong among the logical subjects along with proper names, but my agreement does not extend to thinking of proper names as equivalent to definite descriptions or to 'clusters' of them. If I were pressed to say whether proper names had anything resembling what Frege took to be their senses, I would answer in the affirmative, having in mind what Frege thought the main function of the sense of a proper name to be. For Frege held that the sense of a proper name presents its referent, and that different proper names could present the same referent in different ways. If one holds that proper names are pronominal, then it is plausible to think that the sense of a proper name is somehow to be associated with the background propositions that fix its reference. Just here, Kripke's distinction between fixing the reference and giving the meaning is important. For Kripke is right in denying that a descriptive expression that fixes the reference is equivalent to one that gives the meaning of the name whose reference is fixed by the expression. So while 'a man who taught Alexander the Great' may figure in the background of propositions that serve to fix the reference to Aristotle (of 'Aristotle'), it will not do for the meaning of

---

[6] Peter Geach flatly recognizes Frege's position; Michael Dummett and David Wiggins are at pains to reinterpret Frege to avoid Kripke's critique of descriptionism.

'Aristotle'.[7] Nevertheless, we have argued that the actual background propositions correspond systematically to ascriptive propositions. So, even if we agree that the background propositions do not give the meaning of the proper name, we may recognize that 'an S' will yield to a pronominal 'the S' and that this in turn corresponds to 'the thing said to be (or taken for) an S' and this latter expression may be legitimately counted as part of a longer expression that is the meaning of the proper name. So for example, the ascription 'the man said to have taught Alexander the Great' expresses a part of the meaning of 'Aristotle' as this expression is used by one who has learned his 'Aristotle' by way of a description 'a man who taught Alexander the Great'. The watered down ascriptive sense of 'sense' does not appear to have been what Frege had in mind but it conforms well enough to the crucial condition that the sense of a name should present its reference. Indeed, when we confine ourselves to the ascriptive forms of the referential background for the use of a name (moving directly from 'an S' to 'thing said to be an S'), the distinction between fixing the reference and giving the meaning of a name becomes wholly idle and Kripke's arguments for a no-sense theory of proper names fall harmlessly to the side.

In leaning to Frege on the doctrine of the sense of proper names, the proterm theory is at odds with Kripke's doctrine that the meaning of a proper name is wholly exhausted by its referential role. In holding to this doctrine, Kripke finds it necessary to appeal to a chain of intentions to refer to the thing initially baptized by the name. That a chain of intentions can be forged is nowhere argued for and Kripke acknowledges that he takes the intention of B to refer to what A has referred to as a primitive act whose success is not in question. The proterm theory is free of this assumption. In place of Kripke's chain of intentions we have the initial act of introducing a proterm to denote the individual referred to in the original epistemic context of reference. The proterm is contextually defined but once it has been defined it can be applied like any other term. This is not to say that we have a full explanation of what happens in the initial act of pronominalization. But the

---

[7] I here follow Kripke's usage and do not distinguish between 'giving the meaning' and 'being the meaning'.

problems that remain are not peculiar to proper names; we do not, in addition to assuming the success of pronominalization, need to assume anything about the chain of users of the proper name that replaces the proterm. The use of a proterm is in no worse a case than the use of a general non-anaphoric term like 'philosopher'. If one doesn't know what 'philosopher' denotes one can ask and find out and if one doesn't know what 'it' refers to (because one does not know what its proterm denotes), then one can ask and find out. Similarly, if one doesn't know who Aristotle is, one can ask and be told. But even when B has learned the meaning of the proterm of a pronoun or of a proper name from A, his subsequent use of the pronoun or the name will not require his successful intention to use it as A has used it.

To sum up: if we view the difference between Frege and Kripke in extreme terms—Frege holding that proper names are equivalent in sense to definite descriptions and Kripke holding that the logical subject is devoid of sense, although its reference may be fixed by a connotative expression—then by the present account both are wrong. A proper name is senseless in being non-descriptive. So one must remove descriptive expressions from the category of proper names. Nevertheless a proper name does have sense: it has the sense conferred on it by its ascriptive background and is in fact equivalent in meaning to a definite ascription.

Finally we argued that Kripke misses the point when he thinks of the contrast between rigid and non-rigid designators as a contrast between essential and accidental designators. (See the passage quoted at the beginning of this chapter.) If proper names are pronouns their rigidity is more lightly accounted for: having antecedently referred to a certain individual, one forms a proterm for denoting that individual in every subsequent context of reference including counterfactual contexts in which it is stipulated that the individual in question exists. So while it is necessarily true that Margaret Thatcher cannot but be Margaret Thatcher in any context where one refers to her, this is not because being identical with Margaret Thatcher is an essential (relational) property of her's but simply because of the convention that pronominal reference is always to 'the individual in question' to which antecedent reference was made.

Just here the views of the proterm theorist diverge sharply

from Kripke's views on identity, naming and necessity. In the next chapter we adopt the pronoun theory of proper names and the non-relational theory of identity in examining the doctrine that true identity propositions are necessary. Rejecting the idea that being identical to Phosphorus is any kind of relational property of Hesperus (let alone an essential one) we shall nevertheless find that 'Hesperus is Phosphorus' is necessarily true because the discovery that Hesperus is Phosphorus has conferred new ascriptive sense to the name 'Hesperus'. And generally, for proper names 'a' and 'b' a true identity pro-postition 'a is b' will be necessary because being b is an ascriptive characteristic of a for anyone who recognizes the truth of the identity. Ironically enough it is just because proper names *have* (ascriptive) sense that true identities of form 'a = b' are necessarily true.

We have, in this chapter, proposed that most, if not all, definite subjects are pronouns. The "rigidity" of pronouns needs neither argument nor defence, and one may well ask (a) why Kripke who saw so clearly that proper names are rigid did not see them as pronouns and (b) why he did not see that most definite descriptions are rigid because of *their* pronominal nature. Very probably the answer is that Kripke was unable to see these things because (1) he views pronouns the way most Fregeans view them—as variables *syntactically* bound by their antecedents—and (2) because he views proper names the way most Fregeans view them—as the logical subjects of the most basic propositions. The first doctrine excludes all definite subjects not bound by antecedent quantifiers from having pronominal status. This means that syntactically independent sentences of form 'the S is P' and 'α is P' cannot be construed as having pronominal subjects. The second doctrine is more positive: proper names are the primitive and complete subjects of atomic propositions. Not being pronouns their rigidity needs to be argued for and defended, which Kripke proceeded to do.

12

The Anaphoric Background

1. In the last chapter, I have made some effort to put the proterm theory of proper names in sight of some familiar landmarks. Doubtless, my account of current views has done violence to their subtlety but it should not be so far from the mark as to vitiate my purpose. I shall now proceed with some confidence that the theory will be understood in a contemporary context.

In TFL, the elementary propositions are of form 'some/every X is Y' and there are no elementary propositions of the kind postulated by Frege. In particular, there are no propositions of form 'Pa' where 'a' is a simple designator. In a TFL type of language, there are no simple name subjects, no simple demonstratives, no free or bound variables of the kind familiar to MPL. Instead, every logical subject consists of a sign of quantity followed by a positive or negative term.[1] Whenever a subject of this kind refers to an individual it does so because of the specificity of the term itself. The referring expression will, if it is a proper name, be anaphoric. If it is a definite description it would appear that it could sometimes be non-anaphoric. For it seems that we may initiate talk about an individual by means of an expression of form 'the so and so' by introducing a descriptive term that happens to be uniquely applicable to that individual, e.g. I could initiate talk about the moon by forming the expression 'satellite of the Earth' and then forming the expression 'the satellite of the Earth' without a background of propositions to which 'the satellite of the

---

[1] In the more primitive language of PTL (chapter 9, section 4) there is no opposition of quantity and the basic sentences consist of two terms concatenated by a symmetric functor. The terms may be general or singular and they are interchangeable grammatically: they do not correspond to Frege's 'object words' or to the logical subjects of atomic propositions.

Earth' bears anaphoric reference. As against this it could be argued that all definite singular subjects must always be understood anaphorically with an implicit, if not explicit background of indefinite reference. I have no firm position on this question. There may be good reason for giving some special occurrences of 'the so and so' a non-anaphoric interpretation. But on the whole contemporary philosophers have erred in the opposite direction in treating anaphoric definite subjects as if they had no propositional backgrounds that focused attention on the thing referred to by them. Demonstrative subjects are a case in point. Suppose that, pointing to an object in the sky, I say 'that is a planet'. The syntactic rules for elementary sentences in a termist framework precludes the use of 'that' as a simple designator; they require instead that we parse 'that' as a subject of form '*∅' with '∅' as a U-term associated with several determinate features of a thing to which attention is being directed. The object to which we are being directed in the present instance has the features of Shape, Mass, and Motion; it is a physical object. In forming the U-term associated with these physical features we implicitly refer to a background of categorial propositions like 'there is a physical object in the sky' and the proterm of the pronominal sentence will have that much descriptive content; it is a term that denotes a certain *physical* object. More generally, 'that thing' will always have a meaning like 'that physical thing', 'that animal' and so forth because of the background propositions that inform the demonstrative pronoun.[2] There will, in addition, be conventions for determining a unique object and one requirement for the use of a demonstrative pronoun for a physical object is that the object being referred to must be present to the speaker. The doctrine that demonstrative pronouns are anaphoric contrasts with a Russellian view of them as simple subjects that refer immediately. At one time Russell thought of demonstratives as the ultimate logical subjects and though few philosophers have agreed with him that only demonstratives have this privileged status, there are many who hold that demonstratives are, along with proper names, nonanaphoric subjects and it is this general view that

---

[2] For a discussion of categories and categorial features see below chapter 13, section 4.

needs to be criticized in the light of a termist analysis of definite subjects.

1.1 A background proposition for a demonstrative will typically contain a personal pronoun or some other indexical word. Looking at an animal in the zoo I may say 'that is a bobcat' and 'that' refers to the animal I am looking at and is indeed equivalent to the 'the animal I'm looking at'. The background proposition for 'that is an animal' is something like 'I am looking at an animal' or some similar proposition containing a reference to me. The personal pronoun parses in the prescribed manner—with wild quantity and a uniquely denoting term whose denotation of me has been contextually determined. An anaphoric interpretation of the personal pronoun is not precluded. According to perhaps the majority of psychologists and philosophers the use of 'I' comes after one has learned to command the use of expressions that refer to persons other than oneself. At a very early stage the infant learns to distinguish between those things in the environment that respond to its cries and other verbal behaviour and those that do not. The former things are by far more important to it since the latter can only be moved physically in ways impossible for the child. So the child soon learns to recognize a class of objects subject to 'symbolic' manipulation for which it vaguely forms the concept of 'person'. At a later stage it learns to include itself among the persons for it too responds to verbal manipulation by others and by itself. According to this sort of picture, the background for 'I' consists of propositions concerning a particular person, who is distinguished by being invariably present and by other characteristics that make him or her very important to the infant. The pronoun '*I' refers to the person in question, and its proterm uniquely denotes it. 'I' is always used by many others to refer to themselves and the conventions for its use are far more strict than the conventions for some other term (say 'Fred') that denotes me. In this respect the personal pronoun is less like a proper name and more like an indexical expression. But in my use of 'I' the reference to me is invariant. In this respect 'I' differs from 'here' or 'he' which I may use to refer to many different things. Pronouns like 'he' and 'it' differ also in having B-type pronominal uses but even when they are strongly referential the conventions governing them are less strict than those governing the personal pronoun.

1.2 Anaphoric interpretations of indexicals can also be given. The background for a sentence like 'here is a good place to camp' might be something like 'we have arrived at a place near a brook'. And 'here' will then have proterm denoting the place in question. The additional requirement for the use of 'here' is that the user be in the presence of the place being referred to. In this respect 'here' differs from 'the place in question' ; the latter expression may be used in a greater variety of contexts to refer to the place in question but for that reason its reference may sometimes be in doubt while the reference of 'here' will not be to anyone in the presence of the speaker. I have not shown that all indexicals turn out to be anaphoric nor that the attempt to argue for the anaphoric character of both indexicals and personal pronouns will not lead to circularity. If the circularity could be shown, then certain expressions of form '*J' will have direct and unmediated reference to persons, places or times. Since the syntax of termist language requires that even immediately referring expressions must have the forms 'some /every S', the burden of unmediated reference to individuals will fall on the U-term. Whether reference of this kind will prove to be required by theory is at present an open question.

2. We have distinguished between two kinds of pronouns. In 'Socrates owned a dog and it bit him', the pronoun 'it' is descriptive; the expression 'a dog' not having been uttered by a contemporary speaker in an epistemic situation who took or mistook something for a dog, 'it' is equivalent to 'the dog'. In 'there's a dog on the roof . . . well it may not be a dog', the pronoun is non-descriptive since it is not equivalent to 'the dog' but to 'what I took to be a dog'. In such cases the pronominal reference is 'incorrigible' : I may have been wrong in taking it to be a dog but it cannot be wrong that I referred to something I took to be a dog. Pronominals of either type are equivalent to expressions of form 'some/every S' or 'the S', 'S' being ascriptive in the case of incorrigible pronouns. In either case, the pronoun gets its sense from the antecedent background. In the next few sections, we take a closer look at how this comes about for the incorrigible pronouns that may be replaced by proper names.

2.1 The theory of the proterm and its application to proper names and other anaphoric expressions both descriptive and ascriptive has been presented somewhat schematically. The actual situation, once one leaves the neat cases where the antecedent background is immediately given, is complicated by the diversity of possible backgrounds for any given pronoun or proper name. Very often, the use of a pronoun is characterized by a cumulative enrichment of its sense. Consider the following sequence of corrigible pronominalizations:

> an abominable snowman lives somewhere on a mountain in Tibet
> he must be quite savage
> he is probably very hairy
> very probably he lives in a cave
> I suppose he eats the flesh of goats and other animals that venture up the mountain

The first 'he' has a proterm that denotes the abominable snowman who lives on a mountain in Tibet. The proterm of the second 'he' denotes the abominable snowman who lives on the mountain and who must be quite savage. The next proterm denotes what satisfies the above and in addition satisfies the condition of being very hairy. And so on. All of the pronouns refer to the same individual but they do so in different ways— each later one being more comprehensive than its predecessor.

Consider a similar sequence where the pronouns are incorrigible:

> a senator is on the phone (or is it the vice president?)
> he wants to talk to Robert
> he says it's about next Thursday

Here we begin with an epistemic situation and the first 'he' refers to someone taken to be a senator on the phone. The second 'he' refers to someone taken to be a senator on the phone and said to be desirous of talking to Robert. The third accumulates yet another ascriptive property to 'he'. We may also imagine that one hearer misses the second sentence while another catches all three. The first hearer will then understand the second occurrence of 'he' differently. And, in more complicated and realistic cases, the ascriptive properties for a given occurrence of a pronoun will differ widely for different hearers and speaker even though the denotation of the proterms will not differ. The possibilities for different and cumulative connotations are myriad.

In view of the complexity and diversity of backgrounds in the actual use of pronouns and proper names, it is sometimes hard to see how we achieve the needed consensus in the application of the proterms. I am far from seeing my way clear into this matter and what I have to say is tentative and schematic. Part of the problem is quite general: no term has a single background that determines its meaning for all who know its meaning. This applies to terms like 'philosopher' as much as to terms like 'Socrates'. But the problems of the meaning of proper names are peculiar to terms whose meaning is fixed by the process of pronominalization. And it seems to me that we can learn much about the different ways that a pronoun gets its antecedent backing by attending to situations in which there is a whole or partial failure to understand what a pronoun refers to or purports to refer to. When this happens, the one who hears the pronoun being used may ask for information needed to understand the pronoun and the speaker will normally grant this. For example, I may overhear the following fragment of conversation:

he loved his second wife very much and before he died he willed her all of his possessions which was very unusual at that period in Greek history,

and ask the speaker who he was talking about ('who is he?') and be told about a certain man who lived in Athens in the fifth century BC and who was the first to write about the syllogism and who taught Alexander the Great—'that is the man we have been talking about'. When I receive this answer, I learn that 'he' refers to the man in question as determined by the background sentences about a certain man, etc. This sort of answer is wholly appropriate. Before getting it, I simply did not have the information one usually has when listening to sentences that contain 'he' and this has now been supplied me in the form of sentences that now serve me as background for the back reference for the pronoun ('a certain man who lived in Athens . . . *he* loved his second wife . . . ').

Suppose that never having heard of Aristotle I overhear the same utterance about loving his second wife, etc., but with 'Aristotle' in place of 'he'. I interrupt and ask 'who is Aristotle?' Clearly, the same answer will serve. For 'Aristotle' like 'he' is pronominal and I was in want of information about its pronominal background. The sentences supplied give me a pronominal background and I can move from them to the use of 'Aristotle' as the one referred to. The remarks I overhear augment my command of 'Aristotle' for I have learned further that the man said to have done these things is also being said to have been twice married and to have loved his second wife and so forth. Being experienced in my use of proper names, I am quite prepared for the possibility that any sentence serving as background of my use of 'Aristotle' is false. It could, after all, be false that Aristotle taught Alexander, that he was the first to write on the syllogism or that he loved his second wife. Even so, I should still have my use of 'Aristotle' to name the man in question because the man in question is the person possessing the corresponding ascriptive properties.

For every sentence of form 'someone did Q', there is an ascriptive sentence of form 'someone was said to have done Q'.For example, the name 'Aristotle' taken as a singular term denotes the person said to have taught Alexander the Great. My use of 'Aristotle' need not have the same ascriptive background as your use of 'Aristotle'. But there must be some common elements. Some go without saying and they appear trivial. We both have as background the proposition that some individual was taken to be a male child and subsequently called Aristotle. The first part of this ascription is epistemic, the second may be called nominal. On hearing any personal name NN, I immediately assume that (a) something has been taken for a human being and (b) and called NN. In addition to the epistemic and nominal parts of the ascriptive background for NN, there will be attributions of one kind or another: the individual taken for a male (female)and called NN will be said to have done P, Q, R and so forth. This third part of the ascriptive ground may be called the attributive part. If my ascriptive background for 'Aristotle' differs from yours, it will be in the attributive ascriptions but even there we may assume a good deal of overlap in the attributions. The Kneales have observed that 'is called NN' is always part of the meaning of NN and Kripke has criticized this as trivial and circular. But Kripke's criticism assumes that the Kneales' thesis is meant to be given the whole meaning of NN. I see no reason to assume that they meant to give so much weight to the nominal part of the ascriptive background and in any case the whole meaning of NN is fixed by the full ascriptive background comprising epistemic and attributive as well as nominal ascriptions to determine the person in question.

Quite generally then, if I command the use of a proper name, I am able to supply on demand some ascriptive proposition that could serve as backing for the thing in question. The general form of a proposition of the required kind is

Something has been taken for an S and has been called NN and has been said to be P.

Let us suppose that my ascriptive background for 'Aristotle' consists of the proposition 'someone has been taken for a human male and been called Aristotle and has been said to have taught Alexander the Great for a brief period'. The ascription defines the meaning of Aristotle as 'the one taken for . . . called Aristotle . . . and said to have . . .' This leaves room for the open question concerning any part of the attribution. In the present case, it leaves room for 'did Aristotle ever teach Alexander?' Even the epistemic part is open to question for we may inquire whether Aristotle was a human being. Might he not have been from outer space sent by a superior extra-terrestial race to teach us logic? None of these questions touches the truth of the ascriptive propositions. They are all consistent with it.

2.2 To be told that Aristotle never existed is to be told that the ascriptive proposition is false. This could happen in different ways. It may be that there was no individual that was both taken to be a human male and called Aristotle. (Some peripatetic archivist might have created him out of whole cloth as the mythological founder of his school.) Or it may be that the epistemic parts of the ascriptive proposition are correct but that the attributive part is false. This would happen if it turns out that the one taken for a human male and called Aristotle was never said to have taught Alexander the Great. Perhaps Theophrastus was said to have taught Alexander but, by a proof reader's mistake,the name 'Aristotle' was substituted. In a case of this kind, we may be prepared to acknowledge that a man called Aristotle really existed but that he was not the man we meant. If we still wished to continue to use the name 'Aristotle' for the man we meant, we should have to say that the Aristotle we were talking about was really Theophrastus. We should then recognize that 'Aristotle' is used for two different people one of whom is also known as Theophrastus. (Thus one might say that Shakespeare is really Bacon.)

If there is still some lingering feeling of paradox about 'Aristotle never existed' (a name that names no one is not a name), then I suspect it is due to the strong hold of the theory that names are like labels of individuals (with sense as their glue).But the proterm theory considers this to be a radical mistake since it sees proper names as creative pronouns of form 'some $\hat{S}$' where '$\hat{S}$' denotes an individual taken to be so and so, called such and such, and said to be thus and so. Since it is never improper to deny a proposition of form 'some X exists', there can be no impropriety in denying that Aristotle ever existed.

3. We have observed that the successive use of a pronoun has the effect of accumulating a more comprehensive antecedent. Thus in 'Jack built a house', it (the house that Jack built) was tall. It (the tall house that Jack built) was strong, the second 'it' has a more comprehensive backing than the first. This happens also in the case of proper names where the backing is ascriptive: a later use of the name may connote more than an earlier.

It is however, not always true that a pronoun or name increases its backing by successive use. Consider the following sequence:

I saw a table
It had just been sold
Had I come ten minutes earlier it would not yet have been sold and I would have tried to buy it for myself.

If one reads the second and third 'it' with cumulative comprehension, it would here mean 'the table I saw that had just been sold'. But in the modal sentence, I may be understood to specify a counterfactual situation in which the table I see has not yet been sold. In that situation, I do come earlier and the table is not yet sold. Let Ci be the counterfactual situation or possible world. Then the third sentence may be understood to say that in Ci, I came at the time t (ten minutes before the time in Ca—the actual situation) and it is not sold. It would appear that my use of 'it' in describing the counterfactual situation does not accumulate the description 'sold table that I saw'. We have here a phenomenon that is quite generally found in the use of pronouns in modal sentences. Having just said 'a certain S is P', I may follow this by 'it might (in other circumstances) not have been P' and if we understand the modal sentence to be equivalent to 'in other circumstances it is not P' the pronoun 'it' cannot be taken as equivalent to 'the S that is P'. In 'an S is P . . . it might not have been P' the pronoun refers to the S under consideration which may or not be P—*that* question is not taken as having been settled by having said 'an S is P' since the move to a counterfactual situation reopens the question of what is true of the S.

Some philosophers hold that certain predicates will accumulate to the meaning of any designator even when that designator occurs in a modal context (in a counterfactual situation). Consider

I saw a table
it is made of wood
it might have been made of ice.

Kripke has argued that the stipulation in the third sentence cannot be made since any designator of the thing in question must designate a wooden thing. Thus, if it is true that the table is wooden, there is no alternative situation in which it is made of ice. In this respect 'wooden' differs from 'sold'; the former term accumulates in every context, including modal contexts, the latter term does not.

More generally, let us say that a term T is modal free if it is the case that anything that is T in the actual world and which is stipulated to exist in some world Wi will also be T in Wi.

According to Kripke, the term 'cat' is modal free. If Felix is a cat then Felix is a cat in every possible world that contains Felix. Also 'wooden' is a modal free term: whatever is wooden in the actual world is so in every possible world in which it is stipulated to exist. Unlike 'cat' and 'wooden' the terms 'philosopher' and 'sold' are not modal free. For if Felix is a philosopher in Wa, he may or may not be one in Wi and if the table was sold in Wa, we may stipulate other circumstances in which it is not sold. Stated in terms of the pronominal theory, a modal free term will always accumulate to the background of a pronoun not only ascriptively but descriptively. So if T is modal free and NN is T then all subsequent uses of NN will refer to what is T.

It is easy to see that proper names are themselves modal free terms. Whoever is Nixon in this world is Nixon in every possible world that is stipulated to contain that person. For Nixon is that person. Clearly the modal free character of proper names is readily understood in the pronoun theory of proper names. When we introduce a proper name for a thing, we lay down a convention that the pronouns used to refer to it may be replaced by the name (so that NN may serve for 'it' or 'that person'). If we can speak at all of that thing as existing in some counterfactual situation then *ipso facto* we can speak of NN as existing in that situation. For that is the convention. Thus, once I have learned that a certain man is Nixon, I am able thereafter to refer to that man by his name or by any of the pronouns that the name may replace. Since pronominal reference can be made in counterfactual situations, so can reference by proper name.

The accumulation of a name is conventional. Having learned that the S is NN, all subsequent references to the S will be references to the S that is NN or simply to NN. It is otherwise with other modal free terms like 'cat' and 'wooden'. When I learn that a certain animal is a cat then, according to Kripke and other essentialists, I have learned what that thing is and not merely what it may be called. The accumulation of 'cat' to the background pronominal reference is thus not due to a conventional stipulation but to a real discovery of essence. For I have not learned to refer to the animal in question as a cat; I have learned that this animal is a cat so what I refer to from now on when I refer to the animal will be the cat in question. (And of course 'the cat in question' is a rigid designator.) Although the reason for accumulating 'cat' to the pronominal background of 'that animal' are less trivial than the reasons for accumulating 'Nixon' to the pronominal background of 'that person' or 'he', the very fact that they are non-trivial in the case of 'cat' leaves room for controversy about what to count as a discovery of essential nature as opposed to a discovery of accident. (Compare 'Felix is hungry' with 'Felix is a cat'.) In the case of proper names the discovery is linguistic and not a discovery of the essence of the thing to which I will be referring.

4. In the next sections we shall be examining some of the consequences of this difference between the two kinds of modal free terms with particular attention to Kripke's thesis that identity propositions and propositions like 'every cat is a mammal' are necessary propositions. Our discussion will apply to the analysis of TFL and the doctrine that proper names are pronouns. We shall confirm the doctrine of necessity for identity propositions but we shall also find that the discovery of an identity is no discovery of essence, so that the discovery, say, that Hesperus is Phosphorus, differs in this respect from the discovery that every cat is a mammal. Identity propositions are especially germane to the discussion of the phenomenon of 'accumulation' since my learning that Hesperus is Phosphorus means that henceforth I understand any reference to Hesperus to be a reference to Phosphorus.

In the doctrine of TFL, identity propositions like 'Tully is Cicero' or 'Hesperus is Phosphorus' have proterms for terms. In chapter 6 we discussed the consequences of treating identity propositions as having the same form as other (non-relational) propositions of the familiar categorical kind. I should now like to examine identity propositions with an eye to the pronominal character of their terms thereby bringing into focus the background propositions that fix their denotations. A particular aim is to illuminate thereby the informativeness of identity propositions which some have found to be paradoxical. Consider:

(1) some number is both even and prime
(2) some number is a successor of zero's successor.

These two propositions could serve respectively as background for the following two pronominal expressions:

(a) the prime number that is even
(b) the successor of zero's successor

With (1) and (2) for background, we may also form identity propositions in several ways:

(i) the successor of zero's successor is the number that is both even and prime
(ii) the number in question (in (2)) is the number in question (in (1))
(iii) the latter number is the former number
(iv) the number referred to in (2) is the number referred to in (1)
(v) *J is I (where 'I' and 'J' are proterms that denote what is non-identifyingly referred to in (2) and (1) respectively.

The first of these identities is the most explicit. But it says no more than what could be said by any of the other four or by 'this number is that number' where the denotations of the proterms are determined by the contextual considerations that fix attention to what was referred to in the respective background propositions (2) and (1).

The terms of (i)–(v) are descriptive. But in 'Hesperus is Phosphorus' the terms are proper names. Pronominals of this kind are subject to the open question for every description associated with them. For example, if 'star seen in the evening' is associated with 'Hesperus', it will still be open to ask whether Hesperus is indeed a star. The predication of non-descriptive names is repugnant to contemporary philosophers who are trained to keep their 'individual constants' in subject position on pain of ill-formation. We have seen how this repugnance gives rise to the view that 'is' is here to be understood as 'equals', and have discussed Frege's difficulty with the relational interpretation of identity propositions according to which 'a is b' and 'a is a' both predicate equality of the very same things which makes it hard to understand why one is informative, the other not. The problem of informativeness may, however, arise even for one who is free of the syntactical scruples of those who are accustomed to obey the formation rules prohibiting the predication of proper names. For it is not clear what is being said when 'is Phosphorus' is said to be true of Hesperus even if no paradox is involved in the assumption that what is said differs from what is said in 'Hesperus is Hesperus'.

To see what information we get in learning that 'Hesperus is Phosphorus', we may set up some plausible background for the names 'Hesperus' and 'Phosphorus' and then examine the information content of their identity proposition taken as a monadic predication.

Let us assume that the background is already in its pure ascriptive form so that we shall not be tempted to confer on the names any descriptive content. Thus, although 'brightest star seen in the evening' may be the actual background for 'Hesperus', we will consider the corresponding ascription 'something taken to be the brightest star seen in the evening'. And similarly for 'Phosphorus'. Assume then that the background for 'Hesperus' is 'a thing taken for a star and called Hesperus and said to be the brightest superlunary body in the evening sky' and that the background for 'Phosphorus' is 'a thing taken to be a star and called Phosphorus and said to be the brightest superlunary body in the pre-dawn sky'. Suppose now that an observer in space concludes that the thing in question in the second instance is the thing in question in the first instance. He conveys this information to us and we learn that Hesperus is Phosphorus. In learning this we learn that the proterm 'Hesperus' denotes what the proterm 'Phosphorus' denotes. So we add to the ascriptive backing for 'Hesperus' the information that Hesperus is called Phosphorus, and is said to be the brightest superlunary body in the pre-dawn sky. Clearly once 'Hesperus' accumulates to its backing the ascriptive propositions that give the meaning to 'Phosphorus', it will retain them in subsequent use. In other words, in every world that contains it, Hesperus will be Phosphorus. This necessity of 'Hesperus is Phosphorus' is due to the manner in which we conventionally make use of names; it is not due to anything about the essence of the things they denote. But this still needs arguing for.

If Hesperus is Phosphorus, 'is Phosphorus' is true of it. What condition must Hesperus satisfy for this to be so? Clearly it must possess the ascriptive property of being called Phosphorus. It must possess as well the ascriptive property of being said to be the brightest superlunary body in the pre-dawn sky. Surely these things are not essential to Hesperus. So nothing essential has been attributed. Nevertheless, due to the conventions governing our use of proper names, the identity is a necessary one. One might still feel that this cannot be correct because being identical with Phosphorus is not an ascriptive property. This appears to be Kripke's view since he is at pains to argue for the objective relational sense of the proposition, in opposition to Smullyan and the early Frege who held that identity propositions assert a relation between names, not things. Also, Kripke seems to hold that identity propositions are metaphysically necessary and not merely conventionally necessary, which would suggest that predicating 'is Phosphorus' of Hesperus attributes to Hesperus an objective non-conventional essential property and not merely some 'ascriptive' property. This objection and Kripke's more particular view that true identity propositions are metaphysically necessary assume that 'Hesperus is Phosphorus' is to be read relationally as a binary proposition. But what if one refuses to see here or elsewhere an 'is' of identity equivalent to a relation 'is identical with'? We should then have no room for the predication of an objective relational property *being identical with* of Hesperus and Phosphorus; all we do have is the reading that makes the claim that being Phosphorus is true of Hesperus and we have already analysed that claim as the attribution to Hesperus that it is Phosphorus, i.e., that it too is called Phosphorus, and it too is said to be the brightest morning star.

In defence of the objective relational view (as against the Smullyan reading), Kripke says that we may define identity as the smallest reflexive relation that a thing bears to itself. Wittgenstein, on the other hand, does not recognize a relation of this kind. One may, of course, define anything one likes but the burden of proof is here on Kripke. For we have no assurance that anything answers to this definition even if it were stated without metaphors. I conclude that the relational view of identity is gratuitous and that identity propositions do not predicate essential and objective properties of their subjects.

If, nevertheless, 'Hesperus is Phosphorus' is a necessary proposition, its necessity will not be the metaphysical necessity of a proposition like 'Felix is a mammal' (where 'Felix' is the name of a cat). And we have seen that 'Hesperus is Phosphorus' is a necessary proposition in the formal sense that there is no possible situation in which it is not true. This is so because the truth conditions for the identity proposition in the actual world carry over to any possible situation. To be true, the proterm of 'Phosphorus' must denote Hesperus. But if it does denote Hesperus, it will do so in every possible context of reference by 'Hesperus' since the denotation of a *proterm* (unlike that of an ordinary term) is conventionally stipulated and not subject to the vicissitudes of the thing denoted in some given situation and considered under a variety of different circumstances. Since the denotation of 'Hesperus' or 'Phosphorus' is fixed for all possible worlds, it will be the same for both if it is the same for them in any single world.

I learn that Hesperus is Phosphorus and the situation is analogous to this: I am talking about the mayor of my town and referring to him by such pronouns as 'he' and 'him'. I then overhear you talking about someone in German using 'er' and 'ihm'. It transpires that we are both talking about the mayor so that who you meant by 'er' is who I meant by 'he'. Here we do not form a proposition of identity 'he is er', but that is irrelevant. For what I have learned is the same as could be expressed by such an identity proposition if the grammar of English or German allowed it. Translating 'er' as 'he' we could say that what we have learned is that *he is he*. And clearly we have learned something since the cross references of the two occurrences of 'he' are different even though both denote the same thing. This shows that informativeness is here due to the knowledge gained about the conventional backing of the terms in the identity proposition; in effect, we learn that the conventions for the use of 'he' in the second occurrence also direct us to the mayor. So each 'he' directs us to the same thing.

The account given explains why some philosophers have thought that identity propositions are about names and not about the things they name. When I say that Hesperus is Phosphorus, I do talk about Hesperus but in saying of Hesperus that it is Phosphorus I am saying among other things that Hesperus is called Phosphorus. Being called Phosphorus is a first level ascriptive property of Hesperus. (Note, I do not say that Hesperus is called by the name 'Phosphorus'; I do not mention the name, I use it.) A property of a thing is ascriptive if it belongs to the thing in virtue of the way the thing is spoken of or thought about. Thus being called NN is ascriptive and being thought of as wise is ascriptive. A property of a thing is descriptive and non-conventional if it belongs to the thing in virtue of what that thing is in itself apart from the manner in which anyone thinks or speaks of it. In predicating a proper name (as we often do in an identity proposition), we predicate only ascriptive properties. Such properties do belong to the thing but they do not belong to it in virtue of what it is but in virtue of what it is said to be, called, and so forth. The account explains the informativeness of identity propositions conceived of as propositions of first level. The success of the account is due to the monadic interpretation. For we do not say of a thing that it bears the relation of identity to itself (that, as Wittgenstein says, would make little sense), but say of a thing that it has a certain property. That the property is ascriptive is peculiar to propositions that predicate proper names and other non-descriptive pronominals. And this serves to explain our feeling—a mistaken one—that identity properties and other similar propositions that predicate non-descriptive terms may well be about the terms and not about things that they denote. Finally, our account confirms the necessity of identity propositions. In its own way, the above way of analysing identity propositions incorporates a number of Kripkean theses concerning them (their necessity, their first level character), but it does so from a standpoint quite far removed from Kripke's more conventional standpoint. For Kripke never questions the Fregean doctrines to which we have taken exception: that the subjects of identity propositions are two in number, that they are syntactically simple names, and that the predicate of identity propositions is the relational expression 'equals'. For arguments against the relational view, I refer the reader to chapter 6. For the positive account of inference with identity propositions construed as monadic and with wild quantity, the reader is referred to chapter 9.

5. We have noted that proper names and natural-kind terms

like 'cat' and 'unicorn' are modal free. One can no more say of a cat that it might not have been a cat than one can say of Nixon that he might not have been Nixon. And whatever is (whoever is) a cat (Nixon) is so in every possible context of reference. In the case of proper names and other pronominal expressions, the terms are defined to denote just the things in question where the things in question are contextually determined by some antecedent context of indefinite reference. It is this that makes them modal free; in using a pronominal we refer to just that and no exception is made for the use of a pronoun in a modal context. Let us call a modal free term 'conventionally closed' if its denotation is restricted in this manner. Thus 'Nixon' is conventionally closed but 'cat' is not. Yet both are modal free. The close relation between 'cat' and 'Nixon' has been noted by Kripke and Putnam and is worth looking at from the standpoint of the theory we have developed.

It may appear that even some pronouns have open terms. Thus consider the following remark:

I've invited some philosophers. They all love wisdom you know.

Here the pronoun 'they' stands in for 'philosophers' and denotes all philosophers. So it is not a conventionally closed term denoting the philosophers in question. We may, however, plausibly discount this use of 'they' as non-pronominal; 'they all' is here just a lazy variant of 'all philosophers'. If 'they' is here a pronoun, it is so only in a surface way. For it is not semantically tied to any previous context of indefinite reference; (if it were, we could not replace it by the non-pronominal subject phrase 'all philosophers'). Another way of expressing this is to say that while 'they' may here be a pronoun, it is not a *pronominal* because it is not a pro-nominalization of any expression that has referred to something and to which we now wish to refer. The assumption that genuine pronouns have closed proterms is therefore unaffected by this example; 'they' in this example is neither creative nor cross-referential. Finally, we note that 'they' is probably not even a modal free term. For 'philosophers' is not a modal free term and 'they' is here a mere surrogate for 'philosophers'.

Consider however the following remark made by an Aztec who has encountered horses for the first time:

Some beasts are on that field. The Spaniards call them horses. They say that they are very numerous in the land across the waters.

Here, the pronoun 'they' is open; it refers to all beasts that are like those in the field in essential ways. The question of essential likeness is a complicated one but for our purposes we need not specify a very precise notion of it. We may suppose that a given beast is essentially like those on the field if it is like them in biological-genetic structures (here one needs a narrower specification but I shall avoid attempting one). And let us call the original group that serves as the paradigm for those essentially akin to it the 'paradigm group'. To be a horse is to be in the 'ilk' of the paradigm—ilkhood being essential likeness. Kripke and Putnam have argued that 'horse', like 'Socrates', has a certain non-connotativeness. For at the time we decide to call anything in the ilk of a paradigm a horse, we may not know what the likeness consists in (except in the most general way). The Aztec may realize that he could even be wrong in characterizing the things on the field as beasts (they could be robots, they and their ilk). The point is that whatever is the nature of the paradigm, we have already decided to call them horses. (In the present example, I assume that the Aztec takes this name from the Spaniards and so 'baptizes' the paradigm and its ilk). In this respect, the denotation of 'horse' is fixed by reference to the paradigm group and 'horse' is, as it were, semantically a proterm in denoting the beasts in question. Clearly 'horse' differs from 'philosopher'. If a given group is indifferent to wisdom its members are not philosophers. But if those in the field turn out to be robots and not beasts, they would still be horses as long as they possess some essential structure in common so that we could use them to generate their ilk. Thus, just as 'Nixon' is what is taken to be a male and called Nixon and said to be human and a president, etc., *whatever* he may be in fact, so too a horse is (for that Aztec in his essential ignorance), *whatever* is the ilk of those in the field. According to Kripke and Putnam, 'cat' and 'horse', like 'Socrates' and 'Hesperus' are names. In the case of proper names, the bearers are the individuals that were baptized. In the case of 'horse', the bearers are the individuals of the paradigm group and all of their ilk. The baptism is blind in *both* cases for we may not know the essential nature of what we have baptized. But in the case of 'horse' and similar sortals, we do not at the time of baptism even know what (how many etc.) we have baptized. Indeed, we may never find this out. The crucial thing is that in both cases we must theoretically be able to trace a history to an epistemic situation in which some actual reference was made.

Seen from the perspective of pronominal theory, the original situation with 'horse' may be something like this:

There are some beasts on that field. Let us call them horses.

Here 'them' refers to those and their ilk. If so, it cannot be possible for a thing to be a horse in one situation and a non-horse in another. For a thing is always and under every circumstance essentially like itself and whatever is a horse in one situation must be one in every situation since it will always be essentially like what it is in the original situation.

We see then how 'horse', like 'Socrates', has back reference to 'the thing(s) in question' non-identifyingly referred to in the background propositions that constitute their antecedents. The difference is that where 'Socrates' or Nixon' hark back to 'a child has just been born to . . .', 'horse' harks back to 'some beasts are grazing . . .'. The name 'horse' denotes the ilk of the sample referred to by 'some beasts . . .'; its denotation is the set of things essentially like the sample (and that includes the sample). In contrast, 'Socrates' directly denotes the thing referred to in the propositions that back it up and define the denotation. In brief, if we ignore the difference between the closed proterm in 'Socrates' and the open term 'horse', we can consider that 'horse' too is a proterm in its semantic role. For 'horse', like 'Socrates', has the denotation it has by reference to some antecedent epistemic situation in which something was referred to. Only in the case of 'horse' the earlier reference serves to fix a denotation that is not coincident with the earlier reference but is merely suggested by it.

There is the oddity of thinking of sortals as non-descriptive terms. But the oddity is only superficial. If 'horse' names a paradigm and its ilk, it is non-descriptive in just the way a proper name is. For when we baptize horses ('these and their ilk') we do not have a descriptive equivalent to 'horse' for we need not know the essence of the paradigm in the epistemic situation. So all questions are open; horses could turn out to be very different from what we think them to be. It is true that when we find out that horses are mammals and so forth, that 'horse' becomes more and more connotative. But this is true also of proper names. Thus we all believe that Socrates was a human being and if this is true, then 'Socrates' has accumulated 'human' as part of its meaning. It is still not outside the bounds of epistemic possibility that Socrates was not human, that horses are not mammals. So we might have to fall back on the incorrigible ascriptions that are the original meaning of 'Socrates' or 'horse'. And even if the later accumulations to the meaning are descriptive, the original meaning is not.

Our argument has once again led to a conclusion that is essentially Aristotelian, this time in giving to strongly referential pronouns, to proper names and to natural kind names a common semantical treatment. Most recently philosophers have noted that both proper names and names of natural kinds are modal free. But they have been hampered in accounting for this by their assumption that proper names and natural kind terms belong to different syntactical categories. According to the pronominal account both kinds of names are U-terms whose denotations are determined in antecedent propositions entertained in some epistemic situation. This explains their modal free character at the price of belying the appearance they give of being non-anaphoric.

6. It is instructive to compare the pronominal theory of names with Kripke's theory on another question: whether propositions like 'Homer never existed' and 'unicorns do not exist' are, if true, necessarily true. Kripke thinks so. Since there was never actually an original sample, the term 'unicorn' cannot be what it purports to be: a name of a species whose denotation is generated by likeness to a paradigm sample in an original 'baptismal' situation. Because of this, it will not merely be true that there are no unicorns, it will be true that there could not possibly be any. Without the paradigm, the term 'unicorn' lacks the indexical component that a sortal term must have if we are to be able to refer to objects of that sort in counterfactual situations. So natural kind names are like proper names in their modal behavior. If 'D' is a name and it is true that D does not exist, then there are no conceivable circumstances in which we can say that in those circumstances D would have existed. So, Kripke. The pronominal theory of names comes to different conclusions.

We consider first the case of negative singular existential propositions. If it is true that Homer never existed, then it will be true that no Greek individual in the eighth century BC was taken for a male and called Homer or some variant of that and was later said to have composed the Iliad and the Odyssey. Now the falsity of a proposition affirming the existence of such an individual does not mean that the pronominalization from the ascription to 'the individual in question' is without basis. For the creation of the pronominal and the name 'Homer', all we need is the fact (which no one denies) that many have believed that an individual with the relevant ascriptive properties existed and that these people pronominalized to the 'individual in question', to 'he', and to 'Homer'. This does not ignore that 'Homer was blind' cannot be true unless the ascriptive proposition is true. For if there is no individual with those ascriptive properties, the reference to Homer will fail and 'Homer was blind' will be false. But this dependence, while important, is not semantically radical: the falsity of the antecedent backing does not affect our ability to use 'Homer' or 'he' any more than the falsity of 'Socrates owned a dog' affects our ability to follow it by 'and he bit him'. For all we need here is cross reference, and in this respect our theory of names is less constricting than Kripke's. For Kripke requires the actual or pretended presence of the thing that is baptized and when that is lacking the historical backing for the use of the name is lacking and the name is semantically defective.

It may still be thought that pronouns too may presuppose the truth of the propositions that back them. One cannot say 'there is no God and Jesus is His Son', precisely because the denial precludes the pronominalization. But here we do not have an antecedent at all. For we need some propositions about a divine being and 'there is no God' does not even purport to refer to a divine being. Contrast the above anomalous use of 'His Son' with the case where there is an antecedent that I believe to be false:

John believes in a divine being who sent down His Son. But I don't believe in a divine being nor do I believe in his son.

Here there is no anomaly in forming the pronoun 'his' even though I do not hold to the truth of the antecedent that is the source of the pronoun. Consider the following exchange:

A Some blue swans have just lit on the pond. They migrated from New Zealand if I'm not mistaken.
B You are mistaken. They don't come from New Zealand. In fact they don't exist anywhere.

The use of 'they' by B is only partly ironic. Of course, B would not himself have formed a pronoun to speak of the blue swans but he is well within his rights in trading on A's use of the pronoun. Similarly, the atheist understands well enough what is meant by 'His Son' even though he would not have initiated talk about Him. In similar fashion, one may say: 'Some say that God watches over us. But I don't believe in Him'. The myriad cases of legitimate uses of a pronoun when the user assumes that the antecedent is false and that the pronoun fails to refer shows clearly that the emptiness of the proterm's denotation does not render it ineffectual. In the move from an antecedent to its pronoun we go from what was previously referred to in an indefinite way to a definite reference to that thing. This is similar to focusing on the thing in question. For example, A first refers to some swans in an indefinite way then speaks of them—the swans in question. One who believes that there was nothing to focus on in the first place may still go on to refer to the thing in question if only to make the point that there is no such thing. So might a professional astronomer adjust a telescope to show the novice that what he thought was a new asteroid was no such thing. ('Your asteroid, where is it now'?)

The anaphoric account of 'unicorns' is no more sympathetic to the view that 'unicorns don't exist' is necessarily true than it is sympathetic to the view that if 'Homer never existed' is true, it is necessarily true. Anyone who thinks of unicorns on the analogy of horses thinks of them as being like those in some hypothetical situation that could have served to generate their ilk from a paradigm group. That the situation never actually obtained does not mean that we could not entertain it for purposes of back reference. For a reference to the individuals in question (and generally to all essentially like them), it suffices that a situation of the appropriate kind has been entertained and focused on. The non-existence of the situation is not fatal to its entertainment and to the subsequent 'pronominal' generation of the sort of thing in question. This I think to be true. But it will need more than I have so far said to give this view substance. For Kripke has raised legitimate questions concerning the identity of the counterfactual individuals that 'might exist' but don't. It will hardly do to ignore Kripke's demand for an explanation of 'Homer does not exist but he might have' or 'unicorns do not exist but they might have' if the world were different in certain respects. In the anaphoric account, the proper name or sortal term $\emptyset$ is available for use in propositions of form '$\emptyset$ might have existed'. But what does it mean to say that Sherlock Holmes might have existed or that he does exist in some possible world very much like ours?

Let us agree that saying Holmes might have existed is equivalent to saying that he exists in some counterfactual but possible world. Since we agree he is not anchored in the real world, the question 'who is he?' is the more pressing. Nevertheless, our answer must be that Holmes is the person who satisfies the ascriptions associated with him, someone taken for a male and called Sherlock Holmes, and who was said to have done those things recounted by Conan Doyle. In that situation, Holmes exists and that is who we mean when we say that Holmes might have existed but does not. It seems to me that an account of modal existential propositions whose subjects are rigid designators is available to anyone who adopts a non-Kripkean theory of proper names.

The defenders of a Kripkean standpoint may here object that we have paid insufficient attention to the important distinction made by Kripke between epistemic and real possibility. Kripke does not deny that it is possible that Conan Doyle may have deceived us into thinking that Holmes was a fictional character. It may, in this sense, be possible that Holmes might exist and that someone *was* taken for a male, called Sherlock, etc. So if we adopt a non-Kripkean theory of proper names we may, it appears, entertain the epistemic possibility of Holmes' existence but even if we did this would not in the least affect the real possibility. For Kripke is pointing out that it makes no sense to allow for the metaphysical possibility of Holmes existing if in fact Holmes does not actually exist.

I hold the metaphysical view that, granted there is no Sherlock Holmes, one cannot say of any possible person that he would have been Sherlock Holmes, had he existed. Several distinct possible people, and even actual ones such as Darwin or Jack the Ripper might have performed the exploits of Holmes but there is none of whom we can say that he would have *been* Holmes had he performed those exploits. For if so, which one?[3]

Kripke has a similar view about unicorns maintaining the 'metaphysical thesis that no counterfactual situation is properly described as one in which there would have been unicorns' and the 'epistemological thesis that an archaeological discovery that there were animals with all the features attributed to unicorns in the appropriate myth would not in and of itself constitute proof that there were unicorns'. In effect 'unicorns do not exist' is, if true, necessarily true. And the reasons Kripke gives are similar to those given for the necessary non-existence of Holmes. 'One cannot say which of several distinct mythical species would have been unicorns', and again: 'Since the myth provides insufficient information about their internal structure to determine a unique species, there is no actual or possible species of which we can say that it would have been the species of unicorns.'

The indeterminacy of the non-existent thus gives rise to an apparently insoluble problem of indicating or specifying it for reference. According to Kripke, what does not exist cannot be sufficiently specified for even the possibility that it might exist. And so no possible world is one in which we can stipulate its existence. On the other hand, if Homer existed, the problem of determining his nature need *not* be solved. It is epistemically possible that Homer was an Andromedan sent down to initiate a great classical period in Greece. So the necessary proposition

---

[3] *NN*, p. 764.

'Homer was a human being' is necessary only if true. But it may not be true since all propositions that we may consider to assert truths of metaphysical necessity are 'corrigible'. The prejudice in favour of the actual is so strong as to rule out even the possibility of the non-actual. It comes down to Kripke's challenge 'if so, which one?' This can be met in the case of an actual thing; we may not know what it is but we can always say which it is. In the case of non-actual things, our inability to say what it is makes it impossible in principle to say which it is.

Before taking up Kripke's challenging question, we shall say a word about affirmative existential propositions whose subjects are rigid designators. Assuming that 'Homer existed' is a true proposition, it might even seem that its truth is necessary. For Kripke has plausibly said that 'when we think of a property as essential to an object we usually mean it is true of that object in any case where it would have existed'. One must agree that Homer cannot but exist in any situation that is stipulated to contain him. But this only means that we have stipulated his existence in that situation; it does not clarify what we could mean by saying that his existence is necessary. And generally, the characterization of 'a is P' as a necessary proposition where 'P' is a modal free term will mean that whenever and wherever we stipulate the existence of a we will have stipulated the existence of what is P. This condition is non-trivially satisfied by 'a is a human being' but only trivially satisfied by 'a exists'. This perhaps was Kant's reason to deny to existence the predicate status he would grant to humanity. The notion of necessity is for Kripke bound up with truth in every possible world that contains the object, but it is not hard to see why he does not include as necessary propositions of the form 'a exists' (for rigid 'a').

The negative form presents different problems. And we now turn again to Kripke's objection to saying Holmes (unicorns) might have existed and the equivalent thesis that 'Holmes (unicorns) does not (do not) exist' is, if true, necessarily true. It can hardly be denied that Conan Doyle might after all have been deceiving us and that he was writing biography and not fiction. In the counterfactual world in which we are so deceived Holmes does exist and even though we may wonder who and what he (essentially) was it would there be possible to discriminate Holmes from all others. To begin with, Holmes will still be someone taken for a male, and called Sherlock, and said to have performed the well known exploits. Let us further suppose that we discover the deception and find out more about Holmes. Let it even be the case that we find out his parentage and genetic make-up, properties unique and essential to him. Call these unique properties Gi. At this point, Kripke objects and notes that we could just as well have chosen another essence for Holmes. Kripke's objection can be made more acute if we first consider Holmes in a situation Wi and assign to him a genetic make-up Gi and then consider Holmes (still understood as the one with the ascriptive character that we began with) in another situation Wj and there assign to him the genetic make-up Gj. It now appears we have two Holmes that are not even counterparts to one another! In each world Wi and Wj, Holmes exists because he satisfies the minimal definition of the ascriptive background. So too with unicorns that might exist. In one world we may discover them to be reptilian, in another mammalian. And the definition we now have from the myth is simply undetermined as between these two radically different species of animals. Yet if we allow that unicorns could exist, there is nothing to choose between the two.

Of course, Kripke does not require a determination of essence for the use of a name. When we first baptize a child or come upon the members of a new species, we do not know (and may never know) what we are naming. But in principle the essence of anything actual is determinable. Kripke's point is that the indeterminacy of non-actual things is radical. It is not just that we do not know the essence of unicorns or of Sherlock Holmes but that there is no way—not even counterfactually—to specify an unchallenged essence for these things.

As against this, it is undeniable that we do imagine ourselves able to determine Holmes's essence in a counterfactual situation. We may, for example, imagine Holmes going to an eminent biologist and getting from him a complete genetic picture of himself, one that is unique to Holmes and definitive of his essence. In imagining this, we are quite aware of the arbitrariness of the determination. It gives us no qualms to realize that someone else, or we ourselves, may just as easily have imagined Holmes going to another biologist and getting another picture. So it appears that *we*, at least, are not seriously intimidated by Kripke's concern with the 'real Holmes'. If Kripke is right, our cavalier attitude to the possibility that Holmes might after all be identified in some counterfactual situation is unwarranted. And if so, our intuition that Holmes might after all have existed (does exist in some counterfactual specifiable situation) needs to be corrected.

I believe that the answer to Kripke can be found in the idea that the discovery of essence accumulates to the meaning of the name of the thing whose essence has been determined. Suppose that Homer in Wi has been determined to have the essence Gi. This is what we imagine him to have in that situation. Kripke now raises the point that nothing is to prevent us from stipulating another situation Wj in which Homer is discovered to have the genetic makeup Gj. In point of fact, a further stipulation is inadmissible. Once we have stipulated that Holmes has Gi, he must have this in every world that is stipulated to contain him. Actual or not, Holmes cannot differ essentially from one situation to the next. So it will *not* be possible to suppose that in Wj, Holmes has Gj. This does not affect our ability to think of the Gi Holmes in different compossible situations. For we may think of him as a friend of Watson in one situation and as never having met Watson in another. But we are not at liberty to think of Holmes as having an essential nature Gi in one world and another essential nature Gj in another world. So once having stipulated that Holmes was found to have Gi in Wi that is how we must think of him in every other situation that is stipulated to contain Holmes. Of course, we might have told the story differently; we might have said that Holmes has the essential nature Gj but the epistemic possibility of incompossible worlds is no more relevant in the case of fictional persons than it is in the case of actual persons. For just as we discover Nixon to be human and so forth while acknowledging that we could just as well have made the opposite and incompossible discovery, so too do we stipulate that Holmes is thus and so while acknowledging that we could just as easily have stipulated otherwise.

The difference between Sherlock Holmes and someone like Babe Ruth is thus not as radical as Kripke would have us believe. True, the essence of Holmes cannot be discovered; it can only be stipulated (or its discovery can be). The essence of Ruth can be discovered and to some extent has been. But if we waive the difference between discovering and stipulating, the logic of naming is the same for both. Of course, we must also get out from under the theory that a name is a historical label of an actual thing. Having done these things, we can easily understand 'Holmes might have existed' to say that Holmes does exist in some counterfactural world Wi and that we may there discover the answer to any question about Holmes' essence that one may care to ask.[4]

All this applies to natural kind sortals as well. Kripke is probably right when he says that we should be loathe to apply the name 'unicorn' to a newly discovered species of horse-like one-horned creatures. But that is due to the fact that when the

---

[4] Michael Lockwood has suggested to me that the idea of different sets of compossible worlds could be used to explicate what Kripke calls epistemic possibility. What is epistemically but not metaphysically possible would then be understood as belonging to a world that is not a member of the set of worlds compossible with the actual world. I do not feel able to judge whether Kripke would find acceptable the idea that epistemic possibility is a kind of second-order metaphysical possibility. As Lockwood notes, Kripke has nowhere suggested a model theoretic account of epistemic possibility. Independently of this I see no reason to object to the idea that espstemic possibility could be explained in the manner indicated. On the other hand I do not see why Holmes' existence could not be stipulated in some non-actual world compossible with our own. It is clear that Kripke would still deny this and even clear why he should wish to do so. It is generally assumed that the actual world determines a single set of compossible worlds. The idea that Holmes might have existed or that he does exist in some possible world, and that he there has an essential character Gi, requires us to drop the assumption of singularity and to entertain many sets of compossible worlds each of which contains the actual world as a member and any two of which are mutually incompossible. For we could have said that his essential character is Gj. The trouble with Holmes is that the multiplicity of compossible sets is unrestricted. Contrast with this a scientific doubt concerning the nature of lightning. We may be entertaining two hypotheses that are incompatible, each of which determines a set of possible worlds. In a case of this kind however only one of the compossible sets could contain the actual world. So the thought of two incompatible possibilities does not affect the assumption that the actual world belongs to a single compossible set of worlds.

One response to this line of reasoning is that the actual world belongs to a single set of compossible worlds only in respect of actual things. It is however a fact that we can think of non-actual things and even stipulate for them an essential character or nature. Our conception of such things is arbitrary and incorrigible and each arbitrary choice of an essence for a non-actual thing determines a new set of compossible worlds that includes the actual world. Nevertheless such a choice is not inconsistent or even *outré*. For the actual world is indeed underdetermined with respect to many non-actual things and each such thing can be conceived of in essentially different ways.

myth was formed, our ways of specifying species were very crude. There would be no such reluctance if prior to the discovery someone had updated the myth elaborating it to include the examination of unicorns by zoologists and their discovery that unicorns are mammalian in nature and have a common ancestry with the horse. We may imagine the specification of unicorns to be as precise as that of the rhinoceros by contemporary zoologists. Suppose that having an elaborated myth of this kind to hand, we then make archaeological discoveries that a creature like that once existed. I see no obstacle to saying that unicorns have been discovered to exist. And prior to a discovery of that kind, there can be no objection to saying that unicorns might have existed or that they exist in a counterfactual world (of the kind described in the updated myth).

13

Primitive Predication and the Logic of Categories

1. We have seen how Fregean and pre-Fregean philosophy of language is divided on the question of whether the subject and predicate of an elementary sentence like 'Socrates is wise' are simple or complex. Mainly our attention has focused on the logical subject but Frege held that the predicate too is syntactically simple and free of logical particles. At times, Frege seems to hold the view, associated with Aristotle, that predicates 'come in contrary pairs'. But this view is inconsistent with his doctrine of atomicity which defines atomic sentences as being devoid of logical elements. If predicates come in contrary pairs, we should have to recognize a part of them that constitutes a positive or negative charge and assign to one member of the pair a negative sign which opposes it to its contrary. For example, we should have to recognize that 'un' in 'unwise' confers a negative character to the predicate of 'Socrates is unwise'. But this could not be reconciled with Frege's view of negation as a *sentential* operator. In any case, Frege is at pains to dispel the impression that the negative particle is part of the predicate. In his article 'Negation',[1] Frege's position is that the 'un' of 'Socrates is unwise' is only a stylistic way of negating 'Socrates is wise'. Strictly speaking then, there are no negative predicates; ' −Pa' is always to be understood as ' −(Pa)', never as '(−P)a'. Thus 'Socrates is unwise' is to be read as saying that it is not the case that Socrates is wise. Similar observations may be made concerning predicates like 'rich and handsome' which give the appearance of being conjunctive predicates. A sentence like 'Tom is rich and handsome' is to be understood as a stylistic variant of 'Tom is

---

[1] In Geach & Black.

rich and Tom is handsome'; the latter defines the former and not the other way round.

1.1 In Frege then, the logical subject and logical predicate of atomic sentences do not possess the familiar features of the elementary 'categorical' sentences of TFL. In the atomic sentence, the subject is without quantity, the predicate without quality. It may appear unduly austere to insist that Frege *could* not think of 'is wise' as being positive in quality. But what would he have opposed it to? We must, I think take seriously his mature admonition not to think of 'is unwise' as a negative predicate; thereby ignoring that sentences like 'Tom is rich and handsome' and 'Socrates is unwise' are truth functional in nature. In particular, negation is truth functional and sentential. And this means that a pair of sentences like 'Socrates is wise' and 'Socrates is unwise' both have the same predicate 'is wise' which is neutral in character and neither positive nor negative. Anyone who talks of 'is wise' and 'is unwise' as contraries views them as correlative and opposed expressions. Aristotle saw them this way but Frege emphatically did not. That predicates seemingly opposed are not so in Frege's logical language is also obvious from the fact that while 'Pa' is atomic, ' − Pa' is not. If the predicates of this pair were correlative and opposed expressions, there would be no reason for Frege to deny atomic status to 'Socrates is foolish' or to 'Socrates is unwise'. But in fact he would treat them both as stylistic variants of 'not Socrates is wise'.

1.2 The issue between Frege and his predecessors goes deeper than this. The two basic modes of opposition recognized by pre-Fregean logic are contrariety and contradictoriness. We have seen that Frege has no use for the doctrine that 'is P' and 'is un-P' are correlative and opposed (contrary) expressions. It is perhaps not so clear that he has *as* little use for the doctrine that 'p' and ' − p' are correlatively opposed expressions. Quite simply, Frege's system of logic does not consider these expressions to be at the same level. For the second is a truth function of the first but the opposite cannot be coherently said. The temptation to think of 'p' and ' − p' as correlatively opposed forms is natural enough and even orthodox Fregeans succumb to it. But it should be viewed as a hangover from the days when contradictory propositions could both be thought of as elementary. Those who ought to know better are perhaps deceived by the standard notation into thinking that things are still the same with contradiction. For the common notation uses a unary sign to effect negation; the pair 'p' and '−p' looks very much like the pair '2' and '−2'. A notation of this kind helps keep the idea of correlative contradiction alive. When the truth functions are given a uniformly binary representation, the idea of correlative contradiction is seen to be an anachronism and foreign to Frege's theory of logic. There is no temptation to think of 'p/p' and 'p' as correlative propositions. In brief, it is inconsistent with Frege's fundamental views on the nature of logical signs to hold that either terms *or* propositions come in opposed pairs. For Frege, and generally for any philosophy of language that takes MPL to be 'canonical', the categorematic elements of a language are uncharged and neutral. In particular, the signs for negation are to be considered as external to the categorematic elements.[2]

Recently several Fregean philosophers have compared Frege's logical subjects to Aristotle's primary subjects (substances) pointing out that Frege, like Aristotle, held to the view that logical subject 'has no contrary'. In chapter 3, I criticized those who make this comparison. But anyone who believes that Frege is Aristotelian in his doctrine of the logical subject ought to go on to say that Frege has gone all the way and has also denied that predicates and propositions have 'contraries'. For Frege does not allow opposition in *any* categorematic expression, not in names, not in predicates, not even in propositions.

[2] Contrast Frege's way with negative particles with DeMorgan's: 'The negative words "not", "no", &c., have two kinds of meaning that must be carefully distinguished. Sometimes they deny and nothing more: sometimes they are used to affirm the direct contrary'.

DeMorgan also holds that 'X is Y' and 'not X is Y' 'are the two forms to which all propositions may be reduced'. This accords with our thesis, developed in chapter 9, sections 4 and 5 that a primitive term logic (PTL) that has no opposition of quantity can be the base of a system of traditional formal logic (TFL). *Formal Logic*, Augustus DeMorgan (London, the Open Court Company, 1926), pp. 2–4.

DeMorgan's Denial and Frege's Negation are semantically similar. For both, ' −p' is read as 'it is not the case that p'. But DeMorgan and other pre-Fregeans viewed 'Socrates is ill' and 'not Socrates is ill' as syntactically opposed even as they recognized that the former refers to *Socrates*, the latter to the *proposition* that Socrates is ill. The semantic asymmetry in contradiction is discussed in Appendix B.

2. In a fundamental contrast to the Fregean view of the material elements of a logical language we have the view of TFL that terms and propositions are essentially charged being implicitly or explicitly opposed to other terms and propositions. The opposition for terms is contrariety, that for propositions is contradiction and the logical signs of the language are signs of opposition. The basic form of a proposition from the logical standpoint is one which perspicuously shows whether it is affirmed or denied (propositionally) that a positive or negative term is predicated of another positive or negative term. The general form of a proposition of this basic kind which represents these possibilities is:

Yes/No: an X/not-X is a Y/not-Y

Classical logicians conventionally ignored the opposition in the subject term. This left four possibilities equivalent to a classical A, E, I, O schedule:

not: an S is a not-P	$-(S+(-P))$
not: an S is a P	$-(S+P)$
yes: an S is a P	$+(S+P)$
yes: an S is a not -P	$+(S+(-P))$

The notation on the right was introduced in chapter 9 where it was shown that all the logical signs of a system equivalent to a standard system of MPL can be represented in a plus/minus way. The interesting thing about the plus/minus notation is that it forcibly suggests the doctrine of TFL that the categorematic expressions of a logical language are positively and negatively charged elements. In chapter 9 it was shown how, beginning with the signs for 'not' and 'is' we can define a plus/minus opposition for 'some' and 'every' making it possible to represent propositions like 'some man is taller than every woman' as '$+M+(t^2-W)$'. We also showed how to define plus/minus forms for 'if . . . then' and 'or' by beginning with a plus sign for 'and' and a minus sign for 'not'. The definitions of plus/minus representations for all the familiar logical signs is possible because (as is well known to very student of logic), once we have a way of representing a proposition of form 'an X is a Y' (as we do in MPL by the use of '$(\exists x)$' and ('&') and a sign for conjunction and negation, we can define all the other logical signs. In MPL one must add 'with the exception of the sign for identity'. But in TFL we need not represent identity as a relation at all (see chapter 6).

Propositions that contain only such signs as are intuitively 'plus' or 'minus' are called primitive. Schedule I above consists entirely of primitive forms. Also compound forms with only 'not' and 'and' are primitive. The assignment of pluses and minuses in the representation of primitive propositions is natural. Thus the use of the minus sign for 'not' is natural. The use of the plus sign for 'and' is no less so. And the representation of 'an X is a Y' as 'X + Y' had occurred to Hobbes, to Leibniz and doubtless to many a philosopher who saw that the algebraic representation could be usefully exploited in exhibiting such common features as commutivity. In non-primitive propositions, the plus/minus representations appear odd. We are unprepared for '− X + Y' as a way of representing the form 'every X is Y' and similarly unprepared for ' − p + q' as a way of representing 'if p then q'. The novel representation of non-primitive forms is justified and grounded by definitions that use primitive definitions. From a purely formal standpoint, we could have done it the other way round taking as 'primitive' 'every X is Y' and 'if p then q' and defining what we now consider to be primitive propositions from these (allowing for 'not' as a primitive sign common to both). Thus we could define 'an X is a Y' as 'not every X is a not Y' and 'p and q' as 'not if p then not q'. But apart from the initial unnaturalness of this way of algebraically representing the 'primitive' propositions, there are compelling philosophical reasons for thinking of 'every X is Y' as defined from 'not an X is a not Y' and not the other way round. We shall come to these presently.

2.1 Primitive propositions are distinguished by the positive or negative quality of their terms or by the positive or negative quality of the proposition itself. There is no primitive opposition of 'quantity'. It is only after we have defined 'every' that we oppose it to 'some' and notationally recognize an opposition of quantity. This happens when we derive schedule II from schedule I.

I		II
−(+S+(P)) not an S is a		
not-P	→	+(−S+P) every S is P

$- (+ S + P)$ not an S is a P $\rightarrow + (- S + (- P))$ every S is
not-P
$+ (+ S + P)$ an S is a P $\rightarrow + (+ S + P)$ some S is P
$+ (+ S + (- P))$ an S is a $\rightarrow + (+ S + (- P))$ some S is
not P not -P

For the purpose of discussing the basic sentences of TFL and MPL, it is useful to confine attention to the positive primitive forms 'an X/not-X is a Y/not-Y' contrasting these with the simple atomic sentences of a standard MPL language. We have noted that the negative sentences of a language of MPL are not basic while those of TFL can be. Other differences are perhaps more profound.

Because both the subject and the predicate of an atomic sentence are simple expressions, there is no reason to factor the predicate into a part that is the predicate term and a part that is the copula. Thus in 'Socrates is wise' the 'concept word' is 'is wise'; as for 'is', it serves only as a grammatical device for forming the concept word, a device that is not needed in 'Socrates runs'. Contrasting this with the traditional analysis we find that the categorematic parts of 'Socrates is wise' are the terms of the proposition: 'Socrates' and 'wise'. Where the terms are not explicit, the traditional logician will regiment the proposition to bring out its logical form. Thus 'Socrates runs' could be regimented as 'Socrates is a runner'. Once we define an opposition of quantity for the subjects of categoricals in TFL, there is the further contrast in the subject. The subject 'Socrates' will then be analysed with an implicit sign of particular quantity. The subject 'Socrates' is distinguished from the term 'Socrates'.

2.2 If we consider the derived quantified forms of categoricals with their complex subjects, then TFL and MPL are in agreement that predication—as a tie between subject and predicate—is asymmetrical. For whether one thinks of the logical subject of 'Socrates is wise' as simple (in the manner of Frege) or whether one thinks of it as complex (in the manner of Leibniz), the rules of syntax will prohibit the predication of the subject expression. But another question concerning symmetry arises when we think of predication as a relation between the terms of a basic sentence. One need not go so far as to say that for the traditional logician the terms are the real parties in predication. For Leibniz, no less than Frege, recognizes the integrity of the whole subject as noun phrase and the whole predicate as verb phrase. But where Frege always takes the subject and predicate to be pure categoremata, Leibniz accords this honour to the terms. And even in the terms of pre-Fregean logician recognized the syncategorematic elements that are responsible for the intentional relation of contrariety. We have then to consider two quite different ways of thinking about elements of basic sentences that are related in predication and hence two quite different ways of thinking about predication itself.

We have, in the first way, a relation that holds between the subject and the predicate of 'Socrates is wise'. This relation is clearly asymmetrical on any account of logical grammar that recognizes 'is wise' and 'Socrates' to belong to different classes of syntactical expressions. And both TFL and MPL do so although TFL recognizes that the subject and predicate have terms as common syntactical parts. We have in the second way a relation that holds between the terms of a proposition. We now think of predication as a realtion between common and interchangeable parts of the proposition. This possibility of thinking of predication as a relation between terms is afforded by TFL and precluded by MPL where the idea of a term, in the classical sense, has no place. If we grant that subjects and predicates have terms in common, then it is natural to think of the copula as a sign for predication. Here we have another difference between TFL and MPL for in MPL there are no syncategorematic signs in the basic sentence and so none that could serve as signs of predication (term connectives).

2.3 If we confine ourselves to primitive predication and ask whether the predicative tie between the two terms is symmetrical or not, the answer is clearly in the affirmative. This would be of little interest if the restriction to primitive forms made it impossible to express equivalents to propositions such as 'every boy loves some girl' and others in which an opposition of quantity figures. It is however always possible to express in primitive form what is more naturally and conveniently expressed with signs of quantity. More important, the epithet 'primitive' is not arbitrarily given to say 'not an X is a not Y' in preference to 'every X is Y'. For we have said (although not yet argued) that there is good reason to consider the latter to be defined by the former and not the other way round. If indeed the unquantified primitive forms are significantly primitive and not merely conventionally so then the symmetry of predication in primitive propositions will also be significant. In the next sections, we give reasons for holding that unquantified propositions are logically more basic than their quantified equivalents. If we find convincing reasons for this, then the contrast between MPL and TFL in the analysis of a basic proposition such as 'Socrates is wise' becomes sharp indeed. Taken as a primitive predication tying the two terms 'Socrates' and 'wise' in a proposition of form 'an X is a Y', the predicative tie is symmetrical in TFL. But in no sense available to MPL can one construe a symmetrical relation of predication between parts of this or any other atomic proposition.

3. Consider the pair of subcontrary propositions:

(1) some blue swan is a carnivore
(2) some blue swan is not a carnivore.

On the standard interpretation, (1) cannot be true unless there are carnivores in the actual world. Similarly (2) cannot be true unless there are non-carnivores in the actual world. The terms of (1) and (2) are then taken to have standard amplitude and we can also show that (1) and (2) have existential import.[3] If so, neither can be true unless there are blue swans. Since there are none, the following two propositions are both true:

(3) no blue swan is a carnivore
(4) no blue swan is a non-carnivore.

So far, all four propositions could be viewed as primitive since no opposition of quantity is used in discriminating one from another. Now consider what happens when we distribute the negative signs of (3) and (4) to get 'equivalent' propositions beginning with 'every':

(5) every blue swan is a non-carnivore
(6) every blue swan is a carnivore.

---

[3] See chapter 10, section 1.

(5) is usually taken to the equivalent of (3), and (6) is taken to be the equivalent of (4). But, unlike (3) and (4), (5) and (6) are, if true, paradoxical. At one time Strawson held a view that would judge all six sentences as not making a statement, treating them all as neither true nor false. Later Strawson held that (3)–(6) are truth valueless while (1) and (2) are false. But neither of these views seems to me correct. Surely it is true that no carnivore is a blue swan and so it is true that no blue swan is a carnivore. If so, (3) and (4) are both true and not 'neither true nor false'. By the same token both (1) and (2) are false and not 'neither true nor false'. As for (5) and (6), they *are* anomalous —for aren't they equivalent to (3) and (4)?

This last question reminds us that the logical sign 'every' may be understood to have been implicitly defined by negative primitive propositions:

every X is Y   = df. no X is non-Y
every X is non-Y   = df. no X is Y

Algebraically these definitional equivalences involve the distribution of the external minus sign into 'an X is a (non) Y', an operation that results in a new kind of subject, opposed to the old, and a qualitatively opposed predicate. In the case of (5) and (6), the equivalence defining 'every . . .' by way of 'no . . .' seem to break down. Indeed the anomalous character of (5) and (6) suggests that they *do* break down in this sort of case. For it appears that 'every X is Y' is defined as equivalent to 'no X is not-Y' *only when it is the case* that one of the two subcontrary propositions 'some X is Y' or 'some X is not-Y' is true. When both subcontrarieties are false, then the obverse 'every' propositions are not defined as equivalent to the 'no' propositions. Thus 'every blue swan is a carnivore' is not defined as equivalent to 'no blue swan is a non-carnivore' since it is here the case that both contrary 'no' propositions are true and neither subcontrary proposition is true.

That 'every X is non-Y' is not defined for the vacuous case may also be seen by attending to category absurd cases. It is surely not the case that some prime number is fed. Let us also grant that it is not the case that some prime number is unfed. This may be granted in a system of TFL which treats 'fed' and 'unfed' as contrary terms. (It will not be granted in an MPL type of language which treats the 'un' of 'unfed' as a sign of negation with sentential scope.) I have heard Ryle say that prime numbers are neither fed nor unfed because they are not the sort of thing for feeding. If Ryle is right (surely he is) then both negative contrary propositions are true: no prime number is fed and no prime number is unfed. If so, no obverses may be defined from them. And indeed we are not tempted to say that every prime number is fed on the ground that none is unfed. Here too, then, our intuitions support the hypothesis that 'no' is prior to 'every' and that the range of equivalences defining 'every . . .' from 'no . . .' is restricted to the cases where one of the two negative contrary propositions is true.

3.1 The priority of the primitive 'no' propositions to the 'every' propositions accounts for the fact that the latter are undefined when both subcontrary propositions are false. This happens in the case of category mistakes and it happens in the case of vacuous ('blue swan') subjects. The proper schedule for propositions with vacuous subjects is the primitive schedule (I).

It is tempting to apply this consideration to propositions whose predicate is 'exists'. Moore once observed that we could say 'some unicorns exist' or 'no unicorns exist' but never 'every unicorns exists'. The explanation seems to be that 'no unicorn exists' and 'no unicorn fails to exist' are both true (or equivalently the 'some unicorns exist' and 'some unicorns fail to exist' are both false). I once thought this to be the right explanation but I now believe it to be unsatisfactory. First, I think it wrong to say that no unicorns fail to exist unless 'fail to exist' is used in a way that guarantees its inapplicability. There seems, however, nothing wrong in saying that some tigers exist while others—for example, those in Kipling's stories—do not exist. Also, as we saw in chapter 10, it is sometimes useful to be able to say 'every tiger exists' for example in inferring 'the animal that first landed on the moon exists' from the premises 'the animal that first landed on the moon was a tiger' and 'every tiger exists'. This second premiss is trivially true in the case where the predicate of the first premiss has standard amplitude (which happens when the truth conditions of the proposition require the existence of things denoted by the predicate term). Explaining why we never use 'every P exists' by appeal to the range of the definition thus breaks down on two counts: first because it is incorrect to say that both subcontrarieties are false and second because we do (or could) in fact find use for 'every P exists' as a trivial proposition indicating the standard amplitude of 'P' in a context. But even if one could somehow plausibly get round these defects, the explanation would not do. For one might hold that 'no unicorn exist' and 'no unicorns fail to exist' are both true and this would explain why we never say 'every unicorn exists'. But it would not explain why we never say 'every tiger exists' which is what Moore asks us to explain.

I now think that the key to understanding propositions whose predicate is 'exists' is to be found in the fact that the term 'existent' or 'member of the actual world' is used with unrestricted amplitude. What exists or fails to exist is not confined to any one possible world. For if we allow talk of existing in a possible world, the predicate 'exists' has the meaning of 'is a member of Wi' where the index 'i' specifies the world or situation under consideration. And the range of this predicate is always unrestricted; what fails to be a member of Wi may be a member of Wj. Where 'exists' means 'is a member of the actual world' propositions of form 'every P exists' will not normally be asserted because they will either be trivially true or trivially false, depending on the amplitude (world range) of 'P'. In 'I saw a tiger yesterday' the term 'tiger' has standard amplitude and 'every tiger exists' is then trivially true. But in 'Mowgli saw a tiger' the term 'tiger' has non-standard amplitude and 'every tiger exists' is then trivially false (for 'exists' = 'is a member of Wa'). The fact that 'every P exists' will generally be either trivially true or trivially false adequately accounts for our avoidance of this form. For the same reason, we never say (as Moore also noticed) 'some P do not exist'. For that is trivially false where 'P' has standard amplitude and trivially true when 'P' has non-standard amplitude.

In 'some tigers exist' the term 'existent' has unrestricted amplitude; so too does the term 'tiger'. So we *can* say that some tigers fail to exist—fail to be members of the actual world. When we say that some tigers (Kipling's inventions) fail to exist, we cannot be taken to say that some members of the actual world are non-existent tigers. On the other hand, when we say that some tigers fail to be fierce, we do mean that some actual tigers are non-fierce. This again indicates that in 'some (no) P exist' the term 'P' ranges over actual and non-actual situations. Those tigers that fail to exist in the actual world are not members of the actual world but may be members of some non-actual world. Narrowly construed a property is something that a thing has or fails to have in a given world under consideration. In that sense existence is not a property; for having and failing to have its ranges over many worlds.

4. We have been examining some of the consequences of thinking about the elements of the basic sentences as 'charged' (TFL) or as 'uncharged' (MPL). In TFL, the charged elements are terms. But Frege's analysis of the basic sentence leaves no room for terms. When a Fregean like Geach inveighs against 'the two-term theory', he may give the impression that Frege's theory is a one-term theory (with the predicate construed as the single term). In fact, Frege's theory is a no-term theory; in MPL there are no terms of the kind familiar to every student of syllogistic (the predicates of MPL are not terms in the classical sense since they implicitly contain the copula). Since the elements of the Fregean analysis are subjects and predicates, there would seem to be no problem concerning their difference. Or, at any rate, it might appear that Frege could have appealed to the standard linguistic way of distinguishing the subject and predicate as noun phrase and verb phrase. If that were so, it would indeed be surprising that so many Fregeans have sought to establish the asymmetry of subject and predicate. But in fact Frege cannot avail himself of the standard linguistic distinction since (a) his logical language is artificial and (b) his noun and verb phrases are simple and give no clues to their syntax. For this reason Frege's distinction between subject and predicate rests wholly on semantic grounds. Where Leibniz could appeal to obvious syntactical clues for distinguishing the subject and predicate of 'an X is a Y' (the predicate has a copula, subject does not; or in the case of overtly quantified subjects, the difference is doubled), Frege was forced to appeal to the different semantic roles of the two parties in the predicative tie. Moreover, as we have seen, neither of these is charged and Frege saw their semantic role as that of designating or referring to the things to which they apply. In the formal interpretation of the subject, we understand it to have an object assigned to it. Frege understood the predicate in a similar way as designating or refering to a concept. In modern model-theoretical interpretations of atomic propositions, the predicate is thought of as defined by sets of ordered n-tuples of things and the reference to concepts is avoided. This, too, is in the spirit of Frege since the extensional idea of the predicate does not involve a positive or negative charge. Here is one typical characterization of the way the predicate is understood to be related to the things it applies to:

The predicate 'is white' may be regarded as true of every white thing and false of everything else. Similarly the predicate 'is greater than' may be regarded as true of every ordered pair $a_1 a_2$ such that a_1 is greater than a_2 and false of every other ordered pair . . . /And generally/we understand the extension of an n-ary predicate # with respect to a domain D to be the set of all n-tuples $a_1, \ldots, a_n$ such that # is true of $a_1, \ldots, a_n$.[4]

Note that in this explanation a predicate is false of *whatever* it is not true of. This also accords with Frege's view that 'true' and 'false' are not intrinsic (Aristotelian) contraries since 'is false' is defined as 'it is not the case that . . . is true'. Frege saw and did not flinch from the consequence that the number four is false (four being a number and not being a true proposition). The thesis that predicates are uncharged is inhospitable to the thesis that a sentence like '4 is false' or 'quadruplicity is unfed' is a category mistake. And if not a category mistake, it is either true or false. Frege would say both of these are true since they are the negations of false sentences.

If, on the other hand, one thinks that the categoremata are charged expressions then the categorematic element of the basic proposition is not its subject or predicate but a term that enters into these. Suppose then that P and Q are two such terms that are contrary to one another. Then the predicates 'is P' and 'is Q' are contrary predicates. It is natural to say that 'is P' is true of certain things and false of certain others , namely those things of which 'is Q' is true of. This is not the same as saying that 'is P' is 'false of everything else'. Consider the term 'red'

4 Gerald Massey, *Understanding Symbolic Logic*, p. 160

and some object, k, to which 'red' may or may not apply. Let us say that k is red if and only if it is sufficiently similar in colour to some standard red object—say a certain sheet of cloth preserved in the Smithsonian Institute. The question whether k is red could be answered by matching its colour to that of the object. There are two outcomes to such a test. On one outcome k tests as M-positive (a positive match) on the other outcome k tests as M-negative. We may understand the relation of 'red' to its logical contrary 'unred' as corresponding to the two possible outcomes of a test on k. Viewed thus we can see why being true of or false of an object does not exclude the possibility that an object may be such that neither of these holds. For there are other objects to which the test cannot be applied. For example, we could not compare an event with the coloured cloth to see whether they match. Nor could one know how to begin testing a number for redness. If a thing is neither M-positive nor M-negative—and this holds of any thing to which the matching test is inapplicable—then it is neither red nor un-red (where 'un-red' is the logical contrary, not the Boolean complement of 'red').

4.1 There is a common ambiguity in the use of 'false' that is worth clarifying. We may decide to use 'false' as a characterization of any proposition that is not true. In that case, '4 is red' and '4 is un-red' will both be false. Also both will be category mistakes for on this use of 'false' any non-vacuous proposition of form 'a is P' is a category mistake if it is false and its contrary is also false. We may, alternatively, have decided to use 'false' to characterize 'a is P' only on condition that its contrary is true. In that case neither '4 is red' nor '4 is un-red' will be said to be false and both will be said to be neither true nor false or meaningless. I prefer to consider them both 'false' and to avoid 'truth value gaps' but the preference is terminological. Ryle and Strawson often used 'false' in the second sense. Quine leans the other way:

There has been concern among philosophers to declare meaningless, rather than trivially false, such predications as 'Quadruplicity drinks procrastination' (Russell) and 'This stone is thinking about Vienna' (Carnap) . . . But since the philosophers who would build categorial fences are not generally resolved to banish from language all falsehoods of mathematics and like absurdities I fail to see much benefit in the partial exclusions they do undertake; for the forms concerned would remain still quite under control if admitted rather like self contradictions as false (and false by meaning if one likes). Tolerance of the 'don't-cares' is a major source of simplicity; and in the present instance it counts double sparing us as it does both the settling of categories and the respecting of them.[5]

Quine is right to criticize those who introduce truth-value gaps without showing how to distinguish between absurdities like '4 is factorable by six' and '4 is coloured'. On the other hand, calling '4 is coloured' false ought not induce in anyone a disrespect for categories. For we may distinguish category mistakes as falsehoods whose contraries are also false. As a consistent Fregean, Quine has no use for contrariety; if '4 is coloured' is false, then '4 is colourless' is its true negation. Properly grounded the idea of a category mistake rests on the foundational thesis that terms have quality and 'come in contrary pairs'. The doctrine of contrariety needs an extensive modern treatment that cannot be undertaken here. The following discussion has the limited purpose of indicating that the notion of ranges of predication and categories is one that clear headed philosophers may find useful and respectable.

If my house is on a hill, the question whether my house is or is not taller than the hill may seem puzzling and the contrary predicates 'is taller than the hill', 'isn't taller than the hill', may be reasonably withheld from the house. It is, on the other hand, just as reasonable to force an answer for we can stipulate circumstances under which a definite answer would be correct. (For example, we may imagine the house removed from the hill and placed alongside for comparative measurement.) So on one way of understanding the opposition between being taller than the hill and failing to be, one of the two contrary predicates will be true of my house but on another way of understanding the opposition, neither predicate will be true of it. Understood this second way, the contrariety defines a limited range of things that are or fail to be taller than the hill. Understood the first way the range of things in the union of the contraries is wider and it includes my house. This example of different contrariety ranges is a familiar phenomenon and we shall examine it more closely.

---

[5] *WO*, p. 229.

In what follows a range of things with respect to a term T will be the class of things that are or fail to be T. A category is one kind of range; part of our objective is to specify the kind of range a category is.[6]

If asked whether $\frac{1}{4}$ is even or odd, a correct response may be that it is neither. $\frac{1}{4}$ does not fail to be an even number, in the sense of failure to be even that is commonly applied to odd integers. Let 'even*' be equivalent to 'odd' and let 'is even*' or 'fails to be even' be understood in the way we normally understand 'is odd'. Then these latter predicables will be truly applied to 7 and withheld from $\frac{1}{4}$. $\frac{1}{4}$ is then neither even nor even*; it does not fail to be even-in this narrow sense of failure to be. In a wider sense of failure, both 7 and $\frac{1}{4}$ fail to be even numbers Let 'even″' apply to all numbers that fail to be even in this wider sense. Let '# even #' represent the compound term 'even or even*' and let '/even/' represent the compound term 'even or even″'. Then the range of things that are #even # is included in but does not include the range of things that are /even/. Analogously, the range of things that are # taller than my house # is included in—but does not include—the range of things that are /taller than my house/. The number $\frac{1}{4}$ is not even* and not #even # but since it fails to be # even # we may say that it is # even #* and ## even ##. The ranges of things that are ## even ## and /even/ are co-extensive for whatever is /even/ is ## even ##. The case of ## even ## things is an instance of nested contrariety. We begin with a limited contrariety and then form a contrary to the term formed by the union of the limited contraries. This nesting of contraries has an upper limit. Should we go on to form the term '## even ##*' we would find that nothing falls under it. For whatever is a candidate for being even is a number, and nothing that is not a number is a candidate for being a number. There is, therefore, no gain in comprehensiveness by a further nesting of contraries: whatever is ### even ### is ## even ##. The upper limit of contrariety is indicated by use of '|P|' to signify the union of things that are P and things that fail (in the widest sense

[6] For a discussion of other kinds of ranges see my article 'Predication and Natural Syntax,' chapter 2 of *Essays in Honor of Yehoshua Bar Hillel*, ed. A. Kasher (D. Reidel, 1978). Other writings on the theory of categories may be found in the bibliography, below.

of failure short of the Boolean complement) to be P.

Consider the question whether Bertrand Russell was appreciated by Cleopatra. Here, too, we are inclined to say he neither was, nor failed to be, appreciated by her since she was not acquainted with him or with his work. But again we sense the difference between saying that Russell was neither appreciated nor unappreciated by Cleopatra and saying that Russell was not even and did not fail to be even. We may explain this by the idea of a test for applying the predicates involved. The test for being appreciated by Cleopatra is applicable to Russell under circumstances that we could stipulate (in say a world in which they were contemporaries). But there are no circumstances factual or counterfactual for applying the test for evenness to Bertrand Russell. Let us suppose that Heideger did not appreciate Russell. Then Russell was appreciated* by Heideger but was neither appreciated nor appreciated* by Cleopatra. On the other hand, he was # appreciated #* by Cleopatra. So Russell was ## appreciated ## by Cleopatra. But Russell was not even, not # even #, not ## even ##. Nor was he ## even ##* (for this term applies to nothing whatever).

The process of nesting contraries has an upper limit. We reach a term that 'has no contrary'. In general any term P has, what may be called a primary contrary P′ whose union with P defines the outermost range of predicability for this term. The term '|P|' is defined as the union of P with its primary contrary, P′, and the range thus determined is a category. I can do no better than give more illustrations of this idea and show how it may be reached by a nesting of limited contrariety until the upper bound is reached. One last illustration then. Suppose we are interested in determining which of several red object is crimson in hue. Here the first pair of contraries will range over crimson and red things that are not crimson (which we shall call 'crimson*' things). We may widen our concerns to include all coloured objects. The range of things that are crimson or crimson* is the range of # crimson # or red things but there are many coloured objects that are # crimson #*. Thus the range of predicability of 'crimson' now includes all coloured objects and it is equivalent to the class of ## crimson ## things. We may widen our concerns still further to include an interest in anything that could possibly be crimson, in the sense that we could test it for being crimson or failing to be. This new range will include colourless objects, for these will fail the test for being crimson. The class of things that are coloured or colourless is the class of # # # crimson # # # things. Equivalently taking 'crimson' and 'crimson'' as primary contraries, it is the class of things that are crimson or crimson', i.e., the *category* of |crimson| things. And once again there is nothing to be gained by any further nesting of contraries. For nothing is privative to being # # # crimson # # #. The upper limit of contrariety was reached immediately by forming the union of a term with its primary contrary. And for logical purposes the opposition of primary contrariety is fundamental.

4.2 In what follows 'contrary' will mean 'primary contrary' unless otherwise qualified. The term formed by the union of contraries will be said to determine an *ontological class* or *category*. The attribute shared by all things in a given category will be called a feature or (ontological attribute). Features are contrasted to properties. For example, the term 'round' corresponds to an ordinary class, the class of round things that have property of roundness. The term '|round|' corresponds to an ontological class that have the feature of Shape or |round|ness. Other ontological features of physical things are Texture (shared by whatever is smooth or smooth'), Motion (shared by whatever is in some state of motion, including the state of zero motion called rest), Extension, Colour (shared by whatever is coloured or colourless) and so forth.

The distinctions set forth are needed for the solution of a problem raised by the Aristotelian doctrine of the natural subject. Aristotle observed that 'some logs are white' and 'some white things are logs', though logically equivalent, differ in an important way. The former he called an instance of natural or real predication, the latter he called accidental, unnatural or unreal predication. It is as if, in a predicative tie of the terms 'log' and 'white (thing)', there was an implicit direction. The term 'log' is the natural subject, the term 'white' the natural predicate of such a tie. As Ryle once said to me: 'log' seems to move to the left where it *belongs*. Here we have the acknowledgement of a symmetry with respect to truth (for the proposition that reverses the order of 'log' and 'white thing' is equivalent to the natural one) but an asymmetry of another kind that philosophers have usually taken for granted and occasionally found puzzling. Why does 'log' belong to the left? In recent times the problem of justifying the natural subject has surfaced in the guise of the so-called paradox of confirmation. Roughly, we should expect that any procedure that confirms a generalization will confirm its logical equivalent. But in that case we should be able to confirm 'every raven is black' by observing instances of things that are non-ravens as well as by observing black ravens. In its modern guise the problem does not come up as a question of what the natural subject is since 'every raven is black' is not construed to have 'every raven' as its subject. Instead the canonical rendering is something like 'every thing is such that it is a non-raven or black' a proposition whose truth conditions would be satisfied if there were no ravens at all.

5. Before the success of MPL and the decline of TFL, the paradox of confirmation would have been seen as the more general problem of saying why 'every non-black thing is a non-raven' embodies a reversal of the natural tie between 'raven' and 'black'—a question that has nothing whatever to do with confirmation for we may take it that confirmation should attend to the natural subject of the proposition to be confirmed. To explain the phenomenon of the 'natural subject' we may begin by accepting the following two principles (acceptable at least to anyone not dogmatically committed to the logical syntax of MPL).

(1) In a predicative tie between X and Y, either X or Y is the term of the natural subject. (The 'or' is here inclusive; in a proposition like 'some Spaniards are philosophers' the predication is natural in both directions.)

(2) If 'some X' is the natural subject of 'some X is Y' then any individual that can be said to be an X can be said to be a Y.

Assuming now that the range of 'raven' does not include skies (so that 'some raven is a sky' is a category mistake) we can explain why 'raven' is subject to 'black' and why 'black' is not subject to 'raven'. For the range of 'raven' is included in the range of 'black thing' but there are things (e.g., skies) in the range of 'black thing' that are not in the range of 'raven'. In general then, given a tie between X and Y, the term that may naturally belong in subject position must have a range that is included in the range of the other term. In other words, the condition for X being the subject term is that whatever is |X| is |Y|. Other examples of unnatural ties are 'some things that last an hour are incoherent lectures' and 'some fascinating things are theorems'. The former is unnatural because what is or fails to be an incoherent lecture does not include all things that last an hour or fail to last an hour. Thus the headache I may get from listening to an incoherent lecture may last an hour but it is not an |incoherent lecture|. The latter is unnatural because many things that are fascinating or fail to be so are neither theorems nor non-theorems.

The following principle is a corallary to the two principles concerning the natural subject:

(3) If a predicative tie between X and Y is not a category mistake then either every |X| is |Y| or every |Y| is |X|.

Rule 3 encompasses unnatural as well as natural predications. When a predication is unnatural the inclusion of the categories of the terms goes the wrong way. In the case of a category mistake there is no inclusion in either direction.

The three principles are plausible and they account for the natural subject. Nevertheless, there appear to be some vitiating exceptions. Consider for example the fact that we can say of a land mass but not of a society that it is sunny and that we can say of a society but not of a land mass that it is democratic. Since it is neither the case that whatever is |sunny| is |democratic| nor the case that whatever is |democratic| is |sunny| it should follow that a predicative tie between 'sunny' and 'democratic' must be a category mistake. Yet Italy can be said to be a sunny and democratic country from which we may infer that something sunny is democratic. But the proposition 'something that is sunny is also democratic' appears to violate the conditions laid down for category correct propositions. Appearances, however, can be deceptive and in this case the deceptions are instructive to one who is finally undeceived.

It is, I think, not to be doubted that we can and do often speak separately of a land mass and a society and that neither can take the other's peculiar predicates. This suggests that when we speak of an entity that takes both sorts of predicates—for example, an entity that appears to be in the range of predicability of both 'sunny' and 'democratic'—that the entity in question is to be thought of as composed of two heterotypical parts. A country differs in this respect from a land mass. The latter may be taken to be an individaul of the ontology but the former is not an individual. We may think of countries as socio-geographical entities that consist of a society in intimate connection with a certain geographical situation. The idea of countries as socio-geographical composites is redolent of Descartes' view of persons as psycho-physical composites. Assume that it is not incoherent to think of persons in the way Descartes thought of them. They would then be understood to be composed of two ontologically different substances in intimate connection. It would not however follow that we could not *literally* say of a person that he both thinks and is tall. For if Descartes is right, 'he' and 'person' almost always denote heterotypical composite entities.

The ontological status of persons is a matter of philosophical controversy. The ontological status of countries is not; that a country is a socio-geographical composite entity could only offend the intuitions of a patriot who believed in the mystical union of people and soil. Reference to composite entities is a fairly common thing and it is not hard to find uncontroversial examples. In saying that the lightning that occurred at midnight was bright blue, we refer to an entity consisting of an event and its physical product. In this sense 'lightning' refers to a natural composite of heterotypical things that are associated in experience. Another example of a natural composite is provided by the use of 'gift' in 'The gift was generous—and very expensive' which refers to an act of giving and to the thing given. Once one recognizes that the entities we refer to by the use of singular terms are not necessarily the ontological individuals that we discriminate in our conceptual scheme, we will not automatically assume that 'some A is B' is instantiated by an *individual* that is A and B. For when neither A nor B satisfies the condition for being the natural subject term in a tie between them, the two terms are seen to denote individuals of different types.

Keeping in mind this distinction between ontological individuals and heterotypical composites we may derive a fourth principle from the first two:

(4) An entity k is an ontological individual if and only if for any two terms P and Q that apply to k it is the case that every $|P|$ is a $|Q|$ or every $|Q|$ is a $|P|$.

This principle is of the utmost importance in evaluating the ontological status of entities in a conceptual scheme. For very often what appear to be individuals turn out to be composite, and many philosophical controversies turn on just this sort of question. Stated in terms of the distinction between categorical features and class properties, the condition for ontological individuality may be formulated thus:

(4*) An entity k is an individual if and only if for any two of its ontological features F_1 and F_2 it is the case that whatever has F_1 must have F_2 or else whatever has F_2 must have F_1.

For example, my pipe has the feature of Weight and Colour so if it is to count as an individual in my conceptual scheme it must satisfy the principle of feature dependence. Although it is not the case that whatever has Colour and Weight (skies and glows for example are /coloured/ but they neither weigh nor fail to weigh a hundred pounds), it is the case that whatever has Weight has Colour.

5.1 Philosophers ideologically insensitive to contrariety are, *ipso facto*, insensitive to a real distinction between ordinary classes and ontological categories. They are equally insensitive to a distinction between a property and an ontological feature. Properties come in pairs; what isn't wet lacks wetness and is dry. But nothing is privative to a feature; what has the feature has it; what does not have the feature does not *lack* it. Thus my ability to see has no Colour. But neither is it Colourless for what lacks Colour would have to be in the range of things that could be tested for having it. Features are *essential* attributes. What has a feature *must* have it. The apple I have is red and smooth. It need not have *those* properties. But it must have Colour and Texture. In the Aristotelian doctrine of physical substance, features are substrata, potentialities for taking on determinations. Thus the Colour of an apple would be its capacity for being red (or green) or some other determinate colour and its being red would be the actualization of this potentiality.

In a classic empiricist argument one is asked to perform the *gedanken* experiment of stripping a thing of its attributes. Having done this the empiricists say we are left with 'something I know not what' (Locke) or with nothing at all (Berkeley and Hume). This line of thought ignores the difference between properties like redness and features like Colour. One can imagine the apple without its colour; one cannot imagine it without its Colour. So the empiricist's gedanken experiment cannot be done. The rationalists were characteristically sensitive to the distinction between features and properties. In his experiment with the bit of wax, Descartes emphasized that certain attributes remained under all the imagined transformations and these attributes Descartes held to be essential to material substance. The rationalists thus agreed with Aristotle's view that substance is something that we know quite a bit about. The substance of a thing is to be conceived under its features and these are attributes essential to it and tied to one another by the principle of feature dependence.

That terms come in contrary pairs is in this way related to the idea of an essential categorial attribute of the kind that plays so central a role in the thought of the rationalist philosophers of the sixteenth and seventeenth centuries. It is known that the empiricists' hostility to this idea, and to essentialism generally, has important roots in the nominalist tradition, a tradition that is congenial to Frege's views concerning the semantic role of the basic elements of the basic propositions. It is more than probable that the question whether terms or other categorematic elements have a valence goes way back. The answer to it is in any case of abiding importance for metaphysics.

5.2 I have tried to show that a respect for contrariety leads to a respect for categories and have tried to indicate why we ought to respect categories and to settle categorial relations in a logically coherent way. Many contemporary philosophers, following Quine, see ontology as answering the question 'what is there?' If that were what ontology is about, it would differ in no important respect from taxonomic zoology or other taxonomic disciplines. Indeed Quine sees ontology and zoology as differing only in breadth of interest. From the traditionalist standpoint, Quine's view misses the crucial difference between a classification internal to an ontological sort of thing and the classification of ontological sorts of thing (categories). Classically, ontology is the science of categories, the science that studies how the different categories of being are related to one another. From a more contemporary perspective, ontology is the science of conceptual structure relating the things we talk about to the sorts of things we say about them. Viewed 'materially' the structure is that of the categories of being. Viewed 'formally' it is a structure in language, of semantic types. Either way it has its logic. I have suggested that the logic of categories is rooted in the classical theory of terms and predication. The suggestion has led to formal ontology and taken further it would lead us to the study of different ontological structures. One question that arises is how we may choose between competing ontologies when both are formally coherent. But formal ontology is a large theme whose elaboration deserves its own space.[7]

We have seen in this chapter how modern and traditional logic differ in their conceptions of the categorematic elements of their respective logical languages. In MPL the atomic sentences are themselves devoid of all logical signs and the categoremata are inert elements upon which logical formatives may operate to form molecular sentences. In TFL there are no such sentences and each term or proposition comes equipped with its sign of positive or negative quality.[8] Indeed one way of expressing the difference between the two logical languages is to say that in TFL the idea of a categorematic element is purely formal. A pair of logical contraries like 'coloured' and 'colourless' could be represented as ' +coloured' and ' −coloured' and we can then go on to isolate the common

---

[7] The application of category theory to such fields as language teaching, literary criticism (including the interpretation of poetry and the understanding of metaphor), and cognitive psychology is in its infancy. But a good start has been made by Frank Keil in his recent book, *Semantics and Conceptual Development* (Harvard University Press, 1979).

[8] See Appendix B.

categorematic element of this pair. But the word 'coloured' denuded of its positive or negative charge never actually occurs in a sentence. In contrast predicables like 'is coloured' or 'evaporates' in atomic sentences like 'water is coloured' or 'water evaporates' are inert, and without quality but they are fully constituted and ready for use in other atomic sentences.

We saw how the MPL attitude toward the categoremata is related to the modern doctrine of negation as essentially a sentence operator so that where the traditional logician contrasts 'wise' with its contrary 'unwise' the post-Fregean philosopher will find the contrast in 'x is wise' and 'not x is wise'. And the philosopher who might be loathe to say of a number that it is unwise, is spared the question; he is less hesitant to say that it is not the case that seven is wise. In this way the theory of the uncharged predicate has led modern philosophers to be dismissive about classical ontology as a science of categories. One sensible exception to this attitude is to be found in the works of Gilbert Ryle. Ryle has no qualms about saying things like 'seven is neither wise nor unwise' or calling 'seven is wise' a category mistake. But Quine who considers the negative particle in 'unwise' to be a stylistic variant of a sentential operator like 'it is not the case that' has no use for categories.

Despite its naturalness the traditional view that the categoremata are positively or negatively charged is not given its due even by linguists who ought to know better. One effect of the uncritical acceptance of the Fregean approach to the categoremata is the common linguistic practice representing the negative particle of a sentence such as 'Socrates was not effeminate' with sentential scope. The consequences—for metaphysics, for logic, for the philosophy of language—of a decision on the question whether the categoremata are charged or uncharged, are widely ramified and virtually uninvestigated. But that decision cannot be made in isolation: it depends on which organon of logic we choose to accept.

14

Laws Excluding the Middle

1. In the famous ninth chapter of *The Interpretations*, Aristotle takes exception to the law that of two singular propositions, 'a is P' and 'a is not P', one must be true. He points out that in certain instances, even of category-correct and non-vacuous propositions, neither is true and both are false. One of Aristotle's example is

> this coat will be cut
> this coat won't be cut

A predicate is true of a subject only if that subject possesses a certain determinate character. For example, 'will die' is true of me because I am *now* mortal and a future dead man. Similarly if 'will be cut' were true of my coat, then the coat would have the determinate character—it would be a future cut thing. Alternatively, if 'won't be cut' were true of the coat, it would have the determinate character of not being a future cut thing (but of being a future burnt thing or worn-out thing, etc.). But, argues Aristotle, the coat is not actually characterized either way unless the universe is so arranged as to have already determined the coat to one or to the the other fate. But this is implausible; surely the coat can be underdetermined with respect to being cut someday or to never being cut. Similarly if someone in 1974 had said of Jimmy Carter that he is a future president then that statement would have been as false as the contrary statement that he would never be president. For we may assume that the situation in 1974 was not settled with respect to Carter's presidential prospects and he was then no more a future president than a future non-president. In contrast to this is the statement then or now that the sun will rise tomorrow. This is true because the sun is so determined; it is a future riser.

Having argued that we can neither truly say of this coat that it will be cut nor truly say of it that it won't be cut Aristotle goes on to assure us that the potentiality for either outcome is actual and determinate in the coat: the coat is a future cut-or-un-cut thing. And, generally, where 'a is P' and 'a is not-P' are category correct non-vacuous propositions then if neither is true and both are false it will still be the case that 'a is P-or-un-P' is true. We have then

(1) it is not the case that the coat will be cut
(2) it is not the case that the coat won't be cut
(3) it is the case that the coat will-or-won't-be cut.

Of the three disjunctive propositions

(i) this coat will-or-won't be cut
(ii) either this coat will be cut or this coat won't be cut
(iii) either this coat will be cut or it is not the case that this coat will be cut

only the second is false.

One may take issue with Aristotle's semantic requirement that the subject of a true singular proposition in future tense must refer to a thing already determined to the predicate. For one may say that even if the coat is not now a future cut thing it could nevertheless be the case that 'will be cut' is true of the coat. I shall not discuss this question; suffice to say that Aristotle held that a subject must always refer to a thing actually determined in a certain way if the predicate is to be true of it. This position may here lead to an uncomfortable thesis but it has much in its favour. The requirement of determination is probably implicit in Aristotle's truth definition in the *Metaphysics*, Book 4, Chapter. 7: 'saying of what-is-P that it is P is true', etc.

2. My present concern is with the crucial formal distinction between 'a is P-or-un-P' and 'either a is P or a is un-P'. For convenience I shall refer to the first as the 'categorial law of excluded middle' (CLEM). Given any category correct and non-vacuous proposition of form 'a is P' it will be true that a is P-or-un-P. I shall refer to the second as the 'predicative law of excluded middle' (PLEM). According to Aristotle, where a is

undetermined with respect to being P or to being not-*P*, the
CLEM will stand up but the PLEM will fail:

Necessarily everything is or is not and will be or will not be but one
cannot divide and say that it is necessary for one or for the other to
be.[1]

Neither the CLEM nor the PLEM should be confused with
the standard sentential law of the excluded middle (SLEM): 'p
or not p', of which (iii) is an instance. Aristotle's doubts in
chapter 9 pertain to the PLEM which is his own standard
formulation of the law of excluded middle in the *Metaphysics*.
Aristotle nowhere formulates the standard sentential law and
nothing in chapter 9 should be taken as remotely suggesting
that he had any doubts about it. That the chapter has been so
interpreted by some commentators is not so much symptomatic of a poor state of Aristotelian scholarship as it is
symptomatic of the pervasive influence of current views about
negation and disjunction which preclude an understanding of
the distinctions that Aristotle is making. It is not hard to see
why the Fregean cannot make out the three distinct formulations of the law of excluded middle. First, as we have
observed, he defines 'a is not-P' as a stylistic variant of 'not:a is
P'. This conflates the predicative law with the sentential law of
excluded middle. Next the Fregean does a similar thing to 'a is
P-or-Q' treating it as stylistic variant of 'a is P or a is Q'. Thus
Geach says:

Connectives that join propositions may be also used to join
predicables and the very meaning they have in the latter uses is that by
attaching a predicable so formed to a logical subject we get the same
result as we should by first attaching the several predicables to that
subject and using the connective to join the propositions so formed
precisely as the respective predicables were joined by that
connective.[2]

This conflates the categorial law with the predicative law of
excluded middle. Anyone who thinks that 'the very meaning' of
'a is P-or-not-P' is that of 'a is P or a is not-P' will be unable to
make out Aristotle's distinction between predicating the
potentiality of two possible outcomes and predicating the

[1] Aristotle, *On Interpretation*, ch. 9, 19a, 26-9.
[2] Geach, *R & G*, pp. 58-9.

actuality of one or the other. If, in addition, he holds that the very meaning of 'a is not-P' is that of 'not:a is P' he will be unable to see that denying an instance of 'a is P or a is not-P' is *not* tantamount to denying an instance of 'p or not p'. Not one of the distinctions needed for an understanding of chapter 9 is available to the interpreter who comes to it with a Fregean 'organon'. It is therefore not surprising that recent comment on that chapter has been bizarre, anachronistic, and generally uncomplimentary to Aristotle. Some have him denying the necessity of 'p or not p'; others have him denying that 'necessarily p or necessarily not p'. The first he never would deny, the second he would not have thought it plausible for anyone to seriously entertain. Neither of these interpretations makes sense of his discussion of determinism.[3]

3. Given the currently familiar ways of defining 'a is not-P' and 'a is P or Q', the three different laws of the excluded middle collapse into the third sentential law. This has had significant consequences for modern philosophy. In chapter 12 we saw how the assumption that 'a is P or not-P' must be treated as 'either a is P or not:a is P' inhibits the development of a theory of categories by not allowing us to characterize a category mistake like 'this coat is married' as a case of a false proposition of form 'a is P' whose contrary 'a is not-P' is also false. In the present chapter we are observing how the collapse of the three different principles into one single sentential law inhibits the understanding of even category correct propositions. Even if one does not agree with Aristotle in saying that the under-determination of the coat renders both 'this coat will be cut' and 'this coat won't be cut' false, the crucial distinction between the CLEM and the PLEM (and the integrity of both with respect to the SLEM) will apply in other cases where underdetermination of the subject makes it impossible for us to affirm either one of a contrary pair of predicates.

Consider the proposition 'Sherlock Holmes was unacquainted with the work of Sigmund Freud'. Since Freud is nowhere mentioned in the stories by Conan Doyle, Holmes is under-determined with respect to being acquainted with him or his

---

[3] For a good discussion of these implausibilities, see Ackrill's commentary on chapter 9 of *De Interpretatione*.

works. Nevertheless, Holmes is in the right category; he is | acquainted with the works of Freud | and a more recent writer arranges for Holmes to read Freud and to meet him.

The works of fiction provide one rich field for the application of the distinction between being potentially P and potentially not-P but being determinately neither. But it is not the only one. In an interesting paper, Michael Dummett has suggested that even singular propositions about the actual past may have an underdetermined subject. Dummett imagines a man Jones, now dead, whose bravery was never put to any test during his lifetime and he considers the sentence 'Either Jones was brave or he was not brave'. Dummett sets up two positions, one maintained by A, the other by B, concerning the validity of this sentence. He assumes that none of the facts available to us would enable us to project how Jones would have behaved in a test situation. According to A, the disjunction is then not valid since neither of its limbs is 'decidable.' According to B, the disjunction is valid since one of the two propositions must be true even though 'its truth may lie in a region accessible only to God which human beings can never survey'. Dummett does not clearly consider the possibility that Jones may actually be underdetermined to either bravery or to its opposite but this possibility is certainly coherent. It may be that even a complete knowledge of Jones' physical and spiritual nature could not furnish the information needed to project how he would have behaved in a test situation. Of course, God could know this if he is omniscient with respect to possible worlds as well as actual ones. But it would then still be the case that even God could not *project* Jones' behaviour from his state. Omniscience of the sort that sees into the future without projecting it from the past by means of some law is here irrelevant. If Jones was brave then he must have had a certain nature or virtue which would dispose him to act so and so; if he had no such nature, then how he would have acted is irrelevant; in particular, we could not call him brave even if we were miraculously informed that he *would* have acted 'bravely' in a test situation since in actual fact he did not act at all. Analogously, if a prescient clairvoyant could tell us that in a moment from now this electron will have taken *that* path in the cloud chamber, it would still be wrong to say of the electron that in the present moment it is determined to take the predicted path.

Dummett does not require a real indeterminacy as a condition for denying the validity of 'either Jones was brave or he was not-brave'; it is enough that *we* have no way of determining whether he was or wasn't for both limbs of the alternation to be undecidable. Decidability is, of course, a characteristic of statements that accrues to them in virtue of the abilities of those who make the statements. From the present Aristotelian standpoint there is no reason to consider 'Jones was brave' undecidable since we could, in principle, find out that nothing in Jones's nature sufficed to determine how he would have acted. We should then view Jones as we now view Holmes. Just as Holmes' story is incomplete and underdetermined with respect to many things not mentioned in the story, so Jones's real-life story may be actually incomplete and underdetermined with respect to properties like bravery. And just as Holmes neither knew Freud nor failed to know him, so Jones was neither brave nor not brave; he was simply incomplete in these respects. Dummett characterizes A's position as a 'small retreat from realism'. This is consistent with his characterization of 'Jones was brave' as an undecidable proposition that is neither true nor false. But one who holds that 'Jones was brave' is not true because he was actually incomplete with respect to a determination of behaviour in a test situation will not regard this as giving any ground to the anti-realist. Similarly, when Aristotle insists that a thing may have potentiality in both directions and be actually determined to neither, his is a realist insistence. And one difference is that the Aristotelian will not find 'Jones was brave' neither true nor false. For if it is true that Jones was determined to act in a way that would have attested to his bravery or lack of it, then the sentence 'Jones was brave or he was not' is true even though we could never know which of the two disjuncts makes it true. On the other hand, if Jones was underdetermined with respect to the kind of test situations that attest to bravery or non-bravery then, by Aristotle's lights, both disjuncts will be false and the whole disjunction false. Moreover, if Jones does have a nature complete in respect to being brave or to being not brave there is no reason to think we could never find this out. But neither is there any reason to think that if Jones was incomplete in these respects we could never know this. In any case, the Aristotelian will not countenance a truth-value gap for 'Jones was brave' and even if he allowed that this proposition is undecidable he would give no ground to the anti-realist. Dummett does not ascribe to A the view that both disjuncts are false. According to A (and apparently to Dummett himself) where we cannot know what Jones would have done in a test situation, both 'Jones was brave' and 'Jones was not brave' are neither true nor false. And this position of A is unrealistic in giving up the idea that Jones was brave or that he was not brave because of the undecidability of the alternatives. Dummett defines realism as 'the belief that for any statement there must be something in virtue of which it or its negation is true'. Having considered 'Jones was brave' in the light of this definition Dummett concludes:

> We thus arrive at the following position. We are entitled to say that a statement P must either be true or false, that there must be something in virtue of which it is true or it is false, only when P is a statement of such a kind that we could in a finite time bring ourselves into a position in which we were justified either in asserting or in denying P: that is, when P is an effectively decidable statement.[4]

I shall presently comment on the idea that decidability is a condition of having a truth value. Of immediate concern is the question why Dummett ignores the possibility that we could be in a position to deny that Jones was brave and to deny that he was not brave and to deny that Holmes was prone to colds and to deny that he was not prone to colds. Nothing in Holmes life story suggests either of these alternatives. So, too, we could find out that nothing in Jones's life story would ever make it possible for anyone to have projected from Jones's nature a kind of behaviour that would have tested him for bravery or non-bravery. To ask the question another way: why doesn't Dummett allow for the possibility that 'Jones was brave' and 'Jones was not brave' are both false simply because Jones' nature was not determined in either of these respects. Clearly this line was not open to Dummett because of his inability to assert the joint negations of these contrary propositions.

[4] M. Dummett, *Truth & Other Enigmas* (Harvard University Press, 1978), p. 16. Hereafter referred to as *TOE*.

Having adopted Frege's organon, Dummett does not see them as contraries but as contradictories whose joint negation would violate the law of excluded middle. It is one thing to say that the law does not apply in a given case or over a given domain giving reasons to withhold truth values from the sentences that appear to violate the law. It is quite another thing to assert a conjunction of negations that Dummett cannot but see as an overt violation of the classical sentential law of excluded middle. It is therefore never really possible for Dummett to say that Jones was neither brave nor not brave: he must instead argue for a truth value gap, never a light matter since nothing less than a theory of meaning is required for the judgement that a *prima facie* meaningful statement is neither true nor false.

In a recent paper, Dummett argues that even the intuitionist logician must appeal to a general theory of meaning to justify his rejection of the classical law of bivalence.[5] And in the present instance Dummett first finds that 'Jones was (not) brave' is undecidable and then argues that undecidable propositions are truth valueless. The situation may be compared with the familiar one faced by those who follow Frege and Strawson in interpreting propositions of form 'the S is P' as atomic but who also wish to refrain from saying that the present king of France isn't bald. To avoid the application of the sentential law of excluded middle which would require him to say that either the present king of France is bald or he isn't bald, Strawson proposes and argues for a truth-value gap for vacuous propositions. The semantic doctrine of existential presupposition is brought in to justify the truth-value gap; it serves the same purpose that Dummett's doctrine of the tie between being effectively decidable and having a truth value serves in connection with the statement that Jones was brave or he was not.

Dummett's second example of an undecidable proposition is reminiscent of Aristotle's coat example.

Consider the statement (C) 'A city will never be built on this spot'. Even if we have an oracle which can answer every question of the kind 'will there be a city here in 1990?, in 2100?', etc., we might never be in a position either to declare the statement true or to declare it false.[6]

---

[5] Dummett, *TOE*, pp. 215–247.   [6] Dummett, *TOE*, p. 16.

Dummett concludes that 'either a city will never be built on this spot or a city will someday be built on this spot' is not a valid statement since neither of the two limbs is effectively decidable. According to Dummett, undecidability of (C) is due to the fact that it contains an 'unlimited generality' which precludes a finite decision procedure.

The Aristotelian analogue to (C) might be (C*) 'this spot is the site of a future city' which, according to Aristotle, would be false on the ground that the spot in question is not characterized truly unless the universe is such that the question is settled. Similarly 'this spot is not the site of a future city' is false unless the spot is in fact doomed to be rural forever. If we may plausibly assume that the future of the spot is in fact open, then both C and its contrary would be judged false.

That unlimited generality is not the point may be seen by contrasting (C) or (C*) with

(S) this sow's ear will never be a silk purse.

Here, too, the oracle will not help us to decide. But the facts will. We know enough about the nature of sow's ears and silk purses to claim that the predicate of S truly characterizes the sow's ear; this sow's ear is determinately not a future silk purse. And again the realist who denies Dummett's disjunction need not retreat. For he may recognize that the spot is underdetermined with respect to a rural or an urban fate. But the denial *will* require a sensitivity to the difference between the predicative law of excluded middle and the sentential law.

The more famous of Aristotle's example of an indeterminate proposition is

(F) a sea battle will take place tomorrow

of which he says:

It is necessary for there to be or not to be a sea battle tomorrow: but it is not necessary for a sea battle to take place tomorrow or for one not to take place tomorrow.[7]

Unlike C, F is decidable by the finite procedure of waiting till tomorrow for news of Aegean naval affairs. Nevertheless, if the real culprit is the indeterminacy of the present situation with

---

[7] Aristotle, 19a, 30–4.

respect to a naval engagement tomorrow, there will be no truth difference between F and C. Both will have truth values and both will be false.[8]

4. Chapter 9 of *The Interpretations* had opened with Aristotle's remark that the law of bivalence will not cover certain definite singular propositions about the future. And it is fairly evident that Aristotle seems to think that (F) is a prediction on a par with 'this coat will be cut' or 'this spot is the site of a future city'. To spare him familiar troubles with general propositions asserting existence, we may understand Aristotle's view of F or its contrary as equivalent to a definite singular proposition affirming of the current situation; that it will change in a definite way (from peace to war) by tomorrow, or else that it will remain the same in some definite way (not changing from peace to war). A more particular reading of F that treated it as having a definite subject could understand it as affirming of a certain place (the Aegean, say) that it is the site of a battle tomorrow or saying of certain naval forces or naval heroes that they are to be engaged in a battle tomorrow.

The distinction between 'not a is P' and 'a is not-P' was discussed in the preceding chapter. We there observed that the rule of obversion which normally permits the inference of the latter from the former proposition is qualified by the requirement that one of the contrary propositions be true. We have now seen three types of cases where this condition is not satisfied. Each type of case requires us to limit the sway of the law of bivalence according to which one of the two pro-

---

[8] Another example of the failure to exploit the Aristotelian distinctions is found in Hilary Putnam's article 'Is Logic Empirical?' which argues that the sentential law of distribution fails in the face of experiences we encounter in quantum mechanics. For suppose that p is a proposition asserting that a certain particle has a determinate position at time t. And suppose that m_i is a proposition that affirms of the same particle that it has momentum M_i at that time. Then the joint assertion of 'p' and 'm_i' will be false and, generally, it will be false that $p \& m_1$ or $p \& m_2$ ... or $p \& m_n$, even though we may be in a position to assert both 'p' and 'm_1 v m_2 v ... m_n'. Since this sort of case appears to support Quine's thesis that logical laws are corrigible it is important to point out that Aristotelian term logic has considerably more 'give' in the face of experience that seems to be in conflict with fundamental logical laws. For while we may here allow that the particle has momentum M_1 or M_2 ... or M_n we are quite free to reject each sentence that affirms a given momentum of the particle. cf. H. Putnam 'Is Logic Empirical?' in *Boston Studies in Philosophy of Science*' V (1969) ed. R. S. Cohen and M. Wartofsky pp. 216–41.

positions 'a is P' and 'a is not-P' is true and the other is false. The three types of exceptions are

(a) where the subject is vacuous
(b) where the predication is a category mistake
(c) where the situation is underdetermined with respect to the contrary predicates.

The vacuous case is discussed by Aristotle in chapter 10 of the *Categories*. He tentatively formulates a version of the PLEM using logical contraries and giving sickness and health as an example:

> If contraries are such that it is necessary for one or the other of them to belong to the things they naturally occur in or are predicated of, there is nothing intermediate between them. For example sickness and health naturally occur in animals' bodies and it is indeed necessary for one or the other to belong to an animal's body.[9]

Later in the chapter Aristotle says of the pair of contraries 'Socrates is sick' and 'Socrates is well' that both are false if it should be the case that Socrates does not exist. It is clear that 'Aristotle recognizes two meanings of 'Socrates is not well' one of which we affirm 'is not-well' of Socrates (equivalent to affirming 'is sick') and the other in which we deny the proposition that Socrates is well. In chapter 10 of *The Interpretations*, Aristotle remarks that if someone asks whether Socrates is wise and the answer is 'no', then we may infer from this that Socrates is 'unwise'. In that chapter, Aristotle assumes that Socrates exists and he then allows that 'Socrates is not wise' is equivalent to 'Socrates is unwise'. But in the tenth chapter of the *Categories*, 'Socrates is not well' is treated as the negation of 'Socrates is well': this latter proposition is judged false in the vacuous case and its negation true. To avoid ambiguity it is useful to have a convention for the use of 'not' where this qualifies the predicate; one way of indicating this is to use the contraction 'isn't'. Thus 'Socrates isn't well' will be false if Socrates does not exist but 'Socrates is not well' will be understood as 'not: Socrates is well' and will be true in the vacuous case. Another convention for treating the ambiguity of 'Socrates is not well' is to read this always as the negation of

⁹ Aristotle, *Categories*, 12a, 2–7.

'Socrates is well' and to use the form 'Socrates is not-well' or 'Socrates is unwell' for the contrary affirmation. If this convention is adopted, the only way of forming a negative predicate will be to use a negative predicate term. In this chapter I have made occasional use of this devise to distinguish the two meanings that could be assigned to 'a is not P'.

5. Consider a schedule of primitive propositions about Socrates:

  (1) Socrates is P
  (2) Socrates is un-P
  (3) Socrates is not P
  (4) Socrates is not un-P

If Socrates does not exist, then (1) and (2) are false and (3) and (4) are true. I shall call (3) the primitive contradictory of (1). Similarly, (2) and (4) are primitive contradictories. And, generally, two propositions are primitive contradictories if both are primitive and one is the negation of the other.

If Socrates does exist, we may form another schedule in which the contradictories of (1) and (2) are not primitive:

  (1) Socrates is P
  (2) Socrates is un-P
  (3) (every) Socrates is un-P
  (4) (every) Socrates is P.

In this schedule, (3) is the *proper* contradictory of (1), and (4) is the proper contradictory of (2). Generally, two propositions are proper or 'diagonal' contradictories if both have the same subject and predicate terms and they differ in the quantity of their subjects and the quality of their predicates.

With the advent of proper contradictories, we must distinguish yet another version of the law of excluded middle. I shall call it the 'diagonal law of excluded middle' (DILEM) since its disjuncts are found at the ends of the diagonals of the traditional square of opposition:

(DILEM) Either some A is B or every A is not-B.

The diagonal law of excluded middle does not apply where a

particular proposition lacks a diagonal contradictory. On the other hand, every proposition has a primitive contradictory and there are no exceptions to the law that either some A is B or no A is B.

Contemporary philosophers who are confined to a logic that does not recognize the traditional oppositions of contrariety and contradictoriness have given up more than they realize. For modern logic makes no room for a truth difference between 'every A is B' and 'no A is not-B'. The schemas 'either some A is B or no A is B' and 'either some A is not-B or no A is not-B' are special cases of the more general schema 'either p or not p' and there can be no good logical reason for rejecting their validity. On the other hand, there are a number of familiar contexts in which we are reasonably reluctant to accept either limb of a DILEM disjunction. If I have no children and someone says 'some of your children are unfed' a proper rejoinder is 'none of my children is unfed'. This may not remove the impression that he evidently has, but I may not care to remove it. I should still have told him the truth. On the other hand, 'every one of my children is fed' is not merely misleading; it is not even a formally correct response. Having responded with 'none of my children is unfed' I could, if I wished, remove the false impression by adding 'because I have no children', thereby giving and excellent reason for my having said that none of them is unfed. On the other hand, not having any children is no reason at all, not even a poor one, for saying that all of them are fed.

The curious doctrine that the absence of A's is reason enough to accept 'every A is B' as true leads to curious theses in the theory of meaning. In a well-known paper *On Likeness of Meaning*, Nelson Goodman shows how it has the consequence that we cannot treat 'picture of a centaur' as a relational expression on a par with 'uncle of a centaur' but must treat it as a single term 'centaur picture', analogous to 'bachelor of arts' which is also non-relational and understood as 'arts bachelor'. Centaur pictures are things in the 'secondary extension' of 'centaur'. The primary extension of centaur is empty; its secondary extension is not. As the following passage shows, the doctrine of secondary extensions has no basis apart from the assumption that 'all centaurs are P' is true.

Since there are no centaurs or unicorns, all centaurs are unicorns and all unicorns are centaurs. Furthermore all uncles of unicorns are uncles of centaurs and all feet of centaurs are feet of unicorns. How far can we generalize this? . . . We have a theorem in logic that if all A's are B's, then whatever bears the relation P to an A will bear the relation P to a B . . . Yet not all pictures of centaurs are pictures of unicorns and not all pictures of unicorns are pictures of centaurs. At first sight this seems to violate the cited theorem of logic. Actually what it shows is that 'picture of' is not always a relational expression like 'foot of' or 'uncle of' . . . 'Centaur-picture' and 'unicorn-picture' apply to different objects just as 'desk' and 'chair' apply to different objects.[10]

Goodman's problem had been that 'unicorn' and 'centaur' have the same (null) extension which on his theory of meaning amounts to having the same meaning. But now the doctrine of secondary extensions shows that this is not true: 'unicorn' and 'centaur' do differ in their secondary extensions. From the standpoint of TFL, the doctrine of secondary extensions is unfounded and the idea that 'picture of a centaur' is non-relational is an *ad hoc* solution to a non-problem. For we can allow that 'picture of a centaur' is a relational expression since there is no reason to accept the truth of 'every centuar is a unicorn' to begin with. This simple and natural option is not open to Goodman or indeed to anyone who has adopted the logical syntax of MPL where contrariety and proper contradiction are all reducible to sentential negation. The *ad hoc* character of Goodman's solution is revealed when we observe that it soon rules out some inferences we do want. Thus, suppose we allowed that the following inference is valid:

(C) since every circle is a figure, everyone who draws a circle draws a figure.

We could not then also block the validity of 'since every centaur is a unicorn, everyone who draws a centaur draws a unicorn'. To block the latter, we should have to treat 'drawer of a centaur' as a single non-relational phrase on a par with 'picture of a centaur' which Goodman does not think of as relational. But this would put us back to the days of Jungius

[10] Nelson Goodman, 'On Likeness of Meaning', in *Semantics and Philosophy of Language* V ed. L. Linsky (University of Illinois Press, 1952), pp. 70–1.

who first tried to formalize (C). It is said that Frege succeeded where Jungius had failed. But if Goodman is right, (C) cannot be formalized: there is no way to get 'every circle-drawer is a figure-drawer' from the premiss of (C). The moral of this discussion is that it is not just harmless paradox to say that the absence of A's is reason for the truth of 'every A is . . .'. For it has pernicious consequences.[11]

[11] The paradox of material implication in the logic of propositions is strictly analogous to the paradox of vacuous universals in the logic of terms. Assuming the adequacy of the standard account of 'if . . . then' and bearing in mind that Gilbert Ryle never read a word of Santayana's works the following proposition is true:

(L) If Ryle read Santayana, he failed to appreciate him.

The paradox here is that the following is also true:

(L*) If Ryle read Santayana, he appreciated him.

Compare (L) with its presumed equivalent:

(M) It is not the case that Ryle read Santayana and that he appreciated him.

There is nothing paradoxical about M or about the corresponding equivalent to L*:

(M*) It is not the case that Ryle read Santayana and that he failed to appreciate him.

To explain why (L) and (L*) are paradoxical while (M) and (M*) are not we attend to the distinction between primitive and derived propositions in the logic of propositions. The primitive signs in propositional logic are 'and' (+) and 'not' (−). Propositions containing 'if then' or 'or' are not primitive and are understood as being defined from the primitive propositions. The latter contain no signs other than 'and' and 'not'. Thus 'if p then q' is defined as 'not: p and not q' and 'not p or not q' is defined as 'not: p and q' and so on for all non-primitive forms.

The examples of (L) and (M) indicate that the forms 'if p then q' and 'not: p and not q' differ in an important way. For the falsity of p is a non-paradoxical reason for the truth of the primitive form but not for the truth of the conditional form. Part of the explanation for this is that when someone says 'if p then q' he is interested in the truth or falsity of q on the condition that p is true; we are informed that q is then true and not false. Now it may well be the case that p is in fact false but that is not the case in which we are interested in the truth or falsity of q. We cannot accommodate our conditional interest in the truth value of q if we assume that 'if p then q' is unqualifiedly equivalent to 'not: p and not q'. On the other hand, if we accept the theory of primitive propositions, we can say 'if p then q' is defined as 'not: p and not q' but that this definition is restricted to the case where 'p' is true. So just as 'every A is B' and 'every A is not-B' are not defined for the case where both subcontraries are false, so 'if p then q' and 'if p then not-q' are not defined for the case where 'p' is false and both 'not: p and not q' and 'not: p and q' are false. If the theory of primitive propositions is adopted and a truth table is drawn for 'if p then q' it will look like this:

	if p	then q
t	t	t
f	t	f

Thus the conditional is true if the consequent is true and false if the consequent is false.

So understood, 'if then' is not the same as the sign of the material conditional in standard logic. If one wishes to use the material conditional in translating 'if then' there will be some intensional price to pay. If, for example, one added to a standard system of propositional logic a sign of contrariety so that 'p and "p" ' would be contraries but with 'p″' not equivalent to '-p' then 'if p then q' could be represented as a conjunction of several propositions. For a formulation along these lines see my 1963 paper 'Truth Functional Counterfactuals' (*Analysis Supplement*, January 1963).

6. The lack of an adequate theory of negation shows up in the paradox of vacuous universal propositions; more drastically it shows up in connection with false dilemmas that seem to threaten the law of excluded middle. Consider again the familiar example:

    (K) Either the present king of France is bald or the present king of France is not bald.

According to Russell, K is false; according to Strawson, K is neither true nor false. Even if we put aside Russell's interpretation of 'the present king of France is not bald' as a compound proposition that has a false existential component ('there is one and only one present king of France') we have three formal possibilities of interpreting it:

    (i) as the negation or primitive contradictory of 'the present king of France is bald'
   (ii) as its primitive contrary
  (iii) as its proper contradictory.

On interpretation (i), K is true and valid. On interpretation (ii), K is false. Interpretation (iii) is excluded because no proper contradictory is defined for 'the present king of France is bald' in the vacuous case.

The example of Strawson shows how a philosopher may react when he feels himself confronting a choice between rejecting outright the law of excluded middle and introducing a truth value gap for a proposition that is, *prima facie*, meaningful. The conservative choice is to argue for a truth value gap. A related but different situation occurs in number theory. According to a well-known unproven (and possibly unprovable) conjecture, every even number may be represented as the sum of two prime numbers. Let us call an even number *regular* if it is the sum of two prime numbers and irregular if it is not. And let us consider the disjunction.

    (E) Either some even number is irregular or every even number is regular.

According to intuitionist mathematicians, E is not a valid sentence because neither of its disjuncts is decidable. E is not an anomalous case; in number theory most of the interesting

propositions lack an effective decision procedure. The intuitionist takes the bull by the horns and denies the applicability of 'p or not-p' to the propositions of number theory and
other branches of mathematics where undecidable propositions abound. As Dummett explains him:

Since we cannot, save for the most elementary statements, guarantee
that we can find either a proof for them or a disproof for them we
have no right to assume of each statement that it is either true or
false.[12]

According to this explanation, undecidable statements lack
truth value. But statements of this kind are not anomalous and
this affects the applicability of the classical law of excluded
middle. So we have both a rejection of the logical law of
excluded middle and the semantic law of bivalence.

The rejection of the classical laws is originally made
necessary by what the intuitionists consider to be an illegitimate extension of the interpretation of the universal
quantifier from finite to infinite domains. Referring to propositions like 'every even number is regular' Dummett
remarks:

To conceive of the statement possessing a determinate objective truth
value independently of our being able to prove or disprove it is to
make fallacious assimilation of the infinite to the finite case; our grasp
of the use of mathematical statements cannot supply us with any such
conception of truth for them.[13]

The justification for rejecting the law of excluded middle in
thus tied to quite general considerations concerning the
meaning of statements about all the objects of an unbounded
domain.

In a recent paper, Dummett argues that the intuitionists'
repudiation of the law of excluded middle and several other
classical laws is grounded in 'a thesis in the theory of meaning
of the highest possible level of generality':

To know the meaning of a statement, is to be capable of recognizing
what counts as verifying the statement . . . In the mathematical case

---

[12] M. Dummett, *Elements of Intuitionism* with M. O. Clark (Oxford University
Press, 1977), p. 6.
[13] Dummett, *Elements of Intuitionism*, p. 8.

that which establishes a statement as true is the production of a deductive argument terminating in that statement . . . In the general case a statement is established as true by a process of reasoning not usually deductive in character.[14]

The intuitionists' repudiation of the law of excluded middle thus rests on reasons for rejecting one theory of meaning in favour of another and if Dummett is right, these reasons do not relate specifically to the nature of mathematical objects as some intuitionists claim. Rather they are reasons

. . . in favour of replacing as the central notion of the theory of meaning, the condition under which a statement is true whether we know or can know that that condition obtains, by the condition under which we acknowledge the statement as conclusively established, a condition under which we must, by the nature of the case be capable effectively of recognizing whenever it obtains.[15]

These are rather drastic and far-reaching measures for rejecting E and similar disjunctions that intuitionists find objectionable. It is clear that Dummett sees no alternative to a new theory of meaning justifying the thesis that E has no truth value. As we saw earlier, Dummett believes this theory of meaning to be quite generally acceptable and not necessarily related to any thesis about the specific nature of the objects of mathematical propositions. But whether he is right about this or not, he shares the assumption that rejecting disjunctions of form 'either some x is y or not' will require a theory that justifies a truth-value gap for the disjunction.

Suppose, however, that we could reject E and similar disjunctive propositions whose limbs are undecidable without recourse to a general theory that ties truth values to decidability. We should then have no need to tamper with the sentential connectives and no need to find fault with the law of excluded middle. We could maintain a realist position on undecidable propositions holding that they too are either true or false even where we cannot prove either one of these alternatives. It would, nevertheless, be possible to indulge our intuitionist sympathies by refusing to accept the legitimacy of propositions affirming undecidable predicates of an unboun-

[14] Dummett, *TOE*, p. 227.
[15] Dummett, *TOE*, p. 226.

ded totality. We could do this by maintaining that proper contradictories are not defined for undecidable propositions. Applied to the undecidable proposition 'some even number is irregular' we should allow only the primitive contradictory 'no even number is irregular'; the latter will be false or true depending on whether the former is true or false. On the other hand, 'every even number is regular' will not be defined as a form that is contradictory to 'some even number is irregular' and the use of this form will be banned as illegitimate and without truth value.

To make decidability a condition for having a proper contradictory does not go so far as Dummett who makes it a condition for having a truth value. But it is obviously in the intuitionist spirit. Analogously, those who have respect for categories make category correctness a condition for having a proper contradictory rejecting 'every even number is fed' as the proper contradictory of the category-incorrect proposition 'some even number is unfed'. One who wishes to adopt a modified form of intuitionism that does not commit him to the thesis that undecidable propositions have no truth values may now reject the validity of E while not going so far as to reject that of

E* either some even number is irregular or no even number is irregular.

E* is, of course, an instance of 'p or not p'. But it is distinct from E. Analogously, the category theorist who eschews truth-value gaps will acknowledge the validity of 'either some even number is unfed or no even number is unfed' although he has rejected that of 'either some even number is unfed or every even number is fed'.

One need not, of course, be an intuitionist, not even one as moderate as is allowed for by the recognition of a difference between E and E*. For one may object to making decidability a condition for proper contradiction and insist that 'no even number is irregular' is equivalent to 'every even number is regular'. But for those who have qualms about the use of undecidable predicates in talk about all of the objects in some unbounded domain, a difference between 'no even number is P' and 'every even number is un-P' may be welcome. In saying that no even number is irregular, I need not be understood as making a claim about all even numbers; formally speaking I am doing no more than denying the claim that some even number is irregular, that is, I am claiming that this is false. A similar reservation will not make sense about 'every even number is regular'. So a theory that distinguishes the primitive contradictory form from the proper contradictory form may be accepted by those who feel that affirming a predicate like 'is the sum of two prime numbers' of all even numbers may well be illegitimate, but who are unwilling to pay anything like the price of rejecting standard logic. There may, of course, be other reasons for developing an intuitionist logic. But the desire to rule out unbounded general statements with undecidable predicates can be satisfied in less radical ways.

7. Frege's doctrine that propositions with negative predicates are to be understood as being of form '-p' or as containing components of this form is a source of difficulties, anomalies, and paradoxes that characteristically beset the modern analytical philosopher who works with the Fregean organon. Frege had recommended his doctrine on grounds of economy and when Quine recommends that we dispense with a theory of categories, he too is appealing to our Occamist predilections to get by with less in the way of logical primitives. I have, however, shown that TFL is at least as economical as MPL in its use of logical notions. It would, therefore, appear that we can satisfy our healthy Occamist appetite for less even if we recognize contrariety as a distinct form of negativity. There is, moreover, an overriding reason to accept contrariety or term negation as distinct and independent of contradiction or propositional negation. For we need to be able to distinguish between denying *of Socrates* that he is wise and denying *that* Socrates is wise. If the first is reduced to the second, then we have no way of saying anything negative *about Socrates*. For the second is not about Socrates at all but about the proposition that Socrates is wise. Of that proposition, it says that it is not the case.

It is not always seen that the *exclusive* use of a sentential negation precludes the possibility that a negative proposition can have the same subject as a corresponding positive proposition. If we are to have negative propositions about

Socrates, we cannot avoid the use of negative terms. It is, therefore, vital that logic finds an independent role for term negation. The difficulties that we have discussed in this and the preceding chapter are symptomatic of the principled neglect of just this vital need. The neglect is, for example, responsible for the false dilemma that Russell and Strawson faced. For it is possible to deny that the present king of France is bald without affirming that he is not bald. Russell could only get at this distinction by an elaborate theory of the logical form of propositions whose subjects are definite descriptions. And Strawson overreacted by withdrawing truth values from the present king of France is/isn't bald'.

In conclusion, the discussion of this and the preceding chapter shows how a logic grounded in the traditional oppositions of positive and negative terms and positive and negative propositions can cope with some of the problems that characteristically arise for the analytical philosopher who works with the Fregean organon. More specifically, I hope to have persuaded the reader that the current fashion of making do with sentential negation is an economy that neither the philosopher nor the logician can afford to practice.

15

Referring and Existing

1. In this final chapter, I shall touch on several theses argued for earlier, indicating connections that may not be readily apparent and elaborating further on some comparisons of the logical theories of MPL and TFL.

The theory of reference appropriate to TFL takes indefinite reference by 'some S' to some S (or to something taken for an S) to be primary, holding that definite reference traces its source to indefinite reference. The suggestion is implicit in the very syntax of TFL: so far as logical form is concerned, there is nothing to choose between 'Socrates is wise' and 'some man is wise'. There is in TFL nothing corresponding to the kind of expression known in MPL as an individual constant or individual variable; all elementary TFL propositions are assertions or denials of propositions of form 'some/every S is/isn't P'. The theory of reference that we have developed on this ground considers definite reference to be essentially anaphoric or pronominal: the move from 'an S' to 'that S' is basic.

2. Having argued that the definite subject is 'pronominal' and anaphoric, we went on to say that this applies also to proper names of persons and places and that these should be understood as 'special duty' pronouns introduced for reasons of obvious convenience for referring to the things in question. Our discussion was confined to proper names, that is, to names of things that are ordinarily in the categories to which persons and places belong. But we also name things that are not in such categories and in the case of things in the non-standard categories the process of naming is more codified by conventions. Examples of such names are 'wisdom' (the name of a property), 'the raising of my arm' (the name of an act or movement), 'that snow is white' (the name of a proposition), 'sadness' (the name of a mood). Names for things of these sorts may be called conventional names since the conventions for naming them are fixed. Having discovered an island, I am free to name it as I please. Having raised my arm, I have made a movement but the naming of this movement is conventional: I must refer to it by 'the raising of my arm' or some phrase to that effect. In the case of conventional names the difference, ordinarily important, between a name and a descriptive pronoun, has little purchase. One who insists that 'wisdom' and 'the raising of my arm' are not genuine names but descriptive definite expressions is as much in the right as one who like myself allows himself the latitude of calling them names. In any case what is important is that these definite expressions are introduced for strongly referential D-type pronouns.

The origin of a conventional name in an implicit mediating definite reference and a D-type pronominal expression may be made explicit. The following sequence is an example:

I have raised my arm
(so) I have made a movement
the movement in question is (called) the raising of my arm.

It would be inappropriate to use a baptismal formula for the third step: 'let the movement in question be called the raising of my arm'. This contrasts with

I have just discovered an island
the island in question is (will henceforth be known as) Tamler Island.

Names of properties, acts, propositions, moods and other states, are bestowed in accordance with certain strict conventions. Consider the following sequences:

Tom is wise
(so) Tom has a determinate character (one possessed by all who are wise)
the character in question is (called) wisdom.

Here, too, it would be inappropriate to say 'let it be called wisdom'.

snow is white
(a proposition is being entertained)
the name of the proposition is 'that snow is white'
(or) the proposition in question is that snow is white.

Here the convention stipulates that for a proposition expressible by a sentence 'p' we form the name 'that p'.

Tom is sad
(so) Tom is in a mood
the name of the mood is 'sadness'
(or) sadness is the mood in question

The topic of names for things in the non-standard categories is a large one and I am here concerned to do no more than indicate the approach to it within the theory of reference appropriate to TFL. Characteristically the pronominal move is mediated by a proposition—usually tacit—that refers to a thing or things in the non-standard category under consideration. Thus we saw that the move from 'Tom is wise' to talk about his wisdom is mediated by 'Tom possesses a property' enabling reference to the property in question. Names of states, acts, propositions and other things in the non-standard categories are similarly mediated by the appropriate tacit antecedent.

We may here recall Ramsey's observation that 'Tom is wise' is as much about what Tom is or has, as about Tom himself. Similarly, 'Tom runs' is as much about what Tom does as it is about Tom. The shift of attention from Tom to what he is or does is important for the understanding of adverbs. Here the general theory we have outlined has certain advantages which I shall briefly remark. Consider:

I raised my arm slowly.

The adverb indicates the appropriateness of a Ramseyan shift from talk about me to talk about what I did. I raised my arm—So I did something, and what I did was slow. We may, in fact, analyse 'I raised my arm slowly' as 'I raised my arm and it (the movement in question) (the raising of my arm) was slow'. A similar analysis of 'Brutus killed Caesar with a knife' would represent it as 'Brutus killed Caesar and it (the deed in question) was done with a knife'. The analysis relies on a mediation which leads to the formation of the pronominal 'it' and the possibility of forming the conventional name 'the killing of Caesar by Brutus'.

3. The requirement that a name be traceable to its antecedents is not always possible to satisfy. When it is in *principle* unsatisfiable, the name is illegitimate in the way that 'he' is in 'he is coming soon' when 'he' has been arbitrarily introduced without backing in an antecedent context of reference. Having thus uttered 'he', I could go on to replace it by a name, NN, but the name NN will then be no better than the empty pronoun it replaces. In the case of names conventionally formed, we may violate the requirement that an antecedent be traceable. This happens when I 'say'

what I am now saying is interesting (false, boring, etc.)

intending the statement itself to be the referent of 'what I am now saying'. It is then impossible to find an antecedent for the propositional name 'what I am now saying'. Ryle has here noticed that the attempt to trace one leads to a regress of 'namely riders' (what I am now saying, namely, what I am now saying). The regress is symptomatic of the impossibility of giving the pronominal history of the definite subject 'what I am now saying'. Generally, if 'that p is Q' is to be meaningful, the name 'that p' cannot have been formed by replacing the pronominal expression 'the proposition in question' when that refers to a proposition purportedly expressed by 'p'. More generally, a pronominal sentence cannot serve as its own antecedent. That much is implicit in the pronominal theory of definite subjects as it applies to propositional names.

4. Pronominalization is fundamental to any logic and it is natural to ask whether pronouns can be represented in the primitive unquantified base language of TFL which lacks the notion of 'every'. This question is answered in the affirmative; for example the sequence 'some children are in the yard; they are toddlers' can be represented as ⌊some children⌋$_{Jk}$ are in the yard and *K are toddlers. The second conjunct normally entails 'every K is a toddler'. But where there are no children in the yard, both of the subcontrary sentences 'some K are toddlers' and 'some K are not toddlers' will be false and 'every K is a toddler' will then not be defined as equivalent to 'no K is a non-toddler'. The fact that 'every K is a toddler' is undefined for the vacuous case may give rise to the feeling that pronominals referring to the children in question have no legitimate use. It is this kind of feeling that Strawson appeals to in setting up an existential condition for the use of 'the S'. However, the fact that pronouns are representable in primitive form shows that Strawson's condition is not operative. Consider:

(1) A French king is at the Ritz. He is quite bald.

Since the antecedent sentence of (1) is false, the pronominal sentence is vacuous. But the latter is equivalent to 'the king of France is bald' or perhaps to 'the king of France who is staying at the Ritz is bald'. Clearly all such sentences are false and not 'neither true nor false'. They are false *because* they are vacuous. The existence of S is therefore not in general a condition for 'the S is Q' having a truth value. This is made clear by consideration of the fact that the vacuousness has no effect whatever on the primitive analysis of 'the S is Q' as 'some K is Q'—a proposition that entails 'No K is not Q'.

It might still be argued that 'the king of France is bald is *here* tied to an antecedent but that this is not always, or even normally, the case. Certainly Russell did not think of sentences whose subjects were definite descriptions as normally anaphoric. And if we adopt the view—contrary to the view of this essay—that 'the S is Q' does not have an anaphoric subject, then Strawson's doctrine that statements made by means of such sentences are truth valueless in the vacuous case may seem to be a viable alternative to our own account. I believe, however, that just this line of defence is unavailable to Strawson. For his strongest point against Russell is that 'the S is Q' *is* implicitly an anaphoric form. Strawson himself believed that all statements made by sentences of this form had behind them the presupposition of the truth of 'an S exists', but apart from the fact that he thought of the antecedent proposition as overtly existential, he certainly held that 'the S is Q' had an antecedent backing. Assume then that someone now says 'the present king of France is bald' and that the backing for this is

'France has a king at the present time' or 'the present king of France exists'. We then have

The present king of France exists and he is bald.

The first conjunct is the antecedent sentence and it is false. It is surely wrong to refrain from assigning a truth value to the second (pronominal) proposition on the grounds of the falsity of the first. But that is what Strawson's doctrine of presupposition would have us do.

The thesis that proper names are special duty pronouns replacing common pronouns like 'it' or 'he' in pronominal sentences is perhaps more seriously affected by the vacuousness of antecedent sentences. For it may be argued that a proper name is normally introduced in place of a pronominal subject with wild quantity, and this requires that the pronouns for which we now use the name be of form $*K$, where '$*K$ is P' is understood as a particular proposition that entails its universal generalization, which can only happen when the existence condition is satisfied. Suppose that Homer is understood by me to be someone who was said to have been a blind poet who wrote the Odyssey and the Iliad, and suppose there was no such person. Then although we could form the proterm of the antecedent sentence 'a blind poet wrote the Odyssey and the Iliad' moving from that to 'him' and 'he' and further on to 'Homer' as the proterm denoting the man in question, we could not have formed pronominal subjects of form 'every K'. One might then say: if Homer never existed then 'Homer' is not a genuine proper name since it cannot replace pronominal subjects of form '$*K$'. One would then be maintaining that proper names subjects cannot be introduced in the logically primitive language. The forming of proper names is anyway not a purely logical matter; there may be excellent linguistic reasons for accepting as a condition for the introduction of a genuine proper name in subject position that the background propositions for the pronominals to be replaced not be vacuous.

It would all the same be wrong to see a puzzle in 'Homer never existed'. For we could still allow for 'Homer' as an expression that has replaced the proterm which denotes the person said to have composed the Iliad etc., even as we claim that there is no such person, thereby claiming that 'Homer' cannot serve as a subject with quantity. Here we rely on the distinction between the use of 'Socrates' as a full-fledged subject expression of form '*K' and its use as a mere proterm of form 'K'. In saying that Homer did not exist, we say that there was no such thing as K (or that no K existed); the unavailability of quantified subjects does not affect our ability to use the term 'K'

5. In termist logic the logical forms of 'Homer exists' and 'a creator exists' are not distinguished. Generally, any proposition of form '(a) P exists' (or variants like 'there is a P') will parse as 'some P is an actual thing' or, equivalently, as 'some actual thing is a P'. Whether 'something is P' has existential import depends on the amplitude of the terms. If the terms of 'some thing is P' have standard amplitude the proposition is existential and not otherwise. Even if we assume standard amplitude the modern reader will find 'some thing is a tiger' a strained way of expressing 'there is a tiger' or 'there are tigers'. It is, however, important for TFL that all such expressions can be put into subject-predicate form. Even sentences like 'it is cold', and 'it is raining' are regimented to have the form 'an x is a y' ('a state of cold is obtaining', 'a raining is taking place'). Here we confront the use of such controversial predicates as 'exists', 'obtains', 'takes place'—expressions that many a modern philosopher refuses to call predicates. Bolstering this refusal is Kant's critique of the ontological argument, with its insight that terms like 'existent' or 'occurrent' differ from terms like 'striped' and 'dangerous' in not really characterizing their subjects. All the same these controversial terms can and do occupy subject and predicate positions syntactically. Admittedly when I say (some) tigers exist, I do not characterize tigers in a way that I would if I said that some tigers are dangerous. Similarly if I say that raining is taking place I do not tell you anything about the raining that is taking place (as I would if I told you that it is intense or mild). But this is no reason to deny term status to terms like 'existent' and 'occurrent'. We must here distinguish between two negative theses concerning the status of existence as a predicate. There is the radical thesis which I am concerned to deny. For some say that existence is not a predicate and when asked what it *is* they reply: 'a quantifier'. It is this silly thesis that any advocate of TFL must deny. But others say something less fatuous and less drastic. These latter deny that existence (and obtaining, etc.) are *genuine* predicates. They too seem to me to be wrong but their thesis is not threatening to the logical syntax of TFL. The more moderate sceptics about the status of existence follow Kant in saying that to think of a thing and to think of it as existing is one and the same thing. As Kant uses 'exists' it means 'is a member of some world—actual or not'. But if 'exists = is actual' it will not follow that 'exists' is a trivial thing to say of a thing. For we have observed in chapter 10 that the terms of 'some tigers exist' have unrestricted amplitude. One who tells me that there are tigers probably uses 'tigers' as a term of unrestricted amplitude; he tells me about tigers in the way that an informant may tell me about gold in saying that some gold is in that cave. Of course, existing does not distinguish one actual tiger from another. Nor more does being in the cave distinguish anything that is in the cave from anything else in the cave. But being in the cave does characterize the gold under consideration in locating some of it in the cave. Similarly, existing does characterize the tigers under consideration. For the tigers under consideration in 'some tigers exist' are those in a compossible set of worlds actual and possible. And to be told that some tigers are in the actual world is therefore not trivial. In a similar way, I may be informed that there are no unicorns. This, too, is non-trivial information about the unicorns under consideration; for I learn that none of them is a member of the actual world. In the same way when I hear that it is cold—that some cold obtains—I learn something about cold; I learn that it is present here and now. 'To think of cold and to think of it as a state that obtains (in some possible situation) is one and the same thing'. Yes, but if this is supposed to mean that 'obtains' is a trivial predicate, it misses the point for I needn't think of cold as actual and that is what I learn about cold when told that it obtains.

The informative character of 'exists', 'obtains', and other such predicates as they are ordinarily used comes from their unrestricted amplitude. The information these predicates give is not the usual kind; in one sense they do not characterize the objects that exist (obtain, etc.), but simply tell us where—in the worlds under consideration—things of that kind are to be found. The reader who is uncomfortable with the predicate use of 'exists' will hardly be comfortable with all this intemperate talk of possible worlds. He should not, for all his discomfort, dismiss the predicate use of 'exists' or deny that 'tigers exist' is a subject predicate sentence. For he may choose to say with Kant that 'exist', etc., is not a genuine predicate while acknowledging that it may well be a non-genuine one. I have objected to the man who would deny the syntactical fact that 'exists' is a predicate. It is, to repeat, essential to the point of view that I am advocating to say that 'there are tigers' is construable as a sentence of subject-predicate form. It is not essential to my point of view to insist on any thesis involving possible world semantics or metaphysics.[1]

6. The preceding discussion is something of an aside to those who, like myself, have been trained away from the locutions of the traditional 'subject-predicate logic', locutions which we modern schoolmen find odd and suspect. Even more suspect to our trained sensibility is the theory of reference of TFL which gives priority to 'some man' over 'Socrates' as a referring expression. The contemporary analytical philosopher is by and large a Fregean and to him a view of this kind can only be seen as a reversal of the true and scientific order of things, a sort of ptolemaic revolution. In MPL, reference begins with the logical subjects of atomic sentences and the meaning or truth conditions of all other sentences is inductively stipulated on an atomic base of propositions with definite singular subjects. But in TFL, the original vehicle of reference is the indefinite subject; the definite subject is derivative from the indefinite antecedent. In allowing that 'some S' has genuine reference to

---

[1] Words like 'thing', 'existent', 'actual' suffer from systematic ambiguity of amplitude as they are used in discourse. To reduce confusion in his own writings the philosopher might resolve to use 'exists' and '(is) actual' as synonyms and with unrestricted amplitude. The term 'thing' should be treated as 'horse' and allowed a shifting use relative to different amplitudes depending on context. Pegasus does not exist and is not actual but anyone conversant with the myth knows that something is both a horse and winged. On the other hand if we read the reports of a medieval traveller who says that he has seen a winged horse or that one thing he saw was a winged horse we should interpret 'horse' and 'thing' with standard amplitude and judge his assertion to be false.

an S or to an /S/, TFL ignores the requirement that a logical subject identifies its referent. Implicit in this is the distinction, important to TFL but ignored in MPL, between naming and referring. To refer is not to name; if naming is anything different from christening an object then it is a species of referring. As we have seen, the mode of reference of a name in subject position is very like that of an indefinite subject.

The doctrine of indefinite reference poses a threat to MPL and there are those who saw it as such. Peter Geach was uncommonly alert to the challenge implicit in the view that indefinite subjects do a job of referring and I was forced to spend considerable time in dealing with his attack on this traditional doctrine. It is unfortunate that Geach could not bring himself to take TFL seriously enough to treat it with respect. I shall not here add anything of substance to my discussion of chapters 3 and 4 in defence of the doctrine of indefinite reference. But it is instructive to remind oneself of the ease with which the Fregean, who finds himself considering the traditional alternative, thought he could dismiss it. To be sure, most modern philosophers simply ignored the traditional doctrine. But arguments like the following one—repeated in three of Geach's books—are not atypical of the style and calibre of criticism directed against the logical theories of TFL. As Geach sees it, the doctrine that is fundamental to the theory of reference of TFL, viz., that 'some S' could be said to refer to some S, is not much better than a hoary logical joke.

Jokes about 'no man' as a name are about three thousand years old. And what about 'some man'? We read that this phrase refers to some man.[2]

Or again in *Reference and Generality*:

Many logicians have taken it for granted that 'all men' refers to all men and 'some men' to some men but I have not yet come across the parallel view that 'no men' refers to no men.[3]

And in his latest book:

'Every', 'some' and 'no' belong neither to the category of names nor to that of predicates; they are *quantifiers*. Phrases like 'every man' and

---

[2] Geach, *LM*, p. 115.
[3] Geach, *R & G*, p. 11.

'some man' seem more like names . . . but jokes about 'no man' are about three thousand years old and it's hard to see that whereas 'Socrates' names Socrates, 'every man' does not name every man nor 'some man' some man.[4]

In calling 'no' a quantifier, Geach betrays that he has after all failed to see the point of the three thousand year old joke. The sentences 'not a creature was stirring' and 'no creature was stirring' differ only stylistically; just as 'not' is not a quantifier in the first sentence, so is 'no' not a quantifier in the second sentence. The referring expressions of TFL consist of a word of quantity and a term. The idea that 'no man' refers to no man in the way that 'some man' refers to some man is a joke only to one who playfully pretends that both are expressions of the same syntactical type, i.e., that 'no man' like 'some man' is a subject expression. But Geach is not pretending; he *seriously* holds that 'no man' is an intregal expression of logical grammar.[5] Having assimilated 'no man' to the category of 'some man', he waggishly observes that neither can be referring expressions since 'no man' clearly is not a referring expression. The non-referential character of the non-subject 'no man' is a red herring with no bearing whatever on the referential pretensions of an indefinite subject like 'some man'. The cousin to this fish is the question-begging assumption that any expression that refers to an object is 'naming' that object. Thus 'Socrates' in 'Socrates was wise' names Socrates. Of course, those who hold that 'some man' refers to some man do *not* hold that only names can refer and it is disheartening to see how far the critical standards have been relaxed by one who takes his own position as premiss and proceeds to 'show' that 'some man' cannot be a referring expression because it does not name a man.

None of this is serious criticism of TFL. Unfortunately, it is a fairly representative specimen of the kind of easy going 'bang bang you're dead' style of polemics when the target is TFL. I have, in this essay tried to show that a theory of reference appropriate to the logical syntax of traditional formal logic is an attractive alternative to the standard contemporary theory

---

[4] Geach, *RA*, p. 48.

[5] Geach also considers 'most' along with 'no' as a quantifier on all fours with 'some' and 'every'. See the remarks at the end of Appendix D.

and deserving of careful consideration. In some respects, my task was easier than it ought to have been; certainly it was easier than I expected it to be. For I expected a body of formidable and detailed criticism of traditional logical theory. But what I found was mainly tendentious dogmatism parading as criticism and a cavalier disregard of the traditional positions.

7. The theory of indefinite reference is implicit in the doctrine that the elementary proposition is general in form. So I have argued, and then proceeded to argue that the definite subject has its origins in indefinite antecedents. Analysis of definite reference reveals that the syntax of a sentence like 'Socrates is wise' does not differ in essential respects from that of a sentence like 'a man is wise' or 'every man is wise' so far as the form of the subject is concerned. Here we touch again on the controversy concerning the syntax of the logical subject. For Frege had opened a grammatical gulf between 'genuine' logical subjects like 'Socrates' and the quasi-subject forms like 'a man'. In this respect, the logical syntax of TFL is closer to the linguist's idea of what a logical grammar should be like. It is to be expected that the linguist will sometimes betray his traditional sympathies and, equally to be expected, that the vigilant Fregean will chastize him for back-sliding. We remind ourselves here of Geach's objections to Chomsky's reasonable and straightforward approval of the manner in which traditional logical grammar classifies proper names along with other referring expressions under the one general head of Noun Phrases.

Geach expects the linguist to respect the syntactical insights of modern predicate logic. Yet why should the linguist be respectful of a point of view that summarily dismisses his basic classifications? Dummett has correctly characterized Frege's attitude to the *prima facie* structures of natural language and the reasons for it.

Frege has solved the problem [of explaining inferences involving multiple generality] which has baffled logicians for millenia by ignoring natural language . . . Indeed Frege came later to the conclusion that natural language is in principle incoherent . . . All that can be at issue is how deep the incoherence lies, that is how fundamental are the principles governing its structure which would need to be modified if the incoherence were to be removed. Frege believed it to be very deep indeed. Undoubtedly his predisposition to adopt such a belief was formed by the experience which the discovery of the quantifier variable notation had given him.[6]

Recent efforts on the part of philosophically sophisticated linguists to incorporate the logical syntax of Frege in a theory of deep structure ignore this warning. My own belief is that all such efforts must fail and that they are in any case quite gratuitous. For there is at hand a logical syntax that is not at odds with the linguists' basic intuitions, one that has developed historically alongside of the classical grammar which in Chomsky's words 'is by and large correct as far as it goes'. The linguist who is concerned to understand the role of logical form in natural syntax will be naturally open to acceptable alternatives to a logical system that was developed in conscious suspicion and disregard of the categories of natural grammar. We have lately discussed some of the implications for logic and for metaphysics of the contemporary treatment of negation as a sentential operator or 'connective'. Jerrold Katz has remarked on the bad fit of the modern logician's conception of negation to the linguistic facts of life:

In natural languague negation is not a mechanism for forming compound propositions. Logicians treat negation as a propositional connective . . . within the orthodox conception of logic there is no choice. These systems have to treat negation as applying to propositions as wholes because their restriction of the vocabulary for expressing logical form to the logical particles precludes the kind of internal term and predicate structure that makes it possible to treat negation as a means of turning around concepts inside the meaning of terms and predicates.[7]

Although Katz is certainly right about the contrast between the modern logician's conception of negation and its actual working in the natural languages I cannot agree with his diagnosis that a conception of logic that restricts the expression of logical form to some finite set of logical particles is the culprit. In any case TFL is not open to Katz's criticism since the

    [6] Dummett, *Frege*, pp. 20–1.
    [7] Jerrold, J. Katz, *Propositional Structure & Illocutionary Force* (T. J. Crowell, 1977), p. 238.

theory of term quality is wholly in keeping with the natural requirement to 'treat negation as a means of turning around concepts inside the meaning of terms and predicates'. We may also mention here our own extensive criticism of MPL's treatment of pronouns as bound variables and the contrast with a traditional treatment that gives better syntactical insight into the working of pronouns in natural language.[8]

The quantifier variable notation of MPL has taught logicians and philosophers much that the linguist cannot allow to be correct. If, for contrast, we consider the algebraic notation of TFL, we find nothing that need disturb the linguist. Moreover, the solution to the problem of multiple generality does not require the quantifier variable notion for we have seen that problem solved in the transcriptive algebraic notation without the usual aspersions about the logically misleading character of the syntax of the natural languages. The difference between transcribing and translating a sentence is relevant here. Where the Fregean sees obscurity in a sentence like 'every boy is an admirer of some girl', advocating its translation or replacement by a form like

$$(x) \, [\text{if } x \text{ is a boy then} (\exists \, y) \, (y \text{ is a girl and } x \text{ is an admirer of } y)]$$

the older logic sees no need to translate the sentence but contents itself instead with transcribing it as

$$-\text{boy} + \text{admirer of} + \text{girl}.$$

The TFL formula preserves the syntax of the original; the MPL formula has dismissed it as suspect, confused, and logically useless. The TFL formula is useful for inference and is concrete evidence that the linguist need not be at odds with his logical self. For those linguists who have enough on their plates without taking on the job of reconciling the claims of a hostile

[8] The recent attempts to impose Fregean models of logical form as conditions of adequacy on linguistic theories of deep structures are beginning to meet some resistance from philosophers. Strawson's recent article criticizing Davidson's analysis of action sentences is an admirable example of the sort of thing that could and should be done. It takes up the thread of Strawson's earlier work in logical theory in which he showed that quantification theory does not provide the right kind of syntactical insights into natural language. Strawson's own attempt to reconcile Fregean ideas of logical form with the intuitions of the linguists does not measure up to the standards he demands of Davidson and others. The proper relation of logic to linguistics is distorted by the assumption of atomicity which Strawson has not freed himself of.

and suspicious logic with what they understand about the underlying structures of the natural languages, the availability of a neutral and inferentially powerful logic that does not translate away from natural syntax but conservatively transcribes the vernacular for logical reckoning should be welcome.

Though the algebraic notation does not teach suspicion of natural language, it teaches other things equally exciting. It, too, casts light on problems that have been around for millenia. The notation forcibly suggests that the basic logical words of a language are words of opposition—positive and negative signs—that confer valence on the material signs, the terms and the propositions. Traditional logic is a logic of oppositions— the old square of opposition is not a misnomer—which sees logical form in terms of contrariety and contradiction. We have seen how these oppositions define the opposition of quantity which is then also representable as a plus-minus opposition. Despite the novelty of the algebraic notation, it is entirely traditional in concept. The textbooks of the past few centuries attest to this by their assignments of 'distribution values' to the terms of the propositions entering into logical reckoning. It turns out that a term is distributed just in case it has a negative value in the algebraic notion and undistributed just in case it has a positive value in that notation. The extension of negative and positive valence to whole propositions in a calculus of propositions is a natural application of the doctrine of distribution to propositions. The contrast with MPL is clear. Where MPL simply enumerates the logical signs and tells us that a logical sign is a sign on the list enumerated, TFL tells us something about what these signs have in common and shows us how their common nature derives from the oppositions that are at the foundation of logic.

I have spoken about the possibility of a sympathetic approach to TFL by the contemporary linguist. But that seems to me to be very much dependent on the degree of acceptance that TFL and the logical theories that are appropriate to it can command among philosophers. Acceptance by philosophers is primary; at any rate as a philosopher it is my primary concern. I should be more optimistic about the prospects for this if the fate of philosophical and scientific theories were determined by simple functions of their adequacy, simplicity or correctness.

In the present instance, matters are made more difficult by the circumstance that philosophers have just got over rejecting TFL. There are few who do not think that TFL has not been decisively refuted and replaced. On the other hand, I am convinced that being right is a distinct advantage. Also, and in any event, there is the fun and fuss of controversy to enjoy. This is no small thing; I have enjoyed writing this book as much for the perverse pleasures of advocacy—in this day and age—of Aristotle over Frege as for the more unexceptionable of pleasures that came from seeing more clearly into the nature of reference and inference and other sparkling things in the realm of philosophical logic. And of course, although I believe I am mainly right about the big things, it is likely I am wrong about many things, including perhaps some big ones. On these I await correction.

Appendix A

Translation Rules

1. In an article entitled *Formal Linguistics and Formal Logic* Janet Dean Fodor observes that 'no precise and explicit translation rules relating a natural language and a system of logic have ever been formulated. In logic textbooks the principles of translation are presented informally . . . only rules of thumb are given . . . The student must rely on his own intuitions'.

The observation is correct and familiar but Fodor adds:

The fact that generations of students in introductory logic courses have picked up the art of translation suggests that the task of formulating an explicit set of translating rules is a possible one. It would be rather implausible to maintain that the implicit principles with which someone operates in exercising his skill at translation could never be explicitly characterized.[1]

This too is right and indeed a set of translation rules is at hand if we restrict ourselves to the canonical fragment of natural language sentences that traditional logic works with.

Let us call a sentence of a natural language that enters into deductive reasoning a *cognitive* sentence. Among cognitive sentences we have 'there are black swans', 'some swans are black', 'only Quakers are pacifists' and 'no non-Quakers are pacifists' but not 'keep off the grass!' or 'welcome back!' That subset of cognitive sentences is *canonical* in TFL which directly transcribes into algebraic notation. The general form of a canonical sentence in transcription is

$$\pm\,(\pm\,X\,\pm\,Y)$$
Yes/not (some/every X is/isn't Y)

[1] *New Horizons in Linguistics*, ed. John Lyons (Penguin, Harmondsworth) p. 207

in which X and Y hold the place of interchangeable terms that may be negative as in 'some non-citizen is a professor', '$+ (-C) + P$', or compound as in 'some citizen is a gentleman and a scholar '$+ C + \langle + G + S \rangle$', or relational as in 'every citizen is an owner of a farm', '$- C + (O^2 + F)$', or singular as in '(some) Tom is a citizen', '$+ T + C$'.

It is a fundamental thesis of traditional (pre-Fregean) logic that any cognitive sentence of a natural language is either itself canonical or else can be paraphrased as a canonical sentence. The task of specifying rules for paraphrasing into canonical form belongs to linguistics. The logician properly confines himself to the characterization of the canonical subset as in any case he must. When the syntax of the canonical subset is fully characterized and supplemented by rules for forming compound sentences (conjunctions, conditionals, etc.) then for all logical purposes the specification of the logical syntax of natural language is complete. We remark, *en passant*, that TFL's preference for 'some swans are black' over 'there are black swans' is a pre-Fregean bias that is in accord with the linguistic idea that sentences whose structure is straightforwardly NP/VP are fundamental.

2. Having characterized the logically canonical sentences of natural language in the traditional manner one may go on to consider the technical question of relating these sentences to the corresponding formulas of MPL. The task now is to specify the rules of translation between the canonical sentences of TFL and their canonical counterparts in MPL. Here we are in a position to give precise rules of correspondence that are applicable in translation or mapping procedures. The following three rules are especially prominent:

(R1) some A is B $\Leftrightarrow + A + B \Leftrightarrow (\exists x)(Ax \& Bx)$
(R2) every A is B $\Leftrightarrow - A + B \Leftrightarrow (x)(Ax \to Bx)$
(R3) α is B $\Leftrightarrow \pm \alpha + B \Leftrightarrow B\alpha$

For example we apply the rules in translating 'every patriarch is father of some male' as

(x) [x is a patriarch $\to (\exists y)(y$ is a male & x is father of y)]
(1) every patriarch is father of some male

(2) $\Rightarrow$ (x) [x is a patriarch $\rightarrow$ x is father of
        some male]   (R2)
(3) $\Rightarrow$ (x) [x is a patriarch $\rightarrow$ some male is
        fathered by x]   (converse)
(4) $\Rightarrow$ (x) [x is a patriach $\rightarrow$ ($\exists$y) (y is a male
        & y is fathered by x)]   (R1)
(5) $\Rightarrow$ (x) [x is a patriarch ($\exists$y) (y is a male &
        x is father of y)]   (converse)

Note that we have twice made use of the converse transformation. This can be avoided if we present the original sentence in 'subject–predicate normal form' (SNF). Every relational sentence has an SNF. A sentence is in SNF when each of its subject expressions is followed by its own predicate. (An expression is a *subject* if it is of form 'some S' or 'every S'.) The rule for writing a sentence in SNF is conveniently given in algebraic notation:

SNF Rule $\pm A_1 + R^m \ldots \pm A_m \Rightarrow \pm A_1 + (\pm A_2 + (\ldots$
              $\pm A_m + R^m) \ldots)$.

For example, the SNF of 'some sailor is giving every child a toy' is got by first straightforwardly transcribing it as ' $+ S + G^3 - C + T$' and then giving each subject its predicate in accordance with the SNF rule:

$+ S + (- C + (+ T + G^3))$.
some sailor (every child (some Toy gives))

Similarly the SNF of 'every patriarch is father of a male' is got by transforming ' $- P + F^2 + M$' into ' $- P + (+ M + F^2)$'. Using the SNF the translation proceeds thus

(x) $(Px \rightarrow (+ M + F^2 x))$ R2
(x) $(Px \rightarrow (\exists y)(My \& F^2 xy))$ R1

On the somewhat more complicated sailor sentence the translation goes like this:

$+ S + G^3 - C + T$
$+ S + (- C + (+ T + G^3))$ SNF
$(\exists x)(Sx \& (- C + (+ T + G^3_x)))$ R1
$(\exists x)(Sx \& ((y)(Cy \rightarrow (+ T + G^3 xy)))$ R2
$(\exists x)(Sx \& ((y)(Cy \rightarrow ((\exists_2)(T_2 \& G^3 xyz)))$ R1

3. Before proceeding it will be useful to present a more complete set of corresponding forms that can be appealed to in re-writing one expression as another in a given translation procedure.

CORRESPONDENCE RULES

I   *'And', 'Or', 'If then'*

p and q $\Leftrightarrow$ p&q $\Leftrightarrow$ $+$p$+$q

p or q $\Leftrightarrow$ p $\vee$ q $\Leftrightarrow$ $--$p$--$q

if p then q $\Leftrightarrow$ p $\to$ q $\Leftrightarrow$ $-$p$+$q

α is A and B $\Leftrightarrow$ $\pm\alpha+\langle+A+B\rangle \Leftrightarrow +[\pm\alpha+A]+[\pm\alpha+B] \Leftrightarrow A\alpha \& B\alpha$

α is A or B $\Leftrightarrow$ $\pm\alpha+\langle--A--B\rangle \Leftrightarrow --[\pm\alpha+A] --[\pm\alpha+B] \Leftrightarrow A\alpha \vee B\alpha$

II

R1(i) Some thing is A $\Leftrightarrow$ $+T+A \Leftrightarrow (\exists x)(Ax) \Leftrightarrow +[+Tx+E]+[\pm X+A] \Leftrightarrow (\exists x)(\pm X+A)$

R1(ii) Some A is B $\Leftrightarrow$ $+A+B \Leftrightarrow (\exists x)(Ax\&Bx) \Leftrightarrow +[+Tx+E]+[+[\pm X+A]+[\pm X+B]] \Leftrightarrow (\exists x)[(\pm X+A)\&(\pm X+B)]$

R2(i) Every thing is A $\Leftrightarrow$ $-T+A \Leftrightarrow (x)(Ax) \Leftrightarrow -[+Tx+E]+[\pm X+A] \Leftrightarrow (x)(\pm X+A)$

R2(ii) Every A is B $\Leftrightarrow$ $-A+B \Leftrightarrow (x)(Ax \to Bx) \Leftrightarrow -[+Tx+E]+[-[\pm X+A]+[\pm X+B]] \Leftrightarrow (x)[(\pm X+A) \to (\pm X+B)]$

In addition to the rules of correspondence there are two very useful rewrite rules:

SNF Rule $\pm A_1+R^m \ldots \pm A_m \Leftrightarrow \pm A_1+(\pm Az+(\ldots \pm A_m+R^m)\ldots)$

The 'X' Rule $(\ldots R^m)x \Leftrightarrow (\ldots R^m x)$.

4. Let us now see how the rules can be applied in an MPL $\Rightarrow$ TFL direction. Suppose we are given the following formula

(1) $(\exists x)[Cx \& (y)[A^{12}xy \vee -Py \vee (z)-(F^{12}zx \& B^{12}zy)]]$

and the legend:

C = (a) critic, P = (a) painting, A^{12} = admires, B^{12} = buys, F^{12} = (is) father of.

We want to know what (1) amounts to as an English sentence. To find out we would work from the inside outwards, first taking the quantified formula of smallest scope. Our aim is to eliminate the quantifiers, variables and connectives as far as we can by replacing the form '$(\exists x)(Sx \ \& \ Px)$' by '$+S+P$' and the form '$(x)(Sx \to Px)$' by '$-S+P$' till we reach a readable algebraic formula. We begin with the expression:

$$(z) - (F^{12}zx \ \& \ B^{12}zy)$$
$$= (z)(F^{12}zx \to -B^{12}zy)$$
$$= (z)[(\pm z + F^{12} \pm x) \to (\pm z + (-B^{12}) \pm y)]$$
$$= -(F^{12} \pm x) + (-B^{12}) \pm y \qquad \text{(R2)}$$
$$= \pm y + (-B^{21}) - (F^{12} \pm x) \qquad \text{(converse)}$$
$$= -[\pm y + B^{21} + (F^{12} \pm x)] \qquad \text{(D.M.)}$$

Taking a bit more from (1) we can eliminate one 'y':

$$-Py \lor (z) - (F^{12}zx \& B^{12}zy)$$
$$= (-[\pm y + P]) \lor [-[\pm y + B^{21} + (F^{12} \pm x)]]$$
$$= -[[\pm y + P] \ \& \ [y + B^{21} + (F^{12} \pm x)] \qquad \text{(D.M.)}$$
$$= -[\pm y + \langle +P + (B^{21} + (F^{12} \pm x))\rangle]$$

Now we consider the longer segment

$$(y)[A^{12}xy \lor -Py \lor (z) - (F^{12}zx \ \& \ B^{12}zy)]$$
$$= (y)[[(\pm x + A^{12} \pm y) \lor -[\pm y + \langle +P + (B^{12} + (F^{12} \pm x))\rangle]]$$
$$= (y)[(\pm y + \langle +P + (B^{21} + (F^{12} \pm x))\rangle) \to [\pm y + A^{21} \pm x)]$$
$$= -\langle +P + (B^{21} + (F^{12} \pm x))\rangle + (A^{21} \pm x) \qquad \text{(R2)}$$
$$= \pm x + A^{12} - \langle +P + (B^{21} + (F^{12} \pm x))\rangle \qquad \text{(converse)}$$

Now taking *all* of (1)

$$(\exists x)(Cx \ \& \ (y)[A^{12}xy \lor -Py \lor (z) - (F^{12}zx \ \& \ B^{12}zy)])$$
$$= (\exists x)[[\pm x + C] \ \& \ [\pm x + A^{12} - \langle +P + (B^{21} + (F \pm x)\rangle]]$$
$$= +C_{(X)} + A^{12} - \langle +P + (B^{21} + (F^{12} \pm x))\rangle$$

Some critic is admirer of every painting and bought by some father of him which reads 'some critic admires every painting bought by his father'.

TFL ⇒ MPL

The mapping of canonical TFL sentences into canonical MPL formulas is perhaps of greater interest than the reverse procedure for decoding the latter. Teachers of MPL will welcome a technique that helps the student to translate, say, 'every tail of a horse is a tail of an animal' as '$(x)[(\exists y)(Hy \,\&\, Txy) \to (\exists z)(Az \,\&\, Txz)]$'. The student can easily learn to transcribe the sentence as '$-(T+H)+(T+A)$' and to transform this transcription into SNF as $-(+H+T)+(+A+T)$. The translation then proceeds mechanically.

Very often the natural language sentence will contain a pronoun. An example is

(2) if a man signs, he is responsible

In translating such sentences we can initially represent the pronoun by the letter 'x' and later show how 'x' is bound in the MPL formula. Thus our transcription of (2) is

$$-[+Mx+S]+[\pm x+R]$$
$$(\exists x)(Mx \,\&\, Sx) \to Rx$$

Now in this formula the letter 'x' in 'Rx' is *not* a free variable so we may apply to it the 'rule of passage' '$(\exists x)(Fx) \to P = (x)(Fx \to P)$' thus binding 'x' in the final formula:

$$(x)((Mx \,\&\, Sx) \to Rx)$$

That this last move is legitimate is evident from the following alternative translation of (2):

$$-[+Mx+S]+[\pm x+R]$$
$$= -[+[+Tx+E]+[\pm x+M]+[\pm x+S]]$$
$$\quad +[\pm x+R] \qquad\qquad\qquad\qquad\qquad \text{(R1 ii)}$$
$$= (+Tx+E)\,\&\,(\pm x+M)\,\&\,(\pm x+S) \to (\pm x+R) \qquad \text{(I)}$$
$$= +Tx+E \to [(\pm x+M)\,\&\,(\pm x+S) \to (\pm x+R)]$$
$$= (x)[(Mx \,\&\, Sx) \to Rx] \qquad\qquad\qquad\qquad \text{(R2 ii)}$$

Let us now consider a fairly complicated example of MPL translation.

(3) Some editor is reading everything written by an author of
     a trilogy

(3T) $+ E + (R^2 - (W^2 + (A^2 + T)))$
SNF $+ E + (-(+(+T+A^2)+W^2)+R^2)$
       $= (\exists x)(Ex \,\&\, (-(+(+T+A^2)+W^2)+R^2 x)$
       $= (\exists x)(Ex \,\&\, (y)(+(+T+A^2)+W^2 y) \rightarrow R^2 xy))$
       $= (\exists x)(Ex \,\&\, (y)((\exists z)((+T+A^2 z)\,\&\, W^2 yz) \rightarrow Rxy))$
       $= (\exists x)[Ex \,\&\, (y)((\exists z)(\exists w)((Tw \,\&\, A^2 zw)\,\&\, W^2 yz)$
       $\rightarrow R^2 xy)]$

The noun phrases of the canonical TFL original are subject
expressions of form 'some/every S'. Note how the SNF
formula, in which the embeddedness of the NP/VP structures
are fully perspicuous, is in exact correspondence to the MPL
translation:

SNF: $+ E + (-(+(+T+A^2)+W^2)+R^2)$

MPL: $(\exists x)Ex \,\&\, (y)(\exists z)(\exists w)Tw \,\&\, Azw \,\&\, Wyz \rightarrow R^2 xy$

The SNF forms are perfectly adapted for MPL translation and
with every little practice the mapping from the SNF forms to
MPL can be done 'on sight'. Take our old friend 'every boy-
loves a girl' whose transcription is '$-B+(L^2+G)$' and whose
SNF is '$-B+(+G+L^2)$'. The first step in translation gives
'$(x)(Bx \rightarrow (+G+L^2 x))$' and the second (final) step gives

$(x)(Bx \rightarrow (\exists y)(Gy \,\&\, L^2 xy)$

but there is no reason to do these two steps on two separate
lines provided we take care to work inward from the outside,
doing the universal translation before we do the existential one.
   The moral of the correspondence of MPL formulas to the
SNF formulas of TFL is clear enough: MPL, albeit covertly, is
no less a 'subject-predicate logic' than TFL. The linguist who
quite properly looks to the logician for guidance on basic
aspects of syntactic structure will welcome another moral: the
linguistically fundamental binary NP/VP structure is not
threatened by the rival syntax of function and argument
represented in the formulas of MPL. On the contrary it is clear
that the MPL formulas must themselves be understood in

relation to the sentences that they purport to translate by revealing their common binary structures however reiterated or embedded or disguised. Thus the MPL formula is now itself revealed as having classical categorical noun phrases of form 'some/every S' with a disguised NP/VP structure.

The double moral is made plain if we simultaneously represent the analyses of the linguist, the modern logician, and the traditional logician of a sentence of natural language. A linguistic phrase marker for the editor-trilogy sentence would be over-long so let us take another sentence of moderate complexity.

(4) anyone who has seen one daffodil has seen them all.

(4) paraphrases as

(4*) every seer of some daffodil is a seer of every daffodil

$$\text{(4*T)} \qquad -(S^2+D) + (S^2-D)$$

$$\text{(SNF)} \qquad -(+D+S^2)+(-D+S^2)$$

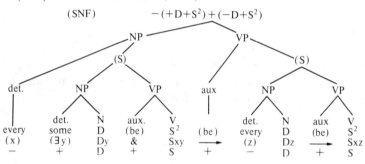

The role of the copula is worth remarking. One often hears (e.g. from Geach) that the copula is superfluous and plays no role in a canonical logical language. Those who say this have MPL in mind and what they say is trivially true if we confine attention to atomic formulas that translate singular sentences. It is non-trivially false if we attend to the structure of the canonical formulas that translate general sentences, including multiply general sentences. In such formulas the role of the copula (in the MPL expressions that translate phrases of form 'some .. is . . .' and 'every . . . is . . .') is very creditably played, in truth-functional drag, by the particles '&' and '→' (respectively).

Appendix B

Quality and Valence

A term or proposition is positive or negative in quality. Thus 'wise' and 'a creature was stirring' are positive in quality; 'unwise' and 'not a creature was stirring' are negative in quality. The valence of a term or proposition may differ from its quality. The valence of a term is its distribution value, the valence of an elementary proposition is its quantity, a particular proposition being positive in valence, a universal proposition, negative. Compound propositions have valences depending on whether they are conjunctious (positive) or disjunctious (negative).

In $'-(+\langle+W+M\rangle+G)'$—'no wise man is a gambler'—the terms 'wise', 'man' and 'gambler' are positive in quality but their valence or distribution value is negative. The sentence $'-(-P+W)'$—'not every player is a winner'—is negative in quality but its valence is positive since it is the negation of a universal sentence and so counts as particular.

Algebraically the valence of an element inside a sentence is determined by driving negation signs in and then seeing whether the element is positively or negatively qualified. The valence of a whole sentence is determined by the first two signs of its explicit algebraic representation: when these are the same the sentence is positive in valence, when they differ the sentence is negative in valence. Thus as we saw $'-(-P+W)'$ is positive in valence ; so too is $'-(-p+q)'$,— 'not:if p then q'. On the other hand $'+(-p+q)'$, the affirmation of a conditional, is negative in valence, as is the universal sentence $'+(-P+W)'$—'every player is a winner'.

For purposes of logical reckoning one attends to the valences of the elements under consideration. Historically TFL looked at the distribution values of the terms and the quantities of the sentences. In the algebraic notation these valences are explicit.

But so too are the valences of the elements in propositional arguments.

Propositions will be said to be either V-positive or V-negative depending on whether their valence is positive or negative. Two propositions of the same valence are said to be *convalent* and two propositions that differ in valence will be said to be *divalent*.

Logically equivalent propositions are convalent; propositions contradictory to one another are divalent. Logical reckoning respects valence constraints that do not govern operations of ordinary algebra. For example, although ' + (+ A + B)' (the transcription of 'some A is B') and ' − (+ (− A) + (− B))' (the transcription of 'not a non-A is a non-B) are algebraically equal, they are not convalent and so not logically equivalent. Similarly even though ' + (+ A + B)' and ' + (+ (− A +) + (− B)' add up to zero they are not divalent and so not contradictory. One can accept the valence constraints of logical algebra as a matter of brute logical fact and leave it at that. Or one can go on to inquire into reasons.

The positive or negative character of a proposition is intrinsic to it and not something we assign to it. Consider for example the pair of contradictory propositions

    (1) a creature was stirring   + C + S
    (2) not a creature was stirring   − (+ C + S).

(1) is V-positive and so is any proposition with the same truth conditions as (1). Similarly (2) is V-negative and so is any proposition with the same truth conditions as (2).

In this respect contradictory propositions are not like contrary terms. Contrary terms, like contradictory propositions, must be divalent but the positive or negative character of a term is not intrinsic to it. Given any positive term it is always possible to find or to define a negative term that denotes what that positive term denotes. Thus 'pure' may be defined as 'uncontaminated' and 'impure' as 'contaminated'. In contrast to this, given any V-positive proposition it is not possible to find or to define a V-negative equivalent. The fact that the opposition of contradictories is not correlative means that V-positive and V-negative propositions are semantically distinct, with different kinds of truth conditions.

This contrast between contraries and contradictories is intriguing. It shows up in the context of the traditional theory which distinguishes between two kinds of negative particles one for signifying the contrary of a term, the other for signifying the denial of a proposition.

But attention to the very distinctions that enhance the contrast will help to explain it. The question is why a proposition's positive or negative character is intrinsic to it in a fixed and absolute way while that of a term is not. I think it is clear why terms have no fixed quality. What needs to be clarified is the reason for the fixed character of propositions. To simplify the discussion I shall restrict attention to primitive contradictories like (1) and (2) whose negative members are overt negations of the positive members. Other forms of contradictories are derived from this primitive form and we shall later see how the argument applies to them.

I can gainsay A, 'Socrates is ill', in two ways:

A′ Socrates isn't ill
− A it is not the case that Socrates is ill

The truth conditions of A′ and − A differ. A′ affirms of Socrates the contrary of the predicate 'is ill'. If A′ is true then Socrates is well. − A, on the other hand, by negating A denies that Socrates is ill, and if − A is true then either Socrates is well or there is no such person as Socrates (in which case A is false and the negation of A is true). The example is taken from Aristotle who says:

'Socrates is ill' is the contrary of 'Socrates is well . . .' if Socrates exists one will be true, the other false but if he does not exist both will be false. (*Cat.* chap. 10, 13b, 14–19.)

And generally (in Aristotle's words)

[I]n the case of affirmation and negation whether the subject exists or not, one is always false and the other true . . . (13b, 26–9.)

And he adds that this holds only for contradictories and not contraries:

Thus it is in the case of those opposites only, which are opposites in the sense in which that term is used with reference to affirmation and negation that the rule holds good, that one of the pair must be true the other false. (13b, 32–5.)

The difference between denial of a proposition and affirming its contrary (by replacing its predicate term by a contrary) was second nature to the pre-Fregeans. Thus DeMorgan warns:

The negative words 'not', 'no', and &c., have two kinds of meaning that must be carefully distinguished. Sometimes they simply deny. Sometimes they are used to affirm the direct contrary. (p. 4, *Formal Logic*.)

A standard Fregean language recognizes propositional negation as the sole particle for gainsaying, thereby treating A' as $-$ A. In both A' and $-$ A the predicate is said to be ' $\sim$ x is ill'. Frege himself avoided the problem of the non-existence of Socrates (which raises the possibility of different truth conditions for A' and $-$ A by stipulating a truth-value gap for sentences containing vacuous proper names. The stipulation also made it easy to treat an expression like 'it is not the case that . . . is ill' (and other expressions that are far removed from the syntactic category of verb phrases) as 'predicates' that characterize the objects that are the bearers of non-vacuous names. I will presently argue that ' $-$ (x is ill)' cannot be construed as an expression that characterizes Socrates but this cannot easily be made out in a language that does not distinguish the denial of a sentence from the 'contraffirmation' of a predicate.

A and A' refer to Socrates. To what does $-$ A refer? If it too refers to Socrates then what it says of him is no different from what A' says of him. The pre-Fregeans must give another answer. More generally, in a logic that carefully distinguishes denial from contraffirmation, a sentence of form 'it is not the case that α is p' cannot be construed as having 'α' as its subject. And this means that what a proposition p refers to and what its negation $-$ p refers to are different.

We read ' $-$ p' as 'it is not the case that p' or as 'that p is not the case'. What is 'it is not the case that p' about? The correct answer recognizes that ' $-$ p' belongs among propositions of form 'that p is Q'. If you say that p, then I can refer to what you said by saying 'what you just said is shocking (true, false, the case, etc.)'. But I can also refer to it by saying:

that p is shocking
that p is (not) the case

and so on.

A phrase of form 'that p' is the conventional noun phrase used for forming the subject of a sentence that refers to a proposition under consideration. A sentence of form 'that p is Q' contains the sentence 'p' but it refers to the proposition that p, not to the sentence 'p'. Similarly, on hearing you say that Socrates is ill, I may refer to the state of affairs that Socretes is ill by saying 'the state of affairs in which Socrates is ill is deplorable'. Here the phrase 'the state of affairs in which' is a nominalizing device similar to 'that' in 'that p' which allows us to embed a sentence in a noun phrase without referring to it. Since neither refers to a sentence, both 'that p is Q' and 'the state of affairs in which p is Q' are sentence forms in the object language. The nominalizing devices, 'that . . .', and 'the state of affairs in which . . .', must therefore be sharply distinguished from the device of quotation which is used for referring to a linguistic expression such as a sentence.[1]

Both Frege and Tarski reinterpret certain sentences of form 'that p is Q'. Tarski treats the subject of 'that p is false' as 'p', something he doesn't do for 'that p is deplorable'. Thus Tarski does not think of 'that p is false' as referring to the proposition that p. On the other hand both Frege and Tarski hold that 'that p is not the case', whose symbolic translation is '− p', refers neither to a sentence nor to a proposition. The naturalist standpoint is linguistically more conservative in treating the subject of 'that p is not the case (false)' as 'that p'. Here is another sensitive area in which the dismissive attitude of Frege and Tarski to the structure of sentences in natural

[1] Someone tells me that Tom has fully recovered to which I respond with 'that Tom has fully recovered is false'. That my response does not mention 'Tom has fully recovered' is arguable from the consideration that my (misinformed) informant may have used some other sentence for saying that Tom has fully recovered. Moreover it would seem that 'that Tom has fully recovered is a great relief to me' has the same referring expression but a metalinguistic interpretation that has it referring to a sentence is altogether inappropriate. I hold that sentences of form 'that p is true (false)' are to be analysed as 'the [p] exists (does not exist)'. For an elaboration of this view see 'On Concepts of Truth in Natural Language', *Review of Metaphysics*, Dec. 1969.

language could be challenged by linguists and philosophers. In particular it seems reasonable that 'it is not the case that p' and 'it is false that p' say exactly the same thing. And since ' − p' is an object-language sentence so too is 'it is false that p'. This linguistically conservative position is in accord with the logical theory of TFL which distinguishes between denying 'Socrates is ill' and affirming the contrary predicate 'isn't ill' of 'Socrates'.

Let us now go back to the question posed by the different ways that contraries and contradictories are in opposition. We noted that in the case of contrary terms ϕ and ψ we can have a situation like

ϕ = pure = uncontaminated
ψ = impure = contaminated

which indicates that the positive and negative character of a term is not fixed. And we asked why we cannot do the same with propositions so that we could have the situation:

ϕ = Socrates is ill = − p
ψ = − Socrates is ill = p

The valence restriction prohibits this and we are now in a position to see why there can be no propositions 'p' and ' − p' equivalent respectively to (− A) and (A). Let us say that A denotes the state of affairs in which Socrates is ill and that A′ denotes the state of affairs in which he is well. Let '[ ]' abbreviate the phrase 'state of affairs in which'. Thus A denotes the [A] and A′ denotes the [A′]. To say that A is true (or the case) is just to say that the [A] obtains and to say that A′ is true is just to say that the [A′] obtains. To say that A is false (or not the case) is to say that the A does not obtain and to say that A′ is false is to say that the [A′] does not obtain. Note that − A and − A′ do not denote states of affairs. If Socrates never existed both − A and − A′ would be true since neither the [A] nor the [A′] would obtain. And generally, the *non*-existence of the [p] is the truth condition for − p; we do not, in addition, need to talk of the existence of a negative state. Thus we need not and do not countenance 'the [− p]' as a state of affairs.

The question before us is why we cannot have a positive proposition, p equivalent to − A and a negative proposition − p equivalent to A. The answer is that the truth conditions of

A and − p are essentially different and the two propositions cannot be equivalent unless they have the same truth conditions. The truth condition of A is the existence of the [A]. But − p is non-denotable; *its* truth condition is the *non-existence* of the [p]. An equivalence between − A and some positive proposition p is similarly precluded: the existence of the [p] is the truth condition of p but unless − A is conflated with A' *its* truth condition is simply the non-existence of the [A]. The non-denotability of negations and the related distinction between − A and A' are decisive in accounting for the asymmetry of contradiction. If Socrates never existed neither the [A] nor the [A'] would obtain and neither − A nor − A' would have the existence of some state of affairs as a condition of its truth. In contrast a positive proposition A or A' denotes a state of affairs whose existence is the condition of its truth.

We can in this way account for the asymmetry of primitive contradictions of form p and − p. Another form of contradiction is that between particular and universal propositions of form 'Some S is (not) P' and 'Every S is (not) P'. We call Every S is P' and Some S is not P' 'diagonal contradictories' since these forms appear on the diagonals of the traditional square of opposition. The square reminds us that 'Every S is P' is a derivative form defined by way of 'not some S is not P'. Moreover the definition is restricted to the case where one of the two subcontraries is true. For example of the two propositions 'Some raindrop is colored' and 'Some raindrop is colorless' one is true so these propositions have diagonal contradictions defined by their negations:

every raindrop is colorless = df not some raindrop is colored
every raindrop is colored = df not some raindrop is colorless.

On the other hand since both 'Some raindrop on the moon is colored' and 'Some raindrop on the moon is colorless' are false their negations do *not* define diagonal contradictories and the sentences 'Every raindrop on the moon is colored (colorless)' cannot be assigned truth values.

Diagonal contradictories, like primitive contradictories, are divalent in an asymmetrical way. Given a universal proposition U1 and its diagonal contradictory P1 it will not be possible to find a another contradictory pair P2 and U2 such that the particular proposition P2 is equivalent to U1 and the universal proposition U2 is equivalent to P1. The asymmetry of the divalence of diagonal contradictories must be explained by showing that the truth conditions of particular and universal propositions precludes equivalence. One explanation is to deny that universal propositions are nondenotable thereby treating them in this respect as the primitive contradictories of particular propositions. Another explanation is that a particular proposition such as 'Some raindrop is colored' has as its truth condition the existence of the [Some raindrop is colored]. The truth conditions of any universal proposition is more complex; for 'Every S is P' to be true two conditions must be satisfied: one being the non-existence of the [Some S is not P] the other being the existence of a state denoted by one of the sub-contraries. Though this second condition is shared by particular propositions, the non-existence condition is peculiar to universal propositions.

Propositions of the form 'No S is P' and 'Every S is P' are negative and both are called universal. Strictly speaking 'No S is P' is not about all S or all P but about the proposition that Some S is P saying of it that it is false or not the case. Equivalently 'No S is P' claims the non-existence of the state of affairs in which some S is P. In contrast, 'Some S is P' is a ground level proposition about S things. Prima facie, so is 'Every S is P'. Ground level propositions about individuals will be said to have a semantic level of zero. Propositions about propositions or states of affairs are of higher level. If p is a ground level proposition then, 'the [p] is Q' is first level and 'the [the [p] is Q] is R' is second level, and so forth. Similarly 'It is Q that p' is first level and 'it is R that it is Q that p' is second level. Clearly 'Some S is P' is zero level and by our arguments its negation is a first level proposition. But just as clearly although defined as equivalent to 'Some S is not P', 'Every S is P' is a zero level proposition about S's. As we said, the equivalence holds only where it is the case that some S' is P or some S is not P. Under the conditions stipulated the definition achieves, as it were, a semantic descent to ground level amounting to an equivalence between a first level and a zero level proposition. This is allowable because, under the constraint, 'No S is P' does have the same truth conditions as 'Every S is P'. Equivalences between propositions are not in themselves anomalous. In the simplest cast where P is a ground level proposition we have the equivalence:

p ≡ that p is the case (true)
p ≡ the [p] obtains

The propositions on the right are not ground level but the truth condition for both is the same: that the [p] exist. Note that our argument has established that there can be no unrestricted equivalence between any ground level proposition and 'that p is not the case'. An unrestricted equivalence would mean that 'Every S is P' is true if there are no S. This indeed is how modern logicians understand the truth conditions for such universal propositions. In effect 'Every S is P' is treated by modern logicians as a first level proposition—a stylistic variant of 'No S is not-p'. Term logic distinguishes affirmative universals from negations of particular propositions. The distinction in term logic between 'no S is un-P' and 'every S is P' leaves room for saying that no raindrop on the moon is colorless without being forced to say that every raindrop on the moon is colored.

Throughout our discussion we have been exploiting the Aristotelian distinction between term negation and propositional negation.

Frege opposed the Aristotelian tradition by holding that all gainsaying has propositional scope. 'Negation . . . needs to be completed by a thought'. This meant that he had to extend the notion of a characterizing predicate beyond the grammatical category of verb phrases. For otherwise there would be no way for him to account for a negative characterization of Socrates. In saying that 'it is not the case that . . . is ill' is the predicate of '− Socrates is ill', Frege kept the negation at zero level.

DeMorgan (to use him as a near modern representative of the Aristotelian tradition) who had 'contraffirmation' as a predicative mode of gainsaying distinguishes between 'Socrates isn't ill' and '− Socrates is ill'. The latter is read as 'it is not the case that Socrates is ill', a proposition of form 'that p is (not) Q' which is about a proposition, denying it. And generally '− p' in traditional logic can be placed, where it linguistically seems to belong, among propositions that refer to propositions and are of a higher semantic level than the propositions to which they refer. [2]

Were Frege's negation sign not so overworked, Frege's view of negation would be close to DeMorgan's view of denial. Frege himself saw that 'p' and ' − p' were semantically different since 'p' may be atomic but ' − p' is a truth function of atomic propositions. But he could not think of the difference as one of semantic level on pain of having no way of negatively characterizing the bearers of proper names. Traditional logic faced no such embarrassment since 'Socrates isn't ill' is understood as 'Socrates is non-ill' which affirms a contrary and is not reducible to the denial of 'Socrates is ill'. [3]

In exploiting the Aristotelian distinctions we observed that while the plus-minus opposition of ' + (+ A + B)' and ' − (+ A + B)' is syntactically symmetrical it is semantically asymmetrical because the negative proposition is a first level proposition referring to the positive proposition. As for the

---

[2] C. B. Martin assures me that many a philospher will balk at identifying 'it is true/false that p' with 'it is the case/not the case that p', maintaining that if no one were around to entertain the proposition that snow is white it would still be the case that snow is white, but it would not then be true that snow is white—because what is true or false is something linguistic, something *said*. I have certain qualms about entertaining propositions and then considering them to be unentertained in a counterfactual situation, but even if we accept that 'true' and 'false' apply only to something said or entertained it would not mean a difference of semantic level for 'it is not the case that p' and 'it is false that p'. For myself, I prefer a correspondence version of truth according to which (where p is elementary) saying that p is true is saying that the [p] obtains. If one accepts Martin's point the definition of truth would be at the same level but somewhat more complicated:

that p is true = the [p] obtains and someone has denoted the [p].

What about 'that p is the case'? Perhaps this only means the same as 'the [p] obtains' or perhaps what is the case, like what is true, is something said or thought. In the old melodramatic movie the son begs his clay-footed father to 'say it isn't *so*' and that is no different from begging his father to deny what is being said about him—to say that it is not the case or false. These considerations would tend to put 'true', 'so', 'the case' back in line.

What now of Martin's counterfactual situation in which no one entertains the proposition that snow is white? One should say that in that situation *snow* would still be white but that it is inappropriate for us to describe the situation as one in which it would still be true that snow is white or the case that snow is white. For by hypothesis no one has denoted the state of affairs in which snow is white.

[3] For more on the difference between denying 'some S isn't P' and affirming 'is P' of every S, see chapter 13.

first plus sign of ' + (+ A + B)' that can be dropped so we *needn't* read it as 'it is the case (true) that an A is a B'. The minus sign of ' − (+ A + B)' is more resistant so that proposition is of form 'that p is Q'.

We also noted that there is a semantic asymmetry in the diagonal contradictories ' + (− A + B)' and ' + (+ A − B)'. Here too the fact that both can be simplified as ' − A + B' (or 'every A is B') and ' + A − B' ('some A isn't B') is indicative of their zero level status. Neither need be read as a proposition of form 'that p is Q'. Nevertheless the asymmetry of divalence holds here too since the truth condition of the universal proposition is negative.

Appendix C

'Any'

When a proposition is given arithmetical representation, its terms are seen to occur with positive or negative valence. Terms of negative valence are said to be distributed, terms of positive valence are said to be undistributed. For example the terms 'philosopher' and 'literate' are distributed and undistributed respectively in 'no philosopher is illiterate' as is evident from the transcription '$-(P + (-L))$'. (To get at the valence we drive all minus signs in as far as possible cancelling them when possible.)

According to a meta-theorem of traditional formal logic, the terms of equivalent propositions have the same distribution values. For example in 'if an A is a B then it is a C', the terms A and B are distributed and the term C is undistributed. The same is true of these terms in the equivalent proposition 'every A is either a C or not a B' which again is clear from the algebraic representations of the two propositions:

$$-[+A_i + B] + [\pm I + C]$$
$$-A + \langle - -C - -(-B) \rangle$$

In the simplest cases a term preceded by 'some' is undistributed. But the whole context determines· the distribution of a term and it often happens that in one context a distributed term is preceded by 'every' and in another, equivalent context the same term is preceded by 'some'. Thus, in the above example, the term A is modified by 'every' in 'every A is either a C or not a B' and modified by 'an' (or 'some') in 'if an A is a B then it is a C'. A is distributed in both of its occurrences but in one case it is preceded by a minus ('every') sign, in the other by a plus ('some') sign.

Because 'every' and 'some' are not infallible guides to the distribution value of the terms that immediately follow them, it is useful to have a modifier that indicates the distribution value given the term by the whole context. Precisely this is the role that 'any' and its translations plays in many natural languages. When a term preceded by 'some' (or by the indefinite articles 'a' or 'an') is distributed, linguistic usage allows for its replacement by 'any'. This permits us to change 'if an A is a B then it is a C' to 'if *any* A is a B then it is a C'. And, generally, the use of 'any' is governed by the distribution values of the terms that follow words of quantity in accordance with the following rules:

(i) 'Any' may go proxy for either 'some' or 'every' (and so may be how we read the plus or minus sign that precedes a subject term) when these words of quantity modify a distributed term.

(ii) 'Any' may not be used when the term modified is undistributed in a sentence.

(iii) 'Any' must be used whenever the use of 'some' would leave us in doubt about the distribution value of a distributed term. Its use in those contexts removes the ambiguity and indicates that the term is distributed.

As an example of the application of rule (iii) consider the sentence 'Tom did not answer a question' uttered by someone who means to say that Tom answered none of the questions and not by someone who means to say that there was some question that he failed to answer. The following pair of transcriptions shows that in the first statement 'question' is distributed and in the second it is undistributed.

$$T - (a + Q) \qquad \text{Tom did not: answer a question}$$
$$T - a + Q \qquad \text{Tom did not-answer a question}$$

The first should properly be read as 'Tom did not answer any question' to indicate that here the sign of particular quantity is followed by a distributed term because the scope of the negative particle covers the whole predicate term. Note that 'every' won't do; the word 'any' here stands in for 'some' or 'a' and must be transcribed as a plus sign.

Rule (i) licenses the use of 'any' before a distributed terms, and rule (ii) prohibits its use before an undistributed term. Consider the difference between 'a snarling dog is unfriendly', and 'a snarling dog is in my office'. The first is equivalent to 'no snarling dog is friendly' in which 'snarling dog' is distributed. In the second, 'snarling dog' is undistributed. The article 'a' may be replaced by 'any' in the first sentence but not in the second where the use of 'any' would run afoul of rule (ii). The replacement of 'a' by 'any' in the first sentence is not mandatory; there is no likelihood of mistaking the distribution value of the term in that context: clearly all dogs are being referred to and 'snarling dog' is distributed.

How 'any' is typically employed in subjects of propositions that are antecedents of conditionals is another illustration of the way distribution determines its use. In 'if a man signs a contract he is committed to fulfill it' both 'man' and 'contract' are distributed and 'any' may replace both indefinite articles.

Because 'every' is normally followed by a distributed term it is most commonly replaced by 'any'. But in 'if every man is aboard we can make way' the term 'man' is undistributed and 'any' may not replace it. Clearly 'any' can stand in for either 'some' or 'every' but only when the terms these modify are distributed.

'Not' reverses the distribution value of any term within its scope and where its scope is unambiguous it is the strongest indicator of distribution. Indeed, to say that a term is distributed is just to say that it is originally within the scope of a negation sign; it is to say that the term has negative valence. In 'not a creature was stirring' the term 'creature' is clearly distributed, so we do not replace 'a' by 'any'; the use of 'any' would here be confusing. A similar point may be made about the indefinite article in 'not every boy loves a girl', where the fact that 'girl' is distributed is sufficiently determined by the reversal of truth values effected by the external negation. Contrast these cases with the ambiguity of scope just noted in 'Tom did not answer a question', where 'any' is called for to determine the distribution of 'question' when the intended meaning requires it. We may state as a general rule suggested by these contrasting cases that the 'use' of 'any' is precluded when the distributed term is within the scope of an external negation for the scope of external negation is unambiguous and the term is then originally distributed. On the other hand the use of 'any' is mandatory for disambiguating the scope of a negation to cover a term in a statement whose intended meaning requires the term's distributed occurrence.

There are then three kinds of cases:

(1) Those in which 'any' may not be used;
(2) Those in which 'any' must be used;
(3) Those in which 'any' may be used.

'Any' may not be used to modify a distributed term within the clear scope of an external negation. And it may never be used to modify an undistributed term. 'Any' must be used to determine the scope of a negative particle to include a term in a statement that requires a distributed occurrence of that term. Finally 'any' is optional for contexts in which the term modified is distributed but not through external negation. Thus 'any' may replace 'every' in 'every A is B' and it may replace 'an' in 'if an A is a B then p'.

Hintikka has proposed an alleged counterexample to Tarski's truth formula that is neatly dealt with by the distribution rules for the use of 'any'. According to Tarski, 'if p then "p" is true' always holds. But this seems to be refuted by examples like

T* If any Australian can run a four minute mile then 'any Australian can run a four minute mile' is true.

That T* should cause no concern becomes evident when we transcribe it:

$$-[+A+C]+[\pm'-A+C'+T]$$

Of course this is not an instance of Tarski's formula. For that formula requires that the name in the consequent be that of the sentence used in the antecedent. If we satisfy the requirement we must have

$$-[+A+C]+[\pm'+A+C'+T]$$

If an(y) Austrialian can run a four minute mile then 'an Australian can run a four minute mile' is true

which is not a counterexample but a harmless instance of the Tarski conditional.[1]

---

[1] I am indebted to Hilary Putnam for pointing out Hintakka's counterexample to me and for his suggestion that the resolution is to be found in the option of replacing 'an' by 'any' in the antecedent. The distribution condition for replacing 'an' by 'any' explains *why* this option is available there and unavailable in the consequent.

To sum up: our analysis shows that 'any' is not a word of quantity in its own right but a distribution indicator that goes proxy for either 'some' or 'every'. The fact that 'any' behaves the way it does is an instructive illustration of how distribution values may affect the surface structure of a natural language.

Appendix D

'Some', 'Every', 'Most', 'Just One', etc.

The logical syntax of TFL recognizes only those logical particles which go to indicate positive or negative valence. This includes signs for 'not', 'and', 'some', and 'every', each of which has a plus-minus representation; it excludes such signs as 'Just One' and 'Most' which must be analysed by way of conjunctions of categorical propositions that contain the elementary (plus-minus) logical particles and no others. Thus 'Just one S is M' is analysed as a pronominalization:

$$\llcorner \text{Some S} \lrcorner_i \text{ is M and no } (-I) \text{ is M}$$
$$+ [+S_i + M] + [-(+(-I) + M)]$$

The analysis of 'Most S are M' is more complicated. It includes a part that says how many S there are and a part that says that a majority of them are M. For example in the case where there are three S, the analysis of 'Most S are M' is

there are just three S	$\llcorner$Some thing$\lrcorner_i$ is S and $\llcorner$Some thing$\lrcorner_j$ is S and $\llcorner$Some thing$\lrcorner_k$ is S and *I isn't J and *I isn't K and *J isn't K and every S is either I or J or K.
at least two of them are M	Either *I is M and *J is M or *I is M and *K is M or *J is M and *K is M

The first part tells us how many S there are. The second tells how many of them—a majority—are M:

$$+ [+T_i + S] + [+T_j + S] + [+T_k + S]$$
$$+ [\pm I - J] + [\pm I - K] + [\pm J - K]$$

$$+ [-S + \langle - -I - -J - -K \rangle]$$
$$+ [- -[+ [\pm I + M] + [\pm J + M]] - -[+ [\pm I + M]$$
$$+ [\pm K + M]] - -[+ [\pm J + M] + [\pm K + M]]]$$

And, generally, propositions with quantitative subjects (two S, few S, most S etc.) differ from 'some S' and 'every S' in having a complex analysis calling for unpacking into categorical components. Geach who is interested in quantitative applications has recognized the portmanteau character in 'just one S is M' and 'few S are M', but he makes an unhappy exception of 'Most S are M' treating it as a categorical on a par with 'some S is M' and 'every S is M'. To a logician, the idea that 'most' is a quantifier on all fours with 'some' or 'every' ought to be distasteful but the idea that 'few'; and 'most' do not have the same status is independently objectionable. The assertion that most S are M is the claim that there are more S that are M than S that are not M. Similarly, the assertion that few S are M could be understood to say that there are less S that are M than S that are not M. So understood, 'most' and 'few' are correlative and we could just as well define 'most S are M' as 'some S are M and few S are not M' as we could define 'few S are M' as 'some S are M and most S are not M'. (Geach, who considers 'most S are M' to be logically more primitive than 'few S are M', does the latter and rejects the former.) The idea that 'most', unlike 'few', behaves like 'some' and 'every' seems to him to be supported by the validity of inferences of the following form:

(Y)   every M is P
       most S are M
       ----
       most S are P

According to Geach (Y) is valid by the *Dictum de Omni*. This may be so on Geach's way of construing the *Dictum de Omni* but properly understood the dictum says that *whatever is true of every M is true of whatever is an M*. Note now that the minor premiss of Y is *not* of form '. . . is an M' and that it *cannot* be parsed as a proposition of this form. This ought to give pause to anyone who would treat (Y) as a syllogism. A closer view of the inference reveals the need to unpack 'most S are M' before applying the *Dictum de Omni* to a conjunction of the major premiss with some components of the minor premiss. Assume for the sake of the argument that there are exactly three S's. Then 'most S's are M' unpacks as before into two parts, one of which says that there are exactly three S's, and the other of which says that a majority of them are M. When the major premiss is conjoined to the second part we get 'either every M is P and *I is M and *J is M or every M is P and *I is M and *K is M or every M is P and *J is M and *K is M'. Applying *DDO* to each of the disjuncts yields either *I is P and *J is P or *I is P and *K is P or *J is P and *K is P which conjoins with the part that says there are exactly three S's to give 'most S are P'. From this analysis is clear that (Y) is no syllogism but a more complicated valid argument in which syllogism plays a part.

The more general moral is that 'some' and 'every' have the privileged status of signs that form logical subjects but that 'most', 'few', 'just seven', are not signs of logical quantity, despite the grammatical similarity between 'some S's' and 'seven S's' etc. The failure to recognize the crucial distinction between 'some' and 'most' may be attributed to the Fregean belief that the *genuine* logical subject is definite and singular in which case 'some S' and 'every S' are not genuine logical subjects anyway. Geach calls them 'quasi-referring expressions'. Having given them this dubious status, he has no qualms about putting 'most S' on the same footing with 'some S'.

Geach's cavalier way with quantified subjects extends to 'no S' as well as to 'most S'. In the preface to his recent book, *Reason and Argument*, Geach remarks:

The eccentric but talented Edinburgh philosopher, Sir William Hamilton, must be credited with drawing attention to the obvious fact that 'most' is a quantifier, of the same category as 'all', 'some', and 'no'.[1]

Treating 'no' as a quantifier is an antique howler. 'No' has sentential scope in 'no S is P' just as 'not' has it in 'not an S is a P'. Calling 'no S' a quantified subject is like calling 'and children' a quantifed subject in 'It was sunny and children were playing in the park'.[2]

[1] P. T. Geach, *Reason and Argument*, (University of California Press, 1976), p. ix.
[2] Also see chapter 14, section 6.

Appendix E

by Aris Noah

Quine's Version of Term Logic and its Relation to TFL

1. Quine's Version of Term Logic

1.1 Clarification and support for the termist logic developed in the text can be gained by comparing it with another system of algebraic term logic, Quine's recently developed 'Predicate-Functor Logic'. The parallels are strong and the differences instructive.

Whereas Sommers' traditional termist approach is, from the very start, shaped by the effort to capture as faithfully and as systematically as possible the logic of ordinary language with its prominent subject-predicate forms, Quine is motivated by the desire to study and understand the syntactical forms of classical quantification theory. His predicate-functor logic was developed in an effort, primarily, to understand theoretically the essential functions of the bound variables of quantification.[1] The schemata of his algebraic logic are systematic transcriptions of quantificational schemata from which the bound variables have been completely 'coaxed away' by the use of algebraic devices called predicate-functors; the expressive power of this system exactly coincides with that of first order quantification theory (with identity). The surprising result of

---

[1] Quine's ideas on predicate–functor logic first appeared in fairly mature form in his paper 'Variables Explained Away', *Proceedings of the American Philosophical Society* 104 (1960), p. 343–7 (reprinted in the first edition of *The Ways of Paradox and Other Essays*). His most mature views, however, are set forth in two articles contained in the second edition of *The Ways of Paradox*, namely 'Algebraic Logic and Predicate Functors' and 'The Variable'.

Quine's sustained analysis of quantification theory, specifically its central use of the bound variable, is that, from the theoretical point of view, it is finally to be construed as a *term* logic. This may strike one as odd in view of the Fregean attacks on term logic and the insistence on viewing predicates as unsaturated verb forms (analogous to mathematical functions). In Fregean symbolism, 'Fx' is an indivisible logical unit from which it is not allowed to disengage the 'F', as a *term* (that is, a noun or adjective in syntactical function). The 'Fx' belongs to the syntactical category of a verb, better read as 'xFs', and has no internal logical structure at all. Quine's contribution is, first, to show how bound variables can be systematically eliminated from closed sentence schemata leaving behind them schematic letters 'F', 'G' etc., which belong to the syntactical category of nouns or adjectives (that is, *terms*), and, second to interpret these results in a coherent and theoretically significant way shedding light on quantification theory as well as the whole development of logic from the late nineteenth century to our own time. The net results are: (a) the reinstatement of terms as the fundamental categorematic elements of sentences, (b) the reinterpretation of quantification theory as an implicit term logic and (c) the development of an *explicit* algebraic term logic equivalent to first-order quantification theory.[2]

What follows is a brief restatement of Quine's ideas (contained in his more theoretical essay on 'The Variable') emphasizing his reinstatement of terms as the fundamental material constituents of sentences.

1.2 The fundamental move underlying Quine's reinterpretation of quantification theory is one of striking simplicity and intuitive naturalness. We can explain it by reference to the

---

[2] Quine does not call his 'F' and 'G' etc. terms, but *predicates*. As we shall see in a moment, however, he makes very clear that they belong to the syntactical category of nouns and adjectives, traditionally called terms. Quine reserves the name 'terms' for monadic predicates only, calling the more structurally complicated elements 'predicates': 'Thus the shift which we have made from terms to predicates can be viewed as a case merely of improving and renaming the idea of a term'. (*Methods of Logic*, 3rd edn. p. 146). The reason the traditional terminology is preferable, however, is that we may want to reserve the name 'predicate' for the syntactical (grammatical) predicate of a subject–predicate sentence, which together with a term includes the copula ('is a man' etc.). Apart from terminology, however, the important point is the possibility of disengaging the 'F' from the 'Fx' and recognizing it as an independent and fundamental syntactical element.

simplest possible quantificational schema, namely '$(\exists x)Fx$'. The classical interpretation, in words, runs as follows:

(1) $\dfrac{\overline{\text{There is something x such that}}\ \overline{\text{x is F}}}{\exists x \qquad\qquad\qquad Fx}$

The quantifier is a complex expression with the variable x embedded into it. Quine's insight is that:

the quantitative force of the quantifier, the 'all' and 'some' is irrelevant to the distinctive work of the bound variable and irrelevant to its referential function. The quantitative component needs no variable; it is fully present in the traditional categoricals 'All men are mortal', 'Some Greeks are wise'. (*Ways of Paradox*, second edition, p. 275).

Alternatively, the quantitative component is also present in a Boolean schema like '$F.G \neq 0$', again without use of the variable as a syntactical device. It is natural, therefore, to expel the variable from the quantifier, in which case what we get is the following:

(2) $\underline{\text{There is something (there are)}}\ \underline{\text{x such that Fx}}$

which, intuitively at least, presents a more natural distribution of syntactical elements (the quantifier in (1) was a very complex and heterogeneous expression 'crying' for analysis).

The question now is, what is the syntactical nature of the expression 'x such that Fx'? It is, simply, a relative clause, equivalent to 'which is F' or, unexpectedly, 'F' pure and simple. The next two steps make this explicit.

(3) $\underline{\text{There is something}}\ \underline{\text{which is F}}$
(4) $\underline{\text{There is something (there are)}}\ \underline{\text{F}}$

As Quine says, 'The "such that" construction is the relative clause simplified in respect of word order and fitted with a bound variable to avert ambiguities of cross-reference.' (*Ways of Paradox*, pp. 275–6) And he adds:

It is not a singular term, neither a singular description nor a class abstract; it is *a general term, a predicate*. It has its use where we have a complex sentence that mentions some object *a* perhaps midway, perhaps repeatedly, and we want to *segregate a complex adjective or common noun* that may be simply predicated of the object *a* with the same effect as the original sentence. Where the original sentence is thought of schematically as 'Fa', the relative clause is the *explicit segregation of the 'F'*. (Ibid., p. 275; italics mine.)[3]

Quine believes he has uncovered

a use of the bound variable that is more basic still than its use in quantification. It carries no connotation of 'all' or 'some' or class or function, but shows rather the distinctive work of the bound variable without admixture. This basic and neglected idiom is the relative clause, mathematically regimented as the 'such that' idiom. (*Ways of Paradox*, p. 275)

while

other uses of the bound variables are readily represented as parasitic upon this use . . . Quantification can be thought of as application of a functor '∃' or '∀' to a predicate; and this functor is what carries the pure quantitative import, with no intrusion of variables . . . What brings the variable, if any, is the predicate itself, in case it is a relative clause rather than a simple adjective or perhaps some Boolean compound (Ibid., p. 276).

Ultimately, then, the use of the relative clause is a device for abstracting complex general terms from complex sentential clauses, a device for forming complex general terms, *a term (or*

---

[3] For example, let's take the following sentence about John:

(1) *John* used to work for the man who murdered the second husband of John's youngest sister.

Can we segregate a complex term which, predicated of John, will have the same effect as (1)? Very easily, if we use the relative clause: '*who* used to work for the man who murdered the second husband of his youngest sister', or (more regimented) '*x* such that *x* used to work for the man who murdered the second husband of the youngest sister of *x*'. We now have:

(2) John is an x such that x used to work for the man who murdered the second husband of the younger sister of x

(which is equivalent to (1)).

Thus: $Fa \equiv a$ is (an) $F = a$ is (an) x such that Fx.

If we do not want to use a relative clause, we have to resort to verbal contortions to isolate a complex term predicated of John:

(John is a) 'former employee of own youngest sister's second husband's murderer'

which shows clearly that the relative clause, no matter how complicated syntactically, amounts, simply to a pure *term*. (The example is borrowed from *Methods of Logic*, p. 145.)

predicate) *compounding device.* And the *essential* use of the *bound* variable (which is basically a relative pronoun), according to Quine, is precisely within such relative clauses: thus, the *bound* variables of quantification theory are, essentially, devices for forming complex predicates and *all* their functions can be captured by a suitable list of algebraic devices doing the same work. These algebraic devices are Quine's 'predicate-functors'.

1.3 Quine explains why the relative clause as a syntactical unit, and, with it, the status of pure general terms have not been clearly appreciated by modern logicians from Peano and Russell to the present day:

> One senses in the modern history of logic a distaste for the general term, or predicate. It is partly the effect and partly the cause, I expect, of our slowness to appreciate the schematic status of predicate letters. One tends to conflate such letters with objectual variables, and so reconstrue general terms as abstract singular terms designating properties or classes. Thereby the relative clause or 'such that' clause, becomes class abstraction . . . (*Ways of Paradox*, p. 277.)

> A later logician, alive to schematic letters, reacts with a true calculus of predicates; and it is the familiar quantification logic in its usual modern style of exposition. But he overreacts: he insists on keeping his predicate letters embedded with their arguments, fearing that a predicate floating free and ungesättigt would be a class name again. He has failed to appreciate 'such that' as an ontologically innocent operator for isolating pure complex predicates, representable by free-floating schematic letters . . . (Ibid., p. 281.)

> Predicates have been an uneasy intermediate between abstract singular terms on the one hand and out-and-out sentences on the other. (Ibid., p. 277.)

Clear recognition of the schematic status of predicate letters means that they are simply viewed as place-holders for general terms, the latter being either single adjectives or nouns or Boolean compounds ('rich and powerful', 'rich man') or relative clauses of whatever complexity. And general terms, simple or complex, are not names of any entities but are *true of* objects or sequences of objects. The ontology of sentences with general terms is clear: all objects that satisfy or fail to satisfy the monadic terms within the sentences (or their complements) are included.[4] The road, then, is clear for developing a calculus of terms (or predicates), a *term logic*, without ontological worries of any kind.

1.4 The net result of these reflections is the possibility and desirability of an explicit recognition of pure general terms and thus, also, or relative clauses (which are, really, nothing but complex general terms). This explicit recognition allows us to reconstrue any quantificational schema as a *term schema*. All we have to do is detach the variable from any given quantifier, turning its scope into a relative clause (as we showed in 1.2). For example, the schema

(1) $(x) (Bx \bullet (\exists y)Rxy)$

adopting Peano's notation of the inverted epsilon '$\ni$' for the 'such that' construction, can be reconstrued as:

(2) $(x) (Bx \bullet \exists(y \ni Rxy))$
(3) $\forall(x \ni [Bx \bullet \exists(y \ni Rxy)])$

where '$y \ni Rxy$' and '$x \ni [Bx \bullet \exists(y \ni Rxy)]$' are relative clauses, that is, *terms*. Any quantificational schema of whatever complexity can thus be read as a schema whose basic constituents are *terms* on the one hand (usually complex relative clauses) and *term functors* (or predicate functors) on the other. Notice that the quantifier-functors '$\exists$' and '$\forall$', applied to monadic terms such as '$x \ni [Bx \bullet \exists(y \ni Rxy)]$' yield closed sentences, while applied to open monadic terms with one free variable such as '$y \ni Rxy$' (read 'which x is R to') yield open *sentences* with one free variable such as '$\exists(y \ni Rxy)$' (the latter can be read in English as 'there is something which x is R to' or 'x is R to something').

Thus, quantification theory can be very naturally interpreted as an implicit term logic.

1.5 We have seen in 1.2 how the relative clause 'x such that Fx' collapses into the general term 'F'. This means that the bound variable 'x' is redundant and eliminable. Can bound variables (or their linguistic equivalents, relative pronouns) be systematically eliminated from *any* relative clause of whatever degree of

---

[4] See Quine, *Ways of Paradox*, pp. 304–5.

syntactical complexity? Can we always produce a compact term tantamount to the relative clause at hand? The question is whether there are other devices, besides the relative pronoun, which can do the same job of abstracting pure complex terms (predicates) from sentential clauses, and do it with sufficient sensitivity to logical structure to give us all the inferences we require. The answer is yes, and again the alternative devices are the term or predicate functors. Using predicate functors we can develop an *explicit* (algebraic) term logic as powerful as quantification theory. It is a logic without variables.

Three of the necessary functors are sufficient for monadic quantification theory.

The first we have already seen: it is what is left of the existential quantifier once we expel the 'x such that' from it, namely the expression 'there is something' or 'there are' which, attached to a term 'F', gives the sentence '∃F' ('There are F', 'There are swans'). A dual (but redundant) functor '∀' can be introduced for the universal quantifier, read 'everything is'. Quine calls these two functors *cropping functors*, because they 'crop' any term they are attached to into a term of degree less by one (attached to a monadic term they 'crop' it down to a sentence, that is, a term of null degree).

A conjunctive relative clause such as 'x ∃ Fx • Gx' can be collapsed into a compound term 'F ∩ G', which is the 'Boolean intersection' of the terms 'F' and 'G'. Quine calls '∩' the *Boolean intersection functor*.

The next device is the Boolean complement functor, ' − ', introduced to handle negations:

'x ∃ ∼ Fx' becomes simply ' − F', the *Boolean complement* of the term 'F'.

These three functors, '∃', '∩', and ' − ', are sufficient for the term version of monadic logic (we can, if we wish, define further functors of 'Boolean' inclusion, coextensiveness, union etc.). Monadic logic turns into a *Boolean Algebra of terms*, not classes.[5]

---

[5] 'We are noting how unready logicians have been to think directly in terms of a calculus of complex predicates . . . This bias has long been visible at the most elementary level, indeed, in the attitude towards the perversely so-called Boolean calculus of classes. There is no call for classes there. This bit of logic has its whole utility as an algebra of predicates . . .' (*Ways of Paradox*, p. 280).

If we allow the three basic Boolean functors to operate not only on simple adjectives or nouns, but also on complex relative clauses built by the use of the same three functors, e.g. '$\exists(-B^1 \cap \exists(R^2 \cap \exists(F^3 \cap -G^3)))$', we can produce a polyadic elaboration of Boolean logic, which differs only superficially from the classical monadic Boolean version. The difference is superficial because the same syncategorematic devices (functors) are used, only they are allowed to operate on polyadic as well as monadic terms. As we shall see, this *extended system of Boolean logic* is very significant in the exploration of the limits of decidability in logic.

As we move to more complicated polyadic logic, additional functors have to be introduced to capture permutations and/or recurrences of variables (as in 'Fxy • Fyx' or 'Gyxy').

First of all, we need a functor to capture the familiar conjunction of open sentences:

'x 3($\exists$y)(By • Rxy)' is rendered '$\exists(B^1 • R^2)$', where '$B^1 • R^2$' is a dyadic term. The Boolean intersection functor '$\cap$' compounds only terms of the same degree, whereas our expanded *conjunction functor*, ' • ', can compound terms of different degrees, such as 'B' (monadic) and 'R' (dyadic) above. We may call the Boolean intersection functor, '$\cap$', *homogeneous conjunction functor*, and the newly introduced ' • ' *non-homogeneous conjunction functor*, according as they can compound terms of homogeneous or non-homogeneous degree.[6]

Notice that the introduction of the non-homogeneous conjunction functor already takes us beyond the boundaries of the extended Boolean system of logic defined above.

To deal with recurrences of variables, Quine introduces the *self functor*, 'S':

for example, 'x 3 Lxx'   becomes 'x 3 SLx'
('lover of himself')   ('self-lover')[7]

[6] Quine's Boolean intersection functor '$\cap$' as defined in the essay 'Algebraic Logic and Predicate Functors' (*Ways of Paradox*, pp. 283–307), corresponds to our non-homogeneous conjunction functor, but it is more natural to reserve the term 'Boolean' for the homogeneous conjunction functor.

[7] In 'Algebraic Logic and Predicate Functors,' Quine defines 'S' in terms of the non-homogeneous conjunction functor and the identity predicate 'I'. However, in a new unpublished essay, Quine limits himself to the homogeneous (Boolean) conjunction functor and introduces 'S' as primitive. The latter strategy is preferable, because it isolates the Boolean from the non-Boolean (or combinatorial) functors.

To handle permutations of variables, we need the *permutation functor*, 'P'. This single permutation functor can, as Quine shows, give us any desired permutation, but it can also be used to define a whole slew of more convenient permutation functors 'p_{ij}' which exchange the i-th for the j-th predicate-place of predicates. For example, 'Rxy' can be rewritten as '$(p_{21} R)yx$'. If 'R' is the term (predicate) 'hater of', '$p_{21} R$' is the term (predicate) 'hated by'. In fact, the passive voice construction in natural languages is a simple case of the use of the permutation functor.

Thus far, all the functors introduced are mathematical elaborations of syntactical constructions available in natural language (even though in a limited form). However, two more functors are needed, the first essential, the second useful but redundant: the *padding functor* ' £ ', and the *Cartesian Product* functor, 'X'. Without them, certain very complex relative clauses could not be purged of their variables, but of them there is no trace of parallel devices in natural language. They are creatures of the mathematician, carrying certain tendencies for the avoidance (elimination) of relative pronouns inherent in natural language to a theoretical completion.

Finally, *identity* is not a functor but a special two-place predicate 'I': '$x = y$' is rendered as 'Ixy' (supporting the thesis of chapter 6 that identity is not a primitive logical, syncategorematic particle).

But where do singular terms fit in a language which consists solely of general terms and term functors? The answer is that, indeed, they do not fit in that language; they yield their place to terms (predicates) satisfied uniquely by the object named by the corresponding singular term.

'Fa' becomes '$(\exists x)(Ax \bullet Fx)$', where 'A' is a term uniquely true of the object named by 'a'. Then translation follows: '$\exists(A \bullet F)$'. Alternatively, we can use universal quantification: '$(x)(Ax \supset Fx)$' and '$\forall(A \supset F)$'.[8] In fact, Quine observes:

$$Fa \equiv (\exists x) (Ax \bullet Fx) \equiv (\forall x) (Ax \supset Fx)$$

(thus giving expression to Leibniz's principle of the 'wild' quantity of singular terms in subject position).

---

[8] *See Ways of Paradox*, p. 305, and *The Roots of Reference*, p. 97.

2. The Plus-Minus Version of Term
Logic and the Limits of Decidability

2.1 The upshot of the foregoing is that we have a wide choice in developing a system of term logic: we can leave *all* relative clauses intact (even though we recognize their status as collapsible general terms), going to the extreme of construing even general categoricals such as 'All humans are mortal' in terms of variables (relative pronouns) as '(x) $(Hx \supset Mx)$', in which case we get classical quantification theory; or we can insist on *always* collapsing relative clauses into explicit compound terms (using term functors) in which case we get Quine's predicate-functor logic. If, however, our interest primarily is in eliciting the logical syntax of natural language sentences, we may adopt the course of the text, and choose a middle path: construe general categoricals and simple relational sentences as pronoun-free constructions consisting exclusively of terms and term-functors, and introduce relative pronouns *only* when the pronoun-free syntactical constructions available to natural language become excessively strained and unnatural.

For example, 'All humans are mortal' can be rendered as '$-H+M$' in the plus-minus notation, or '$\forall(H \supset M)$' in Quine's notation. 'Some men are married to a woman' can be rendered as '$+M+(m^2+W)$', or '$\exists(M^1 \cap \exists(W^1 \bullet m^2))$' in Quine's notation. 'Every villager owns and beats some domestic animal' can be rendered as '$-V+(\langle +O^2+B^2 \rangle + \langle +D+A \rangle)$' in the plus-minus notation, or as '$\forall\{V^1 \supset \exists[(D^1 \cap A^1)\bullet(O^2 \cap B^2)]^2\}$'. So far, abstaining from relative pronouns has led to no departure from normal English. But now consider the sentence 'Every man who owns a car washes it'. It can be rendered without the use of relative pronouns as '$-M+(\langle -O^2+W^2 \rangle + C)$' in plus-minus notation or '$\forall\{M^1 \supset \exists[C^1\bullet(O^2 \supset W^2)]\}$' in Quine's notation, both of which have a very strained English equivalent in 'Every man is, if owner then washer of, a car'. Using relative (or B-type) pronouns, the initial sentence can be transcribed in the mixed plus-minus notation as '$-[+M_i+(O^2+C_j)]+[\pm I+W^2 \pm J)]$' or, in English, 'If a man owns a car, he washes it', which is much more natural and systematically related to the syntax of the original.[9] Even at this relatively benign level of syntactical

---

[9] Ch. 4, sec. 5 of the text offers another natural alternative: $- \langle +M+(O^2+C_i) \rangle + W^2 \pm I.$

complexity, avoiding the use of relative pronouns often results in strained English.

It is instructive to note the similarities and differences between the plus-minus and Quine's notation. Obviously, the pair of functors '$\forall(\ldots \supset ——)$' corresponds to TFL's binary functor '$-\ldots +——$' or 'every ..... is ——', while the pair '$\exists(\ldots \cap ——)$' corresponds to TFL's binary functor '$+\ldots +——$' or 'Some ... is ——'. TFL's '$\langle +\ldots +——\rangle$' corresponds to the homogeneous conjunction functor (in TFL, the conjunction functor never compounds terms of different degrees). In both notations, the Boolean complement functor is represented identically as '$-$'. In both systems, again, there is systematic isomorphism between sentential connectives and the corresponding term functors ('$\cap$' doubles as both sentential conjunction and term compounding, and so does '$+\ldots +—$'). Finally, a relational predicate rendered as '$\exists(W^1.m^2)$' in Quine's notation is more naturally but quite similarly rendered in the plus-minus notation as '$m^2 + W$' (the latter is easily transcribed into English as 'married to a woman', whereas the former has reversed the English order of the syntactical elements and at least superficially obscured the intimate association of the quantifier with the monadic term which is the 'object' of the transitive verb). Notice that the use of the plus within relational terms like '$m^2 + W$' corresponds to the pair of functors '$\exists$' and '$\cdot$', i.e. involves implicitly the use of the non-Boolean, non-homogeneous conjunction functor. The similarities extend to the rendering of singular sentences: 'Socrates is mortal' is rendered indifferently as '$\forall(S \supset M)$' or '$\exists(S \cdot M)$' in Quine's notation and as '$\pm S + M$' in the plus-minus notation, where 'S' represents a term uniquely denoting Socrates. The basic difference concerns identity: Quine treats it as a special binary predicate, while TFL considers it a special case of predication where both terms are singular.

The term-functors most conspicuously used in the plus-minus notation are, as we have seen, the equivalents of Quine's two cropping functors, the homogeneous (or Boolean) conjunction functor (and its redundant cognates corresponding to 'if then' and 'either or'), and the complement functor. The only non-Boolean functor implicitly involved in the plus-minus notation, except for the occasional restricted use of simple passive voice constructions (permutation functor), is the non-homogeneous conjunction functor, use of which is made in building relational terms: 'married to a woman', rendered '$m^2 + W$' or, in Quine's notation '$\exists(W^1 \cdot m^2)$'. However, the use of non-homogeneous conjunction is severely restricted in TFL and in natural languages to compounding *always* an n-place relation with a sequence of $n - 1$ *monadic* terms in order to form a single, complex, *monadic* relational term (e.g. 'gives a present to a woman').

It has been shown in chapter 9 of the text how this fundamental group of functors can be given a plus-minus algebraic interpretation, which results in a simple, intuitive and elegant representation of inferences. A formalization of a plus-minus term system is presented in Appendix F, together with proofs of soundness and completeness (the system of Appendix F is somewhat weaker, since it does not include compound relations such as 'owns and washes', but only compound monadic terms such as 'rich man'; however, it can easily be extended).

Beyond the boundaries of this pronoun-free, minimal extension of polyadic Boolean logic, the plus-minus algebra of TFL makes systematic use of relative (B-type) pronouns and its constructions are closer to those of classical quantification theory. Thus, one part of this mixed TFL system is identical with the extended Boolean fragment of predicate-functor logic minimally enlarged by the restricted use of the non-Boolean non-homogeneous conjunction functor '·', while another parallels quantification theory. (see Appendix A.)

2.2. The boundary line between these two subsystems of TFL turns out to be of theoretical significance. It probably coincides with the boundary line of decidability in logic.[10] The extended Boolean system of predicate-functor logic is known to be decidable by a method devised by Herbrand and generalized by Quine for polyadic schemata of this Boolean type.[11] The more extended system, which employs without *any* restrictions the

[10] See the discussion in A. Noah, 'Predicate-functors and the Limits of Decidability in Logic', *Notre Dame Journal for Formal Logic* vol. 21, No. 4, Oct. 1980, pp. 701–7.

[11] See Quine, 'On the Limits of Decision', *Acts of the XIV International Congress of Philosophy* (Vienna, 1968), vol. 3, pp. 57–62, and the paper by A. Noah.

non-homogeneous conjunction functor instead of the homogeneous Boolean one, is not decidable by the same methods and it is very likely undecidable, though this has not yet been definitely established.[12] The introduction of the self-functor and the permutation functor(s) takes us well beyond the limits of decidability in logic. Relative pronouns have to be naturally introduced at pretty much the same point at which the troublesome non-Boolean functors have to be called into unrestricted play; thus relative pronouns hold the key to the issue of decidability in logic.

2.3. Another fundamental thesis of the text is the following: all purely logical signs (functors) have one thing in common, highlighted by the plus-minus notation, namely their purely oppositional character through which they confer valence on the categorematic elements or terms. This thesis assumes that a clear dividing line can be drawn between categorematic and syncategorematic elements. TFL draws a sharp line by recognizing as purely logical only the Boolean set of functors plus the restricted use of non-homogeneous conjunction in relational terms, and using relative pronouns and other devices to handle all further syntactical complexity. TFL's viewpoint is this: all sentences (including pronominal ones) have fundamentally the same syntax; they consist of terms (general, singular, pronominal, relational etc.) joined by oppositional term functors. All purely logical inferences are mediated by the explicit syntactical forms of the sentences entering into them, as represented in the plus-minus notation. However, the semantic peculiarities of certain terms (e.g. singular and pronominal) may license further inferences of a less than purely logical kind. For example, from '(some) Socrates is wise' we move to '(all) Socrates are wise' provided that we recognize that 'Socrates' is a singular term, yet the move is not a purely logical inference, as an inference following the *Dictum de Omni* surely is. The same is

---

[12] Lockwood is more optimistic, holding that the unrestricted pronoun-free subsystem (with heterogeneous conjunction for n-adic terms) is probably decidable. The undecidability of this subsystem can be shown to entail the existence, within the predicate calculus, of axioms of infinity that are *uniformly quantified* (in the sense of Appendix G). Lockwood's conjecture is prompted by scepticism as to the possibility of constructing such formulae, grounded in the observation that departures from uniformity occur essentially in all such axioms of infinity as appear in the literature.

true of inferences involving pronouns: the special semantic nature of the proterms licences certain moves that are not purely logical inferences. These extralogical inferences are similar to the move from 'A is parallel to B' to 'B is parallel to A' via the extralogical (semantic) recognition that 'parallel to' is a symmetric relation.

This thesis gains some support from the results of the discussion in sections 2.1 and especially 2.2, which show that the fundamentally Boolean logical syntax of TFL (unencumbered by further complications ushered in by semantics) has the kind of transparency that lends itself to decision procedures, whereas any enlargement of this basic vocabulary of logical signs appears to lead to undecidability. If we are to draw any boundary line between logic and other more specialized branches, mathematics for instance, why not draw it at the precise point where decidability ends and undecidability begins? Why not attribute undecidability to the introduction of special terms (relative pronouns especially) rather than to new *purely logical* signs? This proposal deserves serious consideration from logicians.

Appendix F

by Clifton McIntosh

In traditional formal logic the two oppositions of contradiction and contrariety are considered basic. An example of contradictory opposition is 'a creature was stirring' and 'not a creature was stirring'. Contrariety is essentially an opposition of terms like 'wise' and 'unwise'. But derivatively two propositions whose predicate terms are contraries are called contrary propositions. Thus, the pair 'every man is wise' and 'every man is unwise' and the pair 'some man is wise' and 'some man is unwise' are contrary pairs. In the traditional square of opposition contrary particular propositions are called 'subcontraries'.

In what follows we shall present a formal logic whose logical particles are signs of opposition. Expressions such as '$(+A)$' and '$(-A)$' will be used to represent terms and '$(+p)$' and '$(-p)$' will be used to represent propositions. The logical signs, '$+$' and '$-$', serve to give a term or proposition letter a positive or negative valence.

Following a suggestion of Leibniz the positive copula is represented by a plus sign. Thus 'an A is a B' could be represented by '$(+A)+(+B)$' and 'no A is a B', or 'not an A is a B', as '$-((+A)+(+B))$'. For convenience we drop the positive sign for terms. The primitive square of opposition then looks like Figure I.

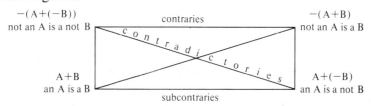

Fig. I

In a primitive version of traditional formal logic 'every' is missing. However, 'every A is B' may be defined by 'no A is un-B' in the following manner

$$-A + B = df - (A + (-B))$$

The definition represents the functor, 'every . . . is . . .' as the pair '$-$, $+$'. We therefore read the minus sign preceding the subject term 'A' as 'every'. Correspondingly the functor 'some . . . is . . .' is better represented by a *pair* of signs to contrast it with 'every . . . is . . .'. 'Some man is wise' now becomes '$+ M + W$' to contrast it with '$- M + W$' ('every man is wise'). The familiar square of opposition for the four categoricals now looks like Figure II.

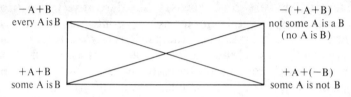

$-A+B$
every A is B

$-(+A+B)$
not some A is a B
(no A is B)

$+A+B$
some A is B

$+A+(-B)$
some A is not B

Fig. II

In Figure II the proposition for 'no A is B' has an external minus sign, the other three are externally positive. A more elegant square would use 'every' for both universal contraries (Figure III). In figure III all propositions are implicitly preceded by an external plus sign.

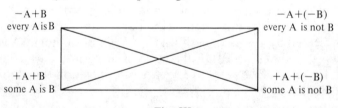

$-A+B$
every A is B

$-A+(-B)$
every A is not B

$+A+B$
some A is B

$+A+(-B)$
some A is not B

Fig. III

The algebraic notation for transcribing propositions into a form for logical reckoning is new. But it is traditional in its treatment of the basic logical signs as signs for the opposition of contradiction of propositions and the contrariety of terms. It is traditional also in assigning to every term a distribution value depending on its negative or positive occurrence. The reader will remember that traditional formal logic assigns the values 'distributed' to the subject terms of A & E propositions and to the predicate terms of E & O propositions. In the algebraic notation distribution is negative occurrence. Thus in 'every A is B' (or ' − A + B') 'A' has negative occurrence and is distributed while 'B' is undistributed.[1] Finally the algebraic transcription repairs the fundamental defect of traditional logic—its inability to handle inferences with relational propositions. Propositions like 'every boy loves some girl' and 'some sailor is giving every child a toy' are transcribed in the algebraic notation respectively as ' − B + (l + G)' and ' + S + (g − C + T)'. We shall show how to reckon logically with expressions like these.

A system of logic with the syncategorematic logical expressions for 'some . . . is . . .', 'not', and 'and' corresponds to a system of modern predicate logic whose logical particles are '∃x', ' ∼ ' and '&'. As is well known, a fair amount of logic can be done with these logical formatives. We have indicated how a plus-minus logic handles 'some is' and 'not', but have not yet given a plus-minus representation for 'and'. 'Not' is a minus sign. If we represent '&' as a plus sign we are able to represent the truth functions algebraically. Thus ' − (p + (− q))' represents ' ∼ (p & (∼ q))'. We find it better to represent 'and' as a pair of signs so that 'p & q' is represented as ' + p + q'. We may proceed to define 'p → q' as ' ∼ (p & (− q))'. Algebraically the definition looks like this:

$$- p + q = df - (+ p + (- q))$$

Our objective then is to present a 'traditional' system of logic in which the primitive plus-minus oppositions of contrariety and contradiction and the primitive operation of conjunction (' + ') supply or define the formative signs. The resultant system is intended to be logically effective in its mapping of inference into algebraic operations.

TRADITIONAL FORMAL LOGIC

In what follows an extension of traditional formal logic is set out in a formalized form and its soundness and completeness is

---

[1] See 'Distribution Matters', *Mind*, 84, 1975.

proved. By traditional formal logic (TFL) we mean a logic of terms, both general and singular. The central characteristics of this traditional framework are its use of the logical notions of quantity (some and all) and quality (positive and negative) and the eschewing of the modern apparatus of free and bound variables. The system to be presented contains the basic framework of the ideas espoused by Fred Sommers in a long series of publications. At the conclusion of this paper, further additions to TFL will be discussed.

The central logical notions of TFL, quantity and quality, are expressed by algebraic signs ('+' and '−') and TFL is given a predominantly algebraic cast. The central aims of TFL are (a) to make the most common inferences a matter of substituting (or adding and subtracting) terms and propositions and (b) to keep the syntax of TFL as close as possible to the surface grammar of English. This second aim requires a subject/predicate approach. It results in making translation from and to English much easier than is the case for quantification theory. The single most important innovation over other traditional subject/predicate approaches lies in the ability of TFL to treat multiply quantified statements. In other words, TFL is able to treat some propositions involving relations and the inferences from them. The limitations on this aspect of TFL and possible extensions to overcome them will also be discussed at the end of this paper.

TFL contains the full logic of propositions, all of syllogistic reasoning, a portion of the logic of identity,[2] and some of the logic of relations. All of this is represented with terms and the two algebraic signs '+' and '−'. This requires '+' and '−' to do many jobs. In fact, they do not less than three jobs each, and have as a result different meanings in different contexts. The semantics to be given will make clear how these different meanings are distinguished and in what contexts they bear one meaning or another.

A few preliminary equivalences between sentences of TFL and quantification theory will help the modern reader to follow the discussion. In the following sentences 'p' and 'q' represent

---

[2] TFL handles identity only for singular terms as it stands. With the addition of a relation sign for identity it can handle some quantified statements involving identity. For details, see the addendum and [3].

sentences, 'A' and 'B' terms, and 'R' a two-place relation.

TFL	Quantification Theory	English
$-p+q$	$p \rightarrow q$	if p then q
$p+q$	$p \& q$	p and q
$-p$	$\sim p$	not p
$-A+B$	$\forall x(Ax \rightarrow Bx)$	Every A is a B
$+A+B$	$\exists x(Ax \& Bx)$	Some A is a B
$-A+R+B$	$\forall x(Ax \rightarrow \exists y(By \& Rxy))$	Every A is R to some B
$+A+R-B$	$\exists x(Ax \& \forall y(By \rightarrow Rxy))$	Some A is R to every B

The formal system to be presented will be called TFL and its language, TL.

Description of TL

Vocabulary:

1. Proposition letters: p, q, r, p', q', r', . . .
2. Term Letters:
   a. General term letters: T, A, B, C, A', B', C', ...
   b. Singular term letters: a, b, c, a', b', c', ...
3. Relation letters (n-place, n > 1): R_1^n, S_1^n, R_2^n, S_2^n, ...
4. Natural numbers (to be used as indices on relation letters)
5. Logical signs: $+ - < > ( )$.[3]

N-Place Relations:

If ξ is an n-place relation letter and $i_1, i_2, \ldots, i_n$ is a sequence of n distinct integers, all less than or equal to n, then $+ \xi^{i_1 i_2 \cdots i_n}$ and $- \xi^{i_1 i_2 \cdots i_n}$ are n-place relations. Nothing else is an n-place relation.

Terms:

1. If α is a term or term letter, then $(+\alpha)$ and $(-\alpha)$ are terms.
2. If α and β are terms, then so are $(\pm \langle \pm \alpha \pm \beta \rangle)$.
3. If ξ is an n-place relation and $\alpha_1, \alpha_2, \ldots \alpha_{n-1}$ are terms, then $(\pm(\xi \pm \alpha_1 \pm \alpha_2 \pm \ldots \pm \alpha_{n-1}))$ are terms.
4. Nothing is a term unless it falls under one of the clauses above.

---

[3] 'T' is really a logical term; it represents the logical property of being a thing.

Df. A term is a *singular term* iff it is of the form $(+\alpha)$ where α is a singular term letter.

Df. A term is a *truth-functionally complex term* iff it is of the form $(\pm\langle\pm\alpha\pm\beta\rangle)$, where α and β are terms.[4]

Df. A term is a *relational term* iff it is of the form $(\pm(\xi\pm\alpha_1 \pm\alpha_2 \ldots \pm\alpha_{n-1}))$ where ξ is an n-place relation and the α_i are terms.[5]

Elementary Sentences:

1. Any proposition letter is an elementary sentence.

2. If α and β are terms, then $(\pm\alpha\pm\beta)$ are elementary sentences.

3. Nothing is an elementary sentence unless it falls under clause (1) or (2).

Sentences:

1. If χ is a sentence or an elementary sentence, then $(+\chi)$ and $(-\chi)$ are sentences.

2. If χ and ψ are sentences then so too are $(\pm(\pm\chi\pm\psi))$.

3. Nothing is a sentence unless it falls under clause (1) or (2).

Model Theory for TL

Df. An *interpretation I of TL* consists of

(a) a non-empty domain D;

(b) an assignment of T or F (but not both) to every proposition letter of TL;

(c) An assignment of an n-place relation on D to every n-place relation of TL in such a way that if $\langle a_1, a_2, \ldots, a_n\rangle$, an n-tuple of elements of D, is an element of the relation on D

---

[4] Such terms represent expressions such as 'both a male and a Democrat' and 'if an animal then owned by Jones'.

[5] Such terms represent such expressions as 'brother of some senator' and 'offspring of some Russian and some American'. The indices are required to indicate which form of the relation is involved (e.g., active or passive) and hence which order the variables in the usual quantified form of the sentence are to be understood. For example, '$L^{2,12}+M$' represents 'one who loves some man' and '$L^{2,21}+M$' represents 'one who is loved by some man'. Thus, the indices function to allow us to represent inverse relations and the like. The most common form of a relation is given the index '123 . . .'. We are indebted to David Bennett for this way of representing the various forms of a relation, which replaced an earlier, clumsier way of doing the same thing.

assigned to $\xi^{n, 123\cdots n}$, then $\langle a_{k_1}, a_{k_2}, \ldots, a_{k_n} \rangle$, a scrambling of the above n-tuple, is assigned to the n-place relation $\xi^{n,k_1k_2\cdots k_n}$ (and vice-versa). The n-place relation, $-\xi^{n,i_1i_2\cdots i_n}$, is assigned the complement of $+\xi^{n,i_1i_2\cdots i_n}$ with respect to D^n;

(d) An assignment of a subset (possibly empty) of D to every term letter, and to every term in such a way that the following hold: [Let $[\alpha]$ be the subset of D assigned to the term or term letter α and let $[\bar{\alpha}]$ be the complement of that subset of D relative to D.]

(i) 'T' is assigned D itself;

(ii) If α is a term or term letter, then $(+\alpha)$ is assigned $[\alpha]$ and $(-\alpha)$ is assigned $[\bar{\alpha}]$;

(iii) If α and β are terms then

$(+\langle +\alpha + \beta \rangle)$ is assigned $[\alpha] \cap [\beta]$, $(-\langle +\alpha+\beta \rangle)$, its complement
$(+\langle +\alpha - \beta \rangle)$ is assigned $[\alpha] \cap [\bar{\beta}]$, $(-\langle +\alpha-\beta \rangle)$, its complement
$(+\langle -\alpha + \beta \rangle)$ is assigned $[\bar{\alpha}] \cup [\beta]$, $(-\langle -\alpha+\beta \rangle)$, its complement
$(+\langle -\alpha - \beta \rangle)$ is assigned $[\bar{\alpha}] \cup [\bar{\beta}]$, $(-\langle -\alpha-\beta \rangle)$, its complement;

(iv) If $\alpha_1, \alpha_2, \ldots, \alpha_{n-1}$ are terms and $+\xi^{n,i_1i_2\cdots i_n}$ is an n-place relation, then $(+(+\xi^{n,i_1i_2\cdots i_n} \pm \alpha_1 \pm \alpha_2 \ldots \alpha_{n-1}))$ is assigned the set of all y such that y satisfies the sentence

'$(Q_1x_1 \in [\alpha_1])(Q_2x_2\in[\alpha_2])\ldots(Q_{n-1}x_{n-1}\in[\alpha_{n-1}])$
$(\xi^{n,i_1i_2\cdots i_n}yx_1x_2\ldots x_{n-1})$'

where Q_i is a universal quantifier if the sign preceding α_i is ' $-$ ', otherwise Q_i is an existential quantifier; if the term is preceded by ' $-$ ', it is assigned the complement of the above specified set. Finally, if ξ is preceded by ' $-$ ', then the sentence to be satisfied is just like the above except that ξ is preceded by a negation sign.[6]

Df: An interpretation I of TL is a *normal interpretation* of TL iff every singular term letter is assigned a subset of the domain D which contains one and only one element of D.

[6] Clause (iv) can be specified without the use of the notion of satisfaction. Basically, the first relational term mentioned is assigned the class of things that bear ξ to some or every α_1, some or every α_2, $\ldots$, and some or every α_{n-1}.

Truth under an Interpretation I

Elementary Sentences:

If α and β are terms, then $(+\alpha+\beta)$ is true under I iff $[\alpha] \cap [\beta]$ is non-empty; $(+\alpha-\beta)$ is true under I iff $[\alpha] \cap [\bar{\beta}]$ is non-empty; $(-\alpha+\beta)$ is true under I iff $[\alpha] \subseteq [\beta]$; and $(-\alpha-\beta)$ is true under I iff $[\alpha] \subseteq [\bar{\beta}]$.

Sentences:

1. If χ is a sentence or elementary sentence then $(-\chi)$ is true under I iff χ is false under I: $(+\chi)$ is true under I iff χ is true under I.

2. If χ and ψ are sentences then $(+(+\chi \pm \psi))$ is true under I iff χ is true and ψ true/(false) under I; $(-(+\chi \pm \psi)$ is true under I iff $(+(+\chi \pm \psi))$ is false under I; $(+(-\chi \pm \psi))$ is true under I iff χ is false or ψ is true/(false) under I; and $(-(-\chi \pm \psi))$ is true under I iff $(+(-\chi \pm \psi))$ is false under I.

The multiplicity of roles played by ' $+$ ' and ' $-$ ' in TL should now be somewhat clear. In front of a sentence, standing alone, or immediately in front of a term, ' $+$ ' and ' $-$ ' function as signs of affirmation or negation, or positive or negative quality for terms. In the context of an elementary sentence of the form $(\pm \alpha \pm \beta)$, where α and β are terms, the initial ' $\pm$ ' signifies 'some' or 'all' and the second signifies 'is' or 'is not'. In the context of compound sentences, $(\pm(\pm \chi \pm \psi))$, with χ and ψ sentences, in the second position ' $+$ ' signifies a conjunction and ' $-$ ' a conditional and in the third ' $\pm$ ' indicates affirmation or negation. The roles played by ' $\pm$ ' in truth-functionally complex terms, $(\pm \langle \pm \alpha \pm \beta \rangle)$, are the same as in compound sentences. Finally, after relations the ' $\pm$ ' indicates 'some' or 'all' when not inside the parentheses around terms.

Df: A sentence χ is a logically valid sentence of TL iff χ is true under every normal interpretation of TL ($\vDash_{TL}\chi$).

Df: A sentence χ is a *logical consequence of a set of sentences* Σ iff χ is true under every normal interpretation of TL which makes all of the sentences in Σ true ($\Sigma \vDash_{TL}\chi$).

Df: A set of sentences of TL, Σ, *has a normal model* iff there is a normal interpretation I under which all of the sentences of Σ are true.

The Formal System TFL

In what follows let α, β, γ, and λ be terms, χ, ψ, and ϕ be sentences, Θ, Ω, and Φ be either terms or sentences, and ξ be an n-place relation letter.

Axioms:

1. $(+(+\alpha+\alpha))$, where α is a singular term.
2. $\ulcorner(+(-\alpha+(+T)))\urcorner$.[7]

Transformation Rules:

1. Duality of singular terms: If λ is a singular term, then $\ldots\ldots\lambda\ldots\ldots/\ldots\lambda\ldots$, where '$\ldots\ldots\lambda\ldots\ldots$' represents a sentence in which λ occurs one or more times as either the subject term of an elementary sentence or as one of the terms in a relational term and '$\ldots\lambda\ldots$' represents the result of reversing the algebraic quantity of one or more such occurrences of λ.

[Thus, $(+(\pm\alpha+\beta))$ entails $(+(\mp\alpha+\beta))$ and $(+(\pm\gamma+(+(+\xi\pm\alpha))))$ entails $(+(\pm\gamma+(+(+\xi\mp\alpha))))$, if α is a singular term].

2. $(+(-\Theta+\Omega))/(+(-(-\Omega)+(-\Theta)))$
3. $(+(+\alpha+\beta))/\ulcorner(+(+(+T)+(+\langle+\alpha+\beta\rangle)))\urcorner$
4. $(+(\pm\alpha+(+\langle+\beta+\gamma\rangle)))/(+(\pm\alpha+\beta))$, $(+(\pm\alpha+\gamma))$
5. $(+(\pm\alpha+(+\langle-\beta+\gamma\rangle)))/(+(-(+(\pm\alpha+\beta))+(+(\pm\alpha+\gamma))))$
6. *Dictum de Omni* (DDO):
   $(+(-\Theta+\Omega))$, $\ldots\ldots\Theta\ldots\ldots/\ldots\ldots\Omega\ldots\ldots$,
   where '$\ldots\ldots\Theta\ldots\ldots$' represents a sentence in which Θ occurs undistributed and '$\ldots\ldots\Omega\ldots\ldots$' represents the result of replacing one or more of the undistributed occurrences of Θ by Ω.

Df: An occurrence of a term or sentence Θ in χ is *undistributed in* χ iff that occurrence of Θ in χ is within the scope of zero or an even number of '$-$' signs, the *scope* of a '$-$' sign being given by the following rules:
   (i) if a '$-$' sign is immediately followed by a '(', or '$\langle$', then

---

[7] We use quasi-quotes to enclose expressions which include expressions of TL and metalinguistic variables. The expression footnoted stands for any sentence of TL formed by concatenating '$+(-$', a term of TL, and '$+(+T)))$'.

its scope is all of the material between that '(' or '⟨' and the corresponding ')' or '⟩';

(ii) otherwise, its scope is whatever immediately follows it.

7. $(+(\pm\alpha_1 + (+(\pm\xi^{i_1 i_2 \cdots i_n} \pm \alpha_2 \pm \ldots \pm \alpha_n))))/$
   $(+(\pm\alpha_{l_1} + (+(\pm\xi^{k_1 k_2 \cdots k_n} \pm \alpha_{l_2} \pm \alpha_{l_3} \ldots \pm \alpha_{l_n}))))$

where $k_1 k_2 \ldots k_n$ is some scrambling of $i_1 i_2 \ldots i_n$, with the terms α_1 to α_n being scrambled in a corresponding fashion (i.e., if i_i and i_k are interchanged then so too are α_i and α_k) *and* in the resulting interchange of terms no α_i preceded by '$+$' is moved to the left of one preceded by '$-$'.

We now need to give definitions of proofs in and theorems of TFL. The definitions and overall structure of what follows is based on Benson Mates's treatment in his *Elementary Logic*. The choice of a framework for TFL is constrained by the awkwardness of the symbolism. It is manageable so long as the sentences and terms do not get too complicated. A straight axiomatization is for this reason unacceptable. A natural deduction system like Mates's avoids the problem to some extent. Further improvements in the presentation of TFL are certain to be made.

Df: A derivation in TFL consists of a finite sequence of consecutively numbered lines, each consisting of a sentence of TL together with a list of numbers, the premiss-numbers of the line, the sequence being constructed according to the following rules:

1. A Any axiom may be entered on any line with the null set of premiss numbers.

2. P Any sentence of TL may be entered on a line, with the line number taken as sole premiss number.

3. T χ may be entered on a line if χ follows from one or two earlier lines by any of the above transformation rules; as premiss numbers take all premiss numbers of lines from which χ is deduced.

4. C $(+(-\chi+\psi))$ may be entered on a line if ψ appears on an earlier line; as premiss numbers take all those of that earlier line, with the possible exception of any that is the line number of a line on which χ appears.

5. ES If $\ulcorner(+(+(+T)+\alpha))\urcorner$ appears on line i, $(+(+\lambda$

$+\alpha$)), λ a singular term, appears on line j as premiss ($j > i$), χ on line k ($k > j$) and if λ occurs neither in χ, α, or any premiss of line k other than $(+(+\lambda+\alpha))$, then χ may be entered on a new line with premiss numbers those of lines i and j, save for j (if desired).

6. Neg χ may be entered on a line if χ is the result of substituting in an earlier line any of the following terms or sentences for the other in the pair; as line numbers take all premiss numbers of the earlier line.

Ω	$(+\Omega)$
$(\pm\langle\pm\alpha-(\pm\beta)\rangle)$	$(\pm\langle\pm\alpha+(\mp\beta)\rangle)$
$(-\langle\pm\alpha\pm\beta\rangle)$	$(+\langle\mp\alpha\mp\beta\rangle)$
$(-(\pm\zeta^n\pm\alpha\pm\ldots$	
$\pm\beta))$	$(+(\mp\zeta^n\mp\alpha\mp\ldots\mp\beta))$
$(-(\pm\Omega\pm T))$	$(+(\mp\Omega\mp T))$
$(\pm(\pm\Omega-(\pm T)))$	$(\pm(\pm\Omega+(\mp T)))$

and, where ζ is a proposition letter, term letter, term or sentence

$$(-(\pm\zeta)) \qquad\qquad (+(\mp\zeta))$$

By applications of the Neg-rule, sentences of TL can be transformed into a simple form which we will call *the canonical form*. A sentence χ is in canonical form iff (i) all '$-$' signs are driven in as far as possible, and (ii) all '$+$' signs that can be eliminated are eliminated. Notice that in particular the second '$\pm$' in an elementary sentence or truth-functionally complex sentence can always be made a '$+$'. In later metatheorems we will need to consider only sentences in canonical form. Once the soundness of the Neg-rule is proved we will know that a sentence and its canonical form are logical equivalents.

Df: A derivation in which the sentence χ of TL appears on the last line and in which all premisses of that line belong to the set Σ of sentences of TL is a derivation of χ from Σ in TFL. If there is such a derivation, we will say that χ follows from Σ, which will be written as $\Sigma \vdash \chi$.

Df: A sentence χ is a theorem of TFL iff there is a derivation of χ from the empty set.

A number of simplifications can be adopted so that the use of TFL in proving theorems is not so cumbersome. No ambiguity will result if some of the many parentheses and '+'s are dropped. In particular, we will often drop outside parentheses and '+'s from positive terms and from positive sentences standing alone. Thus, '$(+(+ (+T) + (+A)))$' would be abbreviated as '$(+ T + A)$'. We also use three derived rules of inference to make the proofs shorter and clearer.

The first derived rule involves an addition to the T-rule. The addition is a correlate of DDO, which we call DDO'. It is

$$(+(-\Theta+\Omega)), \ldots (-\Omega)\ldots/\ldots (-\Theta)\ldots, \quad \text{where} \quad \text{'}\ldots$$
$(-\Omega)\ldots$' and '$\ldots (-\Theta)\ldots$' are as in DDO.

For sentences this rule is just modus tollens or an extension thereof. This rule is easily derived from DDO. One merely uses T(2) to get $(+(-(-\Omega)+(-\Theta)))$ from $(+(-\Theta+\Omega))$ and uses DDO to deduce $\ldots (-\Theta)\ldots$.

The second derived rule allows us to prove things indirectly by reductio. The rule, called RAA, is

χ may be entered on a line if ψ and $-\psi$ appear on earlier lines; as premiss numbers take all those of the lines on which ψ and $-\psi$ appear with the possible exception of any that is the line number on a line on which $-\chi$ appears.

This rule can easily be derived from C and DDO'.

Finally, we introduce a rule to enable us to make use of previously proved theorems. This rule, TH, is

χ may be entered on a line with no premiss numbers if χ is an instance of a previously proven theorem; or χ may be entered on a line if χ follows from earlier lines immediately by an earlier theorem; as premiss numbers take those of the earlier lines.

The use of this rule in any given case is obviously dispensable. One need only insert an appropriate version of the derivation of the theorem.

Derivations are, strictly speaking, done in the object language. We will, however, allow that derivations be done in terms of metalinguistic variables for purposes of convenience. This should cause no problems. Also, and again for convenience, some of the 'theorems' to be proved will be stated in the form '$\chi, \psi \vdash \phi$' rather than as $(+(-(+(+\chi+\psi))+\phi))$.

Before proving the soundness and completeness of TFL, we present some theorems and metatheorems which are necessary for later proofs.

Theorem 1: $(+(-\chi+(-\chi))) \vdash (-\chi)$

1.	$\{1\}$	$(+(-\chi+(-\chi)))$	P
2.	$\{2\}$	$(-(-\chi))$	P
3.	$\{1, 2\}$	$(-\chi)$	1, 2 by DDO'.
4.	$\{1\}$	$(-\chi)$	2, 3 by RAA.

Theorem 2: $\chi, \psi \vdash (+(+\chi+\psi))$

1.	$\{1\}$	χ	P
2.	$\{2\}$	ψ	P
3.	$\{3\}$	$(-(+\chi+\psi))$	P
4.	$\{3\}$	$(+(-\chi+(-\psi)))$	3 by Neg
5.	$\{1, 3\}$	$-\psi$	1, 4 by DDO
6.	$\{1, 2\}$	$(+(+\chi+\psi))$	2, 3, 5 by RAA

Theorem 3: $(+(+\chi+\psi)) \vdash \chi, \psi$

1.	$\{1\}$	$(+(+\chi+\psi))$	P
2.	$\{2\}$	$-\psi$	P
3.	$\{2\}$	$(+(-\chi+(-\psi)))$	2 by C
4.	$\{2\}$	$(-(+\chi+\psi))$	3 by Neg
5.	$\{1\}$	ψ	1, 2, 4 by RAA
6.	$\{6\}$	$-\chi$	P
7.	$\{6\}$	$(+(-\psi+(-\chi)))$	6 by C
8.	$\{6\}$	$(+(-\chi+(-\psi)))$	7 by Neg and T(2)
9.	$\{6\}$	$(-(+\chi+\psi))$	8 by Neg
10.	$\{1\}$	χ	1, 6, 9 by RAA

Theorem 4: $(+(+\chi+\psi)) \vdash (+(+\psi+\chi))$
Immediate from Theorems 2 and 3.

Theorem 5: $(+(-\chi+\psi)), (+(-\chi+\phi)) \vdash (+(-\chi+(+(+\psi+\phi))))$

1.	$\{1\}$	$(+(-\chi+\psi))$	P
2.	$\{2\}$	$(+(-\chi+\phi))$	P

3. $\quad$ {3} $\qquad \chi$ $\qquad\qquad$ P
4. $\quad$ {3, 2} $\qquad \phi$ $\qquad\qquad$ 2, 3 by DDO
5. $\quad$ {3, 1} $\qquad \psi$ $\qquad\qquad$ 1, 3 by DDO
6. $\quad$ {1, 2, 3} $\ (+(+\psi+\phi))$ $\qquad$ 4, 5 by TH(2)
7. $\quad$ {1, 2} $\ (+(-\chi+(+(+\psi+\phi))))$ $\qquad$ 3, 6 by C.

Theorem 6: $\quad +(-\chi+(+(-\psi+\phi)))) \vdash (+(-\psi+(+(-\chi +\phi))))$

Theorem 7: $\quad (+(-\chi+(-\psi+\phi)))) \vdash (+(-(+(+\chi+\psi)) +\phi))$

6 and 7 follow easily from the above.

Theorem 8: $\quad \ulcorner(+(-(+T)+(+\langle-\alpha+\beta\rangle)))\urcorner \vdash (+(-\alpha +\beta))$

1. $\quad$ {1} $\quad \ulcorner(+(-(+T)+(+\langle-\alpha+\beta\rangle)))\urcorner$ P
2. $\quad$ {2} $\quad (-(-\alpha+\beta))$ $\qquad\qquad$ P
3. $\quad$ {2} $\quad (+(+\alpha+(-\beta)))$ $\qquad\qquad$ 2 by Neg
4. $\quad$ {2} $\quad \ulcorner(+(+(+T)+(+\langle+\alpha +(-\beta)\rangle)))\urcorner$ $\qquad$ 3 by T(3)
5. $\quad$ {5} $\quad \ulcorner(+(+(+a)+(+\langle+\alpha+ (-\beta)\rangle)))\urcorner$ $\qquad\qquad$ P
6. $\quad$ Λ $\quad (+(+(+a)+(+a)))$ $\qquad\qquad$ A (1)
7. $\quad$ Λ $\quad (+(-(+a)+(+T)))$ $\qquad\qquad$ A (2)
8. $\quad$ Λ $\quad (+(+(+a)+(+T)))$ $\qquad\qquad$ 6, 7 by DDO
9. $\quad$ {1} $\quad \ulcorner(+(+(+a)+(+\langle-\alpha+\beta\rangle)))\urcorner$ $\qquad$ 1, 8 by DDO
10. $\quad$ {1} $\quad \ulcorner(+(-(+a)+(-\langle+\alpha +(-\beta)\rangle)))\urcorner$ $\qquad$ 9 by T(1) and Neg
11. $\quad$ {1, 5} $\quad (+(-\alpha+\beta))$ $\qquad\qquad$ 5, 10 by RAA
12. $\quad$ {1, 2} $\quad (+(-\alpha+\beta))$ $\qquad\qquad$ 4, 11 by ES
13. $\quad$ {1} $\quad (+(-\alpha+\beta))$ $\qquad\qquad$ 12 by TH(1).

Theorem 9: $\quad (+(-\alpha+\beta)) \vdash \ulcorner(+(-(+T)+(+\langle-\alpha +\beta\rangle)))\urcorner$

1. $\quad$ {1} $\quad (+(-\alpha+\beta))$ $\qquad\qquad$ P
2. $\quad$ {2} $\quad \ulcorner(-(-(+T)+(+\langle-\alpha+\beta\rangle)))\urcorner$ P
3. $\quad$ {2} $\quad \ulcorner(+(+(+T)+(+\langle+\alpha +(-\beta)\rangle)))\urcorner$ $\qquad\qquad$ 2 by Neg
4. $\quad$ {4} $\quad \ulcorner(+(+(+a)+(+\langle+\alpha +(-\beta)\rangle)))\urcorner$ $\qquad\qquad$ P
5. $\quad$ {4} $\quad \ulcorner(+(+(+a)+\alpha))\urcorner$ $\qquad\qquad$ 4 by T(4)
6. $\quad$ {4} $\quad \ulcorner(+(+(+a)+(-\beta)))\urcorner$ $\qquad\qquad$ 4 by T(4)

7. $\{1, 4\}$ $\ulcorner(+ (+ (+ a) + \beta))\urcorner$ 1, 5 by DDO
8. $\{1, 4\}$ $\ulcorner(- (+ (+ T) + (+ \langle + \alpha$
           $+ (- \beta) \rangle))))\urcorner$ 6, 7 by RRA
9. $\{1, 2\}$ $\ulcorner(+ (- (+ T) + (+ \langle - \alpha + \beta \rangle))))\urcorner$ 8, 3 by ES
                                             and Neg
10. $\{1\}$ $\ulcorner(+ (- (+ T) + (+ \langle - \alpha + \beta \rangle))))\urcorner$ 9 by TH(1).

Theorem 10: $(+ (- \alpha + \alpha))$
1. $\{1\}$ $(- (- \alpha + \alpha))$ P
2. $\{1\}$ $(+ (+ \alpha + (- \alpha)))$ 1, Neg
3. $\{1\}$ $\ulcorner(+ (+ (+ T) + (+ \langle + \alpha$
           $+ (- \alpha) \rangle))))\urcorner$ 2 by T(3)
4. $\{4\}$ $\ulcorner(+ (+ (+ a) + (+ \langle + \alpha$
           $+ (- \alpha) \rangle))))\urcorner$ P
5. $\{4\}$ $\ulcorner(+ (+ (+ a) + \alpha))$ 4 by T(4)
6. $\{4\}$ $\ulcorner(+ (+ (+ a) + (- \alpha)))\urcorner$ 4 by T(4)
7. $\{4\}$ $\ulcorner(+ (- (+ a) + (- \alpha)))\urcorner$ 6 by T(1)
8. $\{4\}$ $\ulcorner(- (+ (+ a) + \alpha))\urcorner$ 7 by Neg
9. $\{4\}$ $(+ (- \alpha + \alpha))$ 5, 8 RAA
10. $\{1\}$ $(+ (- \alpha + \alpha))$ 3, 9 by ES
11. Λ $(+ (- \alpha + \alpha))$ 10 by TH(1)

Theorem 11: $(+ (+ \alpha + \beta)) \vdash (+ (+ \beta + \alpha))$
1. $\{1\}$ $(+ (+ \alpha + \beta))$ P
2. $\{2\}$ $(- (+ \beta + \alpha))$ P
3. $\{2\}$ $(+ (- \beta + (- \alpha)))$ 2 by Neg
4. $\{1, 2\}$ $(+ (+ \alpha + (- \alpha)))$ 1, 3 by DDO
5. Λ $(+ (- \alpha + \alpha))$ TH(10)
6. $\{1\}$ $(+ (+ \beta + \alpha))$ RAA

Theorem 12: $(+ (- \alpha + \beta)), (+ (- \alpha + \gamma)) \vdash$
$(+ (- \alpha + (+ \langle + \beta + \gamma \rangle)))$
1. $\{1\}$ $(+ (- \alpha + \beta))$ P
2. $\{2\}$ $(+ (- \alpha + \gamma))$ P
3. $\{3\}$ $(- (- \alpha + (+ \langle + \beta + \gamma \rangle)))$ P
4. $\{3\}$ $(+ (+ \alpha + (+ \langle - \beta + (- \gamma) \rangle)))$ 3 by Neg
5. $\{3\}$ $\ulcorner(+ (+ (+ T) + (+ \langle + \alpha$
           $+ (+ \langle - \beta + (- \gamma) \rangle)))\urcorner$ 4 by T(3)
6. $\{6\}$ $\ulcorner(+ (+ (+ a) + (+ \langle + \alpha +$
           $(+ \langle - \beta + (- \gamma) \rangle)))\urcorner$ P

7. $\{6\}$ $\ulcorner(+(+(+a)+\alpha))\urcorner$ 6 by T(4)

8. $\{6\}$ $\ulcorner(+(+(+a)+(+\langle-\beta$
                     $+(-\gamma)\rangle))\urcorner$ 6 by T(4)

9. $\{6\}$ $\ulcorner(+(-(+(+(+a)+\beta))$
                 $+(+(+(+a)+(-\gamma)))))\urcorner$ 8 by T(5)

10. $\{1, 6, 2\}$ $\ulcorner(+(+(+a)+\beta))\urcorner,\ulcorner(+(+(+a)$
                 $+\gamma))\urcorner$ 1, 2, 7 by
                                             DDO

11. $\{1, 6\}$ $\ulcorner(+(+(+a)+(-\gamma)))\urcorner$ 9, 10 by
                                             DDO

12. $\{1, 2, 6\}$ $(+(-\alpha+(+\langle+\beta+\gamma\rangle)))$ 10, 11 by
                                             RAA

13. $\{1, 2, 3\}$ $(+(-\alpha+(+\langle+\beta+\gamma\rangle)))$ 6, 12 by ES

14. $\{1, 3\}$ $(+(-\alpha+(+\langle+\beta+\gamma\rangle)))$ 13 by TH(1).

Theorem 13: $(+\gamma+\langle+\alpha+\beta\rangle)\vdash(+\alpha+\beta)$

1. $\{1\}$ $(+\gamma+\langle+\alpha+\beta\rangle)$ P

2. Λ $\ulcorner(-\gamma+T)\urcorner$ A(2)

3. $\{1\}$ $\ulcorner(+T+\langle+\alpha+\beta\rangle)\urcorner$ 1, 2 by DDO

4. $\{4\}$ $(-(+\alpha+\beta))$ P

5. $\{4\}$ $(-\alpha+(-\beta))$ 4 by Neg

6. $\{6\}$ $\ulcorner(+a+\langle+\alpha+\beta\rangle)\urcorner$ P

7. $\{6\}$ $\ulcorner(+a+\alpha)\urcorner$ 6 by T(4)

8. $\{6\}$ $\ulcorner(+a+\beta)\urcorner$ 6 by T(4)

9. $\{4, 6\}$ $\ulcorner(+a+(-\beta))\urcorner$ 5, 7 by DDO

10. $\{4, 6\}$ $\ulcorner(-a+(-\beta))\urcorner$ 9 by T(1)

11. $\{6\}$ $(+\alpha+\beta)$ 8, 10 by RAA

12. $\{1\}$ $(+\alpha+\beta)$ 11 by ES.

Theorem 14: $(+\alpha+\gamma)\vdash(+\alpha+\langle-\beta+\gamma\rangle)$

1. $\{1\}$ $(+\alpha+\gamma)$ P

2. $\{2\}$ $(-(+\alpha+\langle-\beta+\gamma\rangle))$ P

3. $\{2\}$ $(-\alpha+\langle+\beta+(-\gamma)\rangle)$ 2 by Neg

4. $\{2\}$ $(-\alpha+(-\gamma))$ 3 by T(4)

5. $\{1\}$ $(+\alpha+\langle-\beta+\gamma\rangle)$ 1, 4 by RAA.

Theorem 15: $(+\alpha+(-\beta))\vdash(+\alpha+\langle-\beta+\gamma\rangle)$

1. $\{1\}$ $(+\alpha+(-\beta))$ P

2. $\{2\}$ $(-(+\alpha+\langle-\beta+\gamma\rangle))$ P

3. $\{2\}$ $(-\alpha+\langle+\beta+(-\gamma)\rangle)$ 2 by Neg

4. $\{2\}$ $(-\alpha+\beta)$ 3 by T(4)

5. $\{1\}$ $(+\alpha+\langle-\beta+\gamma\rangle)$ 1, 4 by RAA.

Metatheorem 1: If α, β, and γ are singular terms then (a) $\vdash$ $(+\alpha+\alpha)$, (b) $(+\alpha+\beta)\vdash(+\beta+\alpha)$, and (c) $(+\alpha+\beta)$, $(+\beta+\gamma)\vdash(+\alpha+\gamma)$. This metatheorem establishes that for singular terms α and β, $(+\alpha+\beta)$ has all of the properties of identity; it is reflexive, symmetric, and transitive. (a) holds by virtue of Axiom 1; (b) is Theorem 11. (c) is obtained by deriving $(-\beta+\gamma)$ from $(+\beta+\gamma)$ by T(1) and using DDO to get $(+\alpha+\gamma)$.

Metatheorem 2: TFL IS SOUND. That is, every theorem of TFL is true under every normal interpretation. The proof of this metatheorem follows a strategy used by Mates in [1]. We show that, for every line l in a derivation K of χ from Σ in TFL, the sentence of TL on line l is a logical consequence of the sentences whose line numbers are the premiss numbers of χ. If χ is a theorem of TFL, it is derivable from Λ and hence is logically valid.

To prove Metatheorem 2 we first prove the following two lemmas.

Lemma 1: If χ appears on the first line of a derivation K, it is a logical consequence of the sentences whose line numbers are the premiss numbers of χ.

Lemma 2: If all previous lines in a derivation K are logical consequences of the sentences whose line numbers are their premiss numbers and χ is derived from earlier lines by the rules T, C, ES, or Neg, then χ is a logical consequence of the sentences whose line numbers are the premiss numbers of the line χ is on.

It should be obvious that Metatheorem 2, the soundness of TFL, is an immediate consequence of Lemmas 1 and 2.

To establish Lemma 1 notice that there are only two rules which allow us to put down the first line of a derivation: A and P. They also allow us to introduce lines anywhere in a derivation. Any line put down by the P rule is clearly the logical consequence of the sentence whose line number is the premiss number of that line, since it is that very line and every sentence is a logical consequence of itself. Since lines put down by the A rule have no premiss numbers, we need to show that all of the axioms are logically valid. Instances of Axiom 1 are simple; they are logically valid iff every singular term has a non-empty extension. This is true by the definition of a normal interpretation. Instances of Axiom 2 are logically valid iff every term is assigned a subset of what '(+ T)' is assigned. Since that is just the whole domain all instances of Axiom 2 are logically valid. Thus, Lemma 1 is proved.

To establish Lemma 2 we need to show that the use of each of the rules C, Neg, ES, and T is truth-preserving. That is, if the sentences on which these rules are applied are true then the results of the applications are also true. Since we are assuming that earlier lines in a derivation are logical consequences of the sentences which are their premisses, if we know that the rules of TFL preserve truth we know that anything derived from earlier lines by those rules will be a logical consequence of its premisses.

(1) Rule C. If χ was entered on a line by the use of C, then χ is $(-\psi + \phi)$ and ϕ was on some earlier line. We are assuming ϕ is the logical consequence of its premisses, which may or may not include ϕ. Since that is true, were some normal interpretation to make all of those premisses (excluding ψ) true, then were that same interpretation to make ψ true it would have to make ϕ true. Therefore, χ is the logical consequence of its premisses.

(2) Rule Neg. That Neg is truth-preserving rests on two facts that are obvious from the semantics for TL: (a) in a truth-functionally compound sentence the truth or falsity of the sentence depends only on the truth values of its components, and (b) in an elementary sentence with terms the truth or falsity of the elementary sentence depends only on the extensions of the terms. Thus, if the interchangeable terms and sentences of the Neg rule have the same extension or truth value, then the Neg rule will preserve truth. We will not bother to go through the cases; they are immediately obvious from the semantics.

(3) Rule ES. The ES rule allows one to derive χ from 'something is α' and other premisses if we can derive χ from 'a is α' and those other premisses, where 'a' does not appear in α or in χ or in any of the other premisses. This rule is truth-preserving because, under the conditions specified, if χ is· a logical consequence of 'a is α', then it is a logical consequence of 'something is α'.

(4) Rule T. This rule is truth-preserving iff each of the seven transformations allowed by it are truth-preserving. Rule 1 is truth-preserving because each singular term has one and only one object in its extention. Therefore, if some or all α are β, then

all or some are, and if something bears some relation to some or all α then it bears it to all or some α, when α is a singular term. Rules 2–5 are obvious from the semantics. Rule 7 is essentially a quantifier exchange rule, for restricted quantifiers. We know from quantification theory that . . . $\exists x \forall y$ . . . (. . xy . .) implies . . . $\forall y \exists x$ . . . (. . xy . .), but not vice-versa, and that within strings of quantifiers of the same type the quantifiers can be arbitrarily interchanged. These are the only sorts of transformations that are allowed by rule 7.

The most difficult rule to prove truth-preserving is Rule 6, DDO, which is the most powerful rule. We prove it by induction on the order of the occurrences of the term or sentence Ω in . . . Ω . . . . We first need to define the order of an occurrence of a term and of a sentence in another sentence.

Df: An occurrence of a sentence χ in a sentence ψ is an occurrence of *order 0* iff χ is ψ; *order 1* iff ψ is $(\pm \chi)$, $(\pm (\pm \chi \pm \phi))$, or $(\pm (\pm \phi \pm \chi))$; and of *order* $n + 1$ iff χ occurs in ϕ with order n and ϕ occurs in ψ with order 1. An occurrence of a term α in a term β is an occurrence of *order 0* iff α is β; *order 1* iff β is $(\pm \alpha)$, $(\pm \langle \pm \alpha \pm \lambda \rangle)$, or $(\pm \langle \pm \lambda \pm \alpha \rangle)$, or $(\pm (\xi^n \ldots \pm \alpha \ldots))$; and of *order* $n + \underline{1}$ iff α occurs in λ with order n and λ occurs in β with order 1. An occurrence of a term α in a sentence is an *occurrence of order n* iff α occurs in β with order $n - 1$ and β is the subject or predicate term of an elementary sentence occurring in χ.

We now prove that DDO preserves truth for the case of sentences. That is, if $(-\chi + \psi)$ and . . . χ . . . are true, then . . . ψ . . . is true, where . . . χ . . . and . . . ψ . . . are as specified in DDO. Some additional terminology will be useful here. Instead of saying that a sentence χ has an undistributed occurrence in ϕ, we will say that χ has a positive occurrence in ϕ. And if . . . χ . . . is ϕ, then . . . ψ . . .will sometimes be represented as ϕ'.

In the following proof we will, for convenience, speak of sentences being true or false, when what is meant is that they are true or false under some unspecified interpretation that is fixed. Suppose χ has an occurrence of order 0 in . . . χ . . . . Then . . . χ . . . is χ, and DDO reduces to modus ponens. Suppose that χ has an occurrence of order 1 in . . . χ . . . . Then there are three cases: $\ldots \chi \ldots$ is (a) $(+\chi)$, (b) $(-\chi)$, and (c) $(\pm(\pm\chi\pm\phi))$ or $(\pm(\pm\phi\pm\chi))$.

(a) If $\ldots \chi \ldots$ is $(+\chi)$, we know that $(+\chi)$ is true iff χ is true. By what was shown for occurrences of order 0 we know that ψ is true and hence that $(+\psi)$ is true.

(b) If $\ldots \chi \ldots$ is $(-\chi)$, then χ has no positive occurrences.

(c) If $\ldots \chi \ldots$ is $(\pm(\pm\ \pm))$, then the only cases in which χ has a positive occurrence are $(+(+\chi\pm\phi))$, $(-(-\chi\pm\phi))$, $(+(\pm\phi+\chi))$, and $(-(\pm\phi-\chi))$. By driving in outside negations, the second reduces to the first and the fourth to the third. We are left with two main possibilities: $\ldots \chi \ldots$ is $(+(+\chi\pm\phi))$ or $(+(+\phi+\chi))$ and $\ldots \chi \ldots$ is $(+(-\phi+\chi))$.

If $\ldots \chi \ldots$ is $(+\chi\pm\phi)$ or $(+\phi+\chi)$, then $\ldots \chi \ldots$ is true iff both χ and ϕ are true. If χ is true, then by DDO for order 0 ψ is also true. Hence, $(+\psi\pm\phi)$ and $(+\phi+\psi)$ are also true.

If $\ldots \chi \ldots$ is $(-\phi+\chi)$, there are two possibilities. If χ is true so is ψ. Hence, regardless of ϕ, so is $(-\phi+\psi)$. If χ is false, then ϕ must also be false for $(-\phi+\chi)$ to be true. Then, regardless of the truth value of ψ, $(-\phi+\psi)$ must also be true. Thus, we have shown that DDO preserves truth for substitutions for occurrences of order 0 or 1.

If DDO fails to hold for all orders of positive occurrences of χ in $\ldots \chi \ldots$, then by the least number principle there must be some least number, n, such that the replacement of a positive occurrence of order n of χ in $\ldots \chi \ldots$ by ψ leads to a falsehood, but all replacements of occurrences of orders less than n lead to truths. From the above we know that $n > 1$. We show that n cannot be greater than 1.

Assume then that $\ldots \chi \ldots$ is a sentence in which χ has at least one positive occurrence of order n, $n > 1$, and that $\ldots \psi \ldots$ is false although $\ldots \chi \ldots$ and $(-\chi+\psi)$ are true. There are three possibilities: $\ldots \chi \ldots$ is (a) $(+\phi)$, (b) $(-\phi)$, or (c) $(\pm(\pm\phi\pm\zeta))$. The first case is simple. If $\ldots \chi \ldots$ is $(+\phi)$, then χ occurs in ϕ with a positive occurrence of order less than n. Hence, by the induction hypothesis, if ϕ is true so is ϕ'. Hence, so is $(+\phi')$ or $\ldots \psi \ldots$. Therefore, $\ldots \chi \ldots$ cannot be $(+\phi)$.

There are three possibilities under case (b), where $\ldots \chi \ldots$ is $(-\phi)$, viz., ϕ is (i) $(+\zeta)$, (ii) $(-\zeta)$, or (iii) $(\pm(\pm\zeta\pm\rho))$. In the first, (i), $\ldots \chi \ldots$ is $(-(+\zeta))$. Then $\ldots \chi \ldots$ is true iff $(-\zeta)$ is true. χ has a positive occurrence of order less than n in $(-\zeta)$, hence, $(-\zeta)'$ is true. Therefore, $(-(+\zeta'))$ or ... ψ ... is true and this case cannot be. In the second, (ii), ... χ ... is $(-(-\zeta))$. Then ... χ ... is true iff ζ is true. χ has a positive occurrence of order less than n in ζ, hence ζ' is true. Thus, $(-(-\zeta'))$ or ... ψ ... is true and this case cannot be. Finally, if ... χ ... is (iii) or $(-(\pm(\pm\zeta\pm\rho)))$, then ... χ ... is true iff $(\mp(\pm\zeta\pm\rho))$ is true, in which χ has a positive occurrence of order less than n. Hence, by the induction hypothesis, $(\mp(\pm\zeta\pm\rho))'$ is true. Thus, $(-(\pm(\pm\zeta\pm\rho)))'$ or ... ψ ... is true. Therefore, ... χ ... cannot be $(-\phi)$.

The final case, (c), is where ... χ ... is $(\pm(\pm\phi\pm\zeta))$ and χ occurs in either ϕ or ζ. By driving in negations whenever possible, we get two main subcases: (i) ... χ ... is $(+\phi\pm\zeta)$ and χ occurs positively in ϕ or ... χ ... is $(\pm\phi+\zeta)$ and χ occurs positively in ζ, and (ii) ... χ ... is $(-\phi\pm\zeta)$ and χ occurs negatively in ϕ or ... χ ... is $(\pm\phi-\zeta)$ and χ occurs negatively in ζ.

In the first subcase, (i), suppose ... χ ... is $(+\phi\pm\zeta)$. χ occurs positively in ϕ with an occurrence of order less than n and by the induction hypothesis ϕ' is true. Hence, $(+\phi'\pm\zeta)$ or ... ψ ... is true. If ... χ ... is $(\pm\phi+\zeta)$ and χ occurs in ζ, then χ occurs positively in ζ with order less than n. Hence, if ζ is true so is ζ'. Hence, $(\pm\phi+\zeta')$ or ... ψ ... is true.

In the second subcase, (ii), suppose ... χ ... is $(-\phi\pm\zeta)$ and χ occurs negatively in ϕ. $(-\phi\pm\zeta)$ is true if $(-(\mp\zeta)+(-\phi))$ is true. χ has a positive occurrence of order less than n in $(-\phi)$. By case (b) above, $(-\phi')$ is true iff $(-\phi)$ is. Hence, $(-(\mp\zeta)+(-\phi'))$ is true and so is $(-\phi'\pm\zeta)$ or ... ψ .... If ... χ ... is $(\pm\phi-\zeta)$ and χ occurs negatively in ζ, then χ occurs positively in $(-\zeta)$ with order n. By case (b) above, $(-'\zeta)$ is true iff $(-\zeta)$ is. Since $(\pm\phi-\zeta)$ is true iff $(\pm\phi+(-\zeta))$ is, $(\pm\phi+(-\zeta'))$ and $(\pm\phi-\zeta')$, or ... ψ ... are true. Therefore, ... χ ... cannot be $(\pm(\pm\phi\pm\zeta))$ and we have shown that DDO holds for the case of sentences.

We now proceed to show that DDO holds for term substitutions. We first show that DDO holds for terms when ... α ... is $(\pm(\pm\gamma\pm\lambda))$. We then use what we have shown for sentences to prove DDO holds for term substitutions in more complex contexts. It makes matters much easier if we first prove a simple lemma. First, some additional terminology.

Df: If α and β are terms and α occurs one or more times in β, then an occurrence of α in β is *a positive occurrence in β* iff that occurrence of α occurs within the scope of 0 or an even number of '$-$'s in β. All occurrences of α in β that are not positive occurrences are negative occurrences.

Lemma: For any interpretation I of TL, if $[\alpha] \subseteq [\beta]$, α occurs in λ, and λ' is the result of replacing one or more occurrences of α in λ by β, then if only positive occurrences are replaced $[\lambda] \subseteq [\lambda']$ and if only negative occurrences are replaced $[\lambda'] \subseteq [\lambda]$.

The proof proceeds by induction on the order of the occurrence of α in λ. If α occurs in λ with order 0, then α is λ, λ' is β, and α has positive occurrence in λ. Clearly, $[\alpha] \subseteq [\beta]$. We now assume that the lemma holds for all replaced occurrences of α of order less than n. We show that it holds for occurrences of order n. We know $n > 0$.

Suppose then that α occurs in λ with one or more occurrences of order n. There are four basic cases: λ is $(+\gamma)$, $(-\gamma)$, $(\pm \langle \pm\gamma \pm v \rangle)$, or $(\pm(\pm\xi^n \pm \gamma_1 \pm \ldots \pm \gamma_{n-1}))$. Assume that λ is $(+\gamma)$. Since $[(+\gamma)] = [\gamma]$ and α occurs in γ with order less than n, the induction hypothesis entails that the lemma holds of γ and therefore of $(+\gamma)$. If λ is $(-\gamma)$, then α occurs in γ with order less than n and the lemma holds of $[\gamma]$ and $[\gamma']$. If only positive occurrences of α in $(-\gamma)$ are replaced, then only negative occurrences of α in γ are replaced, and they are of order less than n. By the induction hypothesis $[\gamma'] \subseteq [\gamma]$. Hence, $[\bar{\gamma}] \subseteq [\bar{\gamma'}]$ and $[(-\gamma)] \subseteq [(-\gamma')]$. Negative occurrences are the reverse.

The third case, λ is $(\pm \langle \pm\gamma + v \rangle)$, reduces to two cases: (a) λ is $(+ \langle +\gamma + v \rangle)$ and (b) λ is $(+ \langle -\gamma + v \rangle)$. This is so because the case of an initial '$-$' sign can be handled by the reasoning just employed for $\lambda = (-\gamma)$. The '$\pm$' between terms can always be made into '$+$', with a '$-$' pushed into the second term, to be handled in the same way as the initial '$-$.'

Suppose then that λ is $(+ \langle +\gamma + v \rangle)$. Then α occurs in γ and v, if at all, with order less than n and $[\lambda] = [\gamma] \cap [v]$. If only positive occurrences of α in λ are replaced, then only positive occurrences of α in γ and v are replaced. Hence, by the induction hypothesis, $[\gamma] \subseteq [\gamma']$ and $[v] \subseteq [v']$. Hence, $[\gamma] \cap [v]$ is a subset of $[\gamma'] \cap [v']$ and $[\lambda] \subseteq [\lambda']$. The reasoning for negative occurrences is just the reverse.

Suppose that λ is $(+ \langle -\gamma + v \rangle)$. Then $[\lambda] = ([\bar{\gamma}] \cup [v])$. If we replace only positive occurrences of α in λ, then we will replace negative occurrences of α in γ and positive occurrences in v. By the induction hypothesis, $[\gamma'] \subseteq [\gamma]$ and $[v] \subseteq [v']$. Therefore, $[\bar{\gamma}] \subseteq [\bar{\gamma'}]$ and $([\bar{\gamma}] \cup [v]) \subseteq ([\bar{\gamma'}] \cup [v'])$ or $[\lambda] \subseteq [\lambda']$. The reasoning for negative occurrences is exactly parallel.

The final case to be treated is where λ is $(\pm (\xi^n \pm \gamma_1 \pm \cdot \cdot \pm \gamma_{n-1}))$. Again, we treat only the case with initial '$+$', since the case with initial '$-$' can be handled by the reasoning used for $\lambda = (-\gamma)$. We need to show that the set of y such that y satisfies the sentence '$(Q_1 x_1 \in [\gamma_1])(Q_2 x_2 \in [\gamma_2]) \cdots (Q_{n-1} x_{n-1} \in [\gamma_{n-1}])(\pm \xi y x_1 x_2 \cdot \cdot x_{n-1})$' is a subset of the set of y satisfying the sentence just like the above save with γ_i' instead of γ_i, when positive occurrences are replaced and vice-versa when negative occurrences are replaced. Assume that only positive occurences of α in λ are replaced. Then only positive occurrences of α in the γ_j preceded by '$+$' will be replaced and only negative occurrences of α in the γ_k preceded by '$-$' will be replaced. Moreover, all occurrences of α in the γ_i will be of order less then n. Consider those terms preceded by '$+$'. By the induction hypothesis, $[\gamma_j] \subseteq [\gamma_j']$. Obviously, the classes of y satisfying $\ldots (\exists x_j \in [\gamma_j]) \ldots$ will include the class satisfying $\ldots (\exists x_j \in [\gamma_j']) \ldots$. Consider now those terms preceded by '$-$'. By the induction hypothsis, $[\gamma_k'] \subseteq [\gamma_k]$. Clearly, the class of y satisfying $\ldots (\forall x_k \in [\gamma_k']) \ldots$ will include the class satisfying $\ldots (\forall x_k \in [\gamma_k]) \ldots$. Hence, $[\lambda] \subseteq [\lambda']$ when positive occurrences only are replaced. The reasoning for negative occurrences is exactly parallel.

Now that the lemma is proved, we can show that DDO holds for term substitutions when $\ldots \alpha \ldots$ is $(\pm (\pm \lambda \pm v))$. That is, if $(-\alpha + \beta)$ and $(\pm (\pm \lambda \pm v))$ are true then $(\pm (\pm \lambda' \pm v'))$ is also true, where λ' and v' are the results of replacing one or more positive occurrences of α in $\ldots \alpha \ldots$ with β.

We can reduce the cases to two by driving in negations as far as possible: $\ldots \alpha \ldots$ is either $(+\lambda + v)$ or $(-\lambda + v)$. If $\ldots \alpha \ldots$ is $(+\lambda + v)$, then it is true iff $[\lambda] \cap [v] \neq \Lambda$. By our lemma we know that $[\lambda] \subseteq [\lambda']$ and $[v] \subseteq [v']$. Hence, $[\lambda'] \cap [v'] \neq \Lambda$, and $\ldots \beta \ldots$ is also true. If $\ldots \alpha \ldots$ is $(-\lambda + v)$, then it is true iff $[\lambda] \subseteq [v]$. Since α occurs positively in v

and negatively in λ, $[v] \subseteq [v']$ and $[\lambda'] \subseteq [\lambda]$ by the lemma. Therefore, $[\lambda'] \subseteq [v']$ and $\ldots \beta \ldots$ is also true.

We have now shown that DDO holds for term substitutions in the simplest term sentences. We now need to show it for term substitutions where $\ldots \alpha \ldots$ is arbitrarily complex. Clearly, any given occurrence of α in $\ldots \alpha \ldots$ will occur in a sentence χ of the form $(\pm(\pm\lambda\pm v))$. We need only replace these sentences one by one with the result of replacing the appropriate occurrences of α by β to get the desired result. There are only two cases: (1) χ occurs positively in $\ldots \alpha \ldots$ and the to-be-replaced occurrence of α occurs positively in χ, and (2) χ occurs negatively in $\ldots \alpha \ldots$ and the to-be-replaced occurrence of α occurs negatively in χ. We can rule out χ occurring positively in $\ldots \alpha \ldots$ and α occurring negatively in χ and vice-versa since we are only interested in positive or undistributed occurrences of α.

Case (1): χ occurs positively in $\ldots \alpha \ldots$ and α occurs positvely in χ. By our proof that DDO holds for term substitutions in simple term sentences, we know that if χ is true, so is χ'. That is, we know that $(-\chi+\chi')$ is true. By DDO for sentences, the result of replacing χ by χ' in $\ldots \alpha \ldots$, which just $\ldots \beta \ldots$, is also true.

Case (2): χ occurs negatively in $\ldots \alpha \ldots$ and α occurs negatively in χ. If we replace the occurrence of χ in $\ldots \alpha \ldots$ with $(-(-\chi))$, then $(-\chi)$ will have a positive occurrence in $\ldots \alpha \ldots$ and α will occur in $(-\chi)$ with a positive occurrence. Hence, by the reasoning for case (1), $\ldots (-(-\chi')) \ldots$ or $\ldots \chi' \ldots$ or $\ldots \beta \ldots$ will be true.

We have now shown that DDO is truth-preserving and that TFL is sound. It is therefore consistent. We proceed to show that TFL is complete.

Completeness of TFL

TL, the language of TFL, is unable to represent many of the sentences of quantification theory (see Addendum, p. 420). That is a problem, but not for completeness. We need merely show that every logically valid sentence of TL is derivable in TFL. The proof that follows is a Henkin-style proof. We show that every derivation consistent set of sentences of TFL has a model by showing that a larger set of sentences containing it has a model. First, we need some definitions and preliminary lemmas.

Df: A set of sentences, Γ, of TFL is *d-consistent* iff there is no χ such that both χ and $-\chi$ can be derived from Γ. A set of sentences, Γ, of TFL is *maximal d-consistent (mdc)* iff Γ is d-consistent and, for every sentence χ of TL, either $\chi \in \Gamma$ or $\Gamma \cup \{-\chi\}$ is d-consistent. A set of sentences, Γ, of TFL is *ω-complete* iff for every sentence in Γ of the form $(+\alpha+\beta)$ there is another sentence in Γ of the form $(+\lambda+\beta)$, where λ is a singular term.

Lemma 1: $\Gamma \cup \{\phi\}$ is d-inconsistent iff $\Gamma \vdash (-\phi)$ and $\Gamma \cup \{(-\phi)\}$ is d-inconsistent iff $\Gamma \vdash \phi$.
Proof: (of the first conjunct) Clearly, if $\Gamma \vdash (-\phi)$ then $\Gamma \cup \{\phi\}$ is d-inconsistent. If $\Gamma \cup \{\phi\}$ is d-inconsistent, then, for some χ, $\Gamma \cup \{\phi\} \vdash \chi$ and $\Gamma \cup \{\phi\} \vdash (-\chi)$. Then $1 \vdash (-\phi+\chi)$, $(-\phi + (-\chi))$. Using contraposition, or T(2), we get $\Gamma \vdash (-(-\chi) + (-\phi))$ and, by DDO, that $\Gamma \vdash (-\chi + (-\chi))$. By Theorem 1 we get that $\Gamma \vdash (-\phi)$. The proof of the other conjuncts is much the same, save that the Neg rule is used also.
Lemma 2: If Γ is a mdc set of sentences of TFL, then, for any sentences ψ, ϕ of TL, the following hold: (i) $\phi \in \Gamma$ iff $(-\phi) \notin \Gamma$, (ii) $\phi \in \Gamma$ iff $\Gamma \vdash \phi$, (iii) $(+\phi+\psi) \in \Gamma$ iff $\phi \in \Gamma$ and $\psi \in \Gamma$, and (iv) $(-\phi+\psi) \in \Gamma$ iff $\psi \in \Gamma$ or $\phi \notin \Gamma$.
Proof: (i) Clearly, not both ϕ and $(-\phi)$ are elements of Γ. We need to show that one of the two is. Suppose neither is. Then $\Gamma \cup \{\phi\}$ and $\Gamma \cup \{(-\phi)\}$ are d-inconsistent. By Lemma 1, $\Gamma \vdash (-\phi)$ and $\Gamma \vdash \phi$, or Γ is d-inconsistent. Therefore, at least one of ϕ and $(-\phi)$ are in Γ. (ii). Clearly, if $\phi \in \Gamma$ then $\Gamma \vdash \phi$. Assume that $\Gamma \vdash \phi$. Then $(-\phi) \notin \Gamma$ and, by (i), $\phi \in \Gamma$. (iii) follows immediately from (ii) by Theorems 2 and 3. (iv). Suppose $(-\phi+\psi) \in \Gamma$. Then $\Gamma \vdash (-\phi+\psi)$. Assume that $\psi \notin \Gamma$ and $\phi \in \Gamma$. But then $\Gamma \vdash \psi$, which contradicts our assumption. Therefore, either $\psi \in \Gamma$ or $\phi \notin \Gamma$. Suppose $\psi \in \Gamma$ or $(-\phi) \in \Gamma$. If $\psi \in \Gamma$ then $\Gamma \vdash \psi$ and, by Rule C, $\Gamma \vdash (-\phi+\psi)$. If $(-\phi) \in \Gamma$, then $\Gamma \vdash (-\phi)$, and, by Rule C, $\Gamma \vdash (-(-\psi) + (-\phi))$. By contraposition, $\Gamma \vdash (-\phi+\psi)$. QED.
Lemma 3: If Γ is a mdc and ω-complete set of sentences of TFL, then (i) $(+T+\alpha) \in \Gamma$ iff, for some singular term λ, $(+\lambda$

$+\alpha)\in\Gamma$, (ii) $(-T+\alpha)\in\Gamma$ iff, for every singular term λ, $(+\lambda+\alpha)\in\Gamma$, (iii) $(+\alpha+\beta)\in\Gamma$ iff, for some singular term λ, $(+\lambda+\alpha)$ and $(+\lambda+\beta)$ are in Γ, and (iv) $(-\alpha+\beta)\in\Gamma$ iff, for every singular term λ, if $(+\lambda+\alpha)\in\Gamma$ then $(+\lambda+\beta)\in\Gamma$.

Proof: (1) The 'only if' holds by definition. If $(+\lambda+\alpha)\in\Gamma$, λ a singular term, then, since $(-\lambda+T)$ is an axiom, $\vdash(+T+\alpha)$ by DDO.

(2) Assume that $(-T+\alpha)\in\Gamma$ and that for some singular term λ $(+\lambda+\alpha)\notin\Gamma$. Then, by Lemma 2, $(-(+\lambda+\alpha))\in\Gamma$. Hence, $(-\lambda+(-\alpha))$ and $(+\lambda+(-\alpha))$ are in Γ. By (1), $(+T+(-\alpha))\in\Gamma$, and Γ is d-inconsistent. Therefore, if $(+T+\alpha)\in\Gamma$, then, for every singular term λ, $(+\lambda+\alpha)\in\Gamma$. Assume that for every singular term λ, $(+\lambda+\alpha)\in\Gamma$ and that $(-T+\alpha)\notin\Gamma$. By Lemma 2, $(+T+(-\alpha))\in\Gamma$. But that cannot be by (1). Hence, if, for every singular term λ, $(+\lambda+\alpha)\in\Gamma$, then $(-T+\alpha)\in\Gamma$.

(3) If $(+\alpha+\beta)\in\Gamma$, then $\Gamma\vdash(+\alpha+\beta)$. By T(3), $\Gamma\vdash(+T+\langle+\alpha+\beta\rangle)$. By (1), for some singular term λ, $(+\lambda+\langle+\alpha+\beta\rangle)\in\Gamma$. Then, by Lemma 2 and T(4), $\Gamma\vdash(+\lambda+\alpha)$, $(+\lambda+\beta)$, and they are in Γ. If, for some singular term λ, $(+\lambda+\alpha)$ and $(+\lambda+\beta)$ are in Γ, then $\Gamma\vdash(+\lambda+\alpha)$ and $\Gamma\vdash(+\lambda+\beta)$. By the duality of singular terms, $\Gamma\vdash(-\lambda+\alpha)$, $(-\lambda+\beta)$. By Theorem 12, $\Gamma\vdash(-\lambda+\langle+\alpha+\beta\rangle)$ and, by T(1) $\Gamma\vdash(+\lambda+\langle+\alpha+\beta\rangle)$. By Theorem 13, $\Gamma\vdash(+\alpha+\beta)$ and $(+\alpha+\beta)\in\Gamma$.

(4) If $(-\alpha+\beta)\in\Gamma$, then $(-T+\langle-\alpha+\beta\rangle)\in\Gamma$ and, for every singular term λ, $(+\lambda+\langle-\alpha+\beta\rangle)\in\Gamma$. Hence, by T(4), $(-(+\lambda+\alpha)+(+\lambda+\beta))$ is in Γ. Therefore, if $(+\lambda+\alpha)\in\Gamma$, then $(+\lambda+\beta)\in\Gamma$, for every singular term λ. Assume that for every singular term λ if $(+\lambda+\alpha)\in\Gamma$, then $(+\lambda+\beta)\in\Gamma$. Suppose $(-\alpha+\beta)\notin\Gamma$. Then $(+\alpha+(-\beta))\in\Gamma$. By (3), for some singular term λ, $(+\lambda+\alpha)$ and $(+\lambda+(-\beta))$ are in Γ. That is inconsistent with our assumption. Hence, $(-\alpha+\beta)\in\Gamma$.

Lemma 4: If Γ is a d-consistent set of sentences of TFL, then Γ is a d-consistent set of sentences of TFL$'$, where TFL$'$ is the system resulting by adding an infinite list, $\mu_1, \mu_2, \ldots\ldots$, of new singular term letters to the vocabulary of TL. We assume this without proof.

Lemma 5: There is an effective enumeration of all terms of TFL and TFL$'$ and of all sentences of TFL and TFL$'$. We again assume this without proof. It would be fairly simple to set up a Gödel numbering for the sentences and terms of TL.

Lemma 6: If Γ is a d-consistent set of sentences of TFL, then Γ can be extended to Γ^*, a mdc and ω-complete set of sentences of TFL'.

Proof: We first extend Γ to Γ' by adding an infinite list of sentences χ_i to Γ, where χ_i is $^\ulcorner (-(+T+\alpha_i)+(+(+\mu_k)+\alpha_i))^\urcorner$, α_i is the ith term in some enumeration of the terms of TFL', and μ_k is the first new singular term letter which does not appear in α_i nor in any χ_j, $j < i$. Then let $\Gamma_0 = \Gamma$, $\Gamma_1 = (\Gamma_0 \cup \{\chi_1\})$, $\Gamma_n = (\Gamma_{n-1} \cup \{\chi_n\})$, and $\Gamma' = \Gamma_\infty$. The product, Γ', is d-consistent. To show this, assume the opposite. Then for some ϕ both ϕ and $(-\phi)$ can be derived from Γ'. Let k be the largest number for which χ_k appears in either derivation. Then Γ_k must be d-inconsistent. This cannot be. Γ_0 is d-consistent by definition, and if Γ_n is d-consistent so is Γ_{n+1}. The only way for Γ_{n+1} to be d-inconsistent is for $\Gamma_n \vdash (-\chi_n)$. But then $\Gamma_n \vdash {}^\ulcorner(+T+\alpha_n)^\urcorner$, $(+(+\mu_m)+(-\alpha_n))$. The only way the latter sentence could be derived from Γ_n, given that $(+\mu_m)$ does not appear in any sentence of Γ_n, is if $\Gamma_n \vdash {}^\ulcorner(-T+(-\alpha_n))^\urcorner$. In that case, Γ_n would be d-inconsistent, contrary to assumption. Therefore, Γ_k and Γ' are d-consistent.

We now extend Γ' to Γ^* by the use of the strategy of Lindenbaum's Lemma. We assume that we have an enumeration of all of the sentences of TFL: $\phi_1, \phi_2, \ldots$ Let $\Gamma_0^* = \Gamma'$, $\Gamma_1^* = (\Gamma_0^* \cup \{\phi_1\})$, if it is d-consistent, Γ_0^* otherwise, and Γ_n^* be $\Gamma_{n-1}^* \cup \{\phi_n\}$ if d-consistent, Γ_{n+1}^* otherwise. Finally, let Γ^* be Γ_∞^*. Notice that by construction each of the Γ_i^* are d-consistent. Therefore, Γ^* is also d-consistent. For if not, then, for some ψ, both ψ and $(-\psi)$ can be derived from Γ^*. Let j be the highest index of any sentence in either derivation according to the above enumeration. Then both ψ and $(-\psi)$ can be derived from Γ_j^*. This cannot be since Γ_j^* is d-consistent.

Γ^* is maximally d-consistent, i.e., for any ψ either $\psi \in \Gamma^*$ or $\Gamma^* \cup \{\psi\}$ is d-inconsistent. Assume there is a sentence ψ such that $\psi \notin \Gamma^*$ and $\Gamma^* \cup \{\psi\}$ is d-consistent. But ψ is ϕ_i for some i and hence, Γ_{i+1}^*, which is a subset of Γ^*, contains it.

Finally, Γ^* is ω-complete. To show this we have to show that if $(+\alpha+\beta) \in \Gamma^*$, then, for some singular term λ, $(+\lambda+\beta) \in \Gamma^*$.

Since $(+\alpha+\beta)\in\Gamma^*$, by T(3), $\ulcorner(+T+\langle+\alpha+\beta\rangle)\urcorner\in\Gamma^*$. By construction, we know that $\ulcorner(-(+(+T+\langle+\alpha+\beta\rangle))$ $+(+(+(+\mu_k)+\langle+\alpha+\beta\rangle))))\urcorner\in\Gamma^*$, for some μ_k. By DDO and Lemma 2, $(+(+\mu_k)+\langle+\alpha+\beta\rangle)\in\Gamma^*$, and, by T(4), so is $(+(+\mu_k)+\beta)$.

We have now shown that any d-consistent set of sentences of TFL can be extended to a mdc and ω-complete set of sentences. The reader will have noticed that our completeness proof is so far little more than a translation of standard proofs into our vocabulary. The only novelties to be found come in the construction of the model and in the details of the proof that it is a model. In fact, the model to be constructed is very like the standard model for quantification theory with identity; this is to be expected since TFL contains some fragments of the theory of identity.

Metatheorem 3: For any mdc ω-complete set of sentences, Σ, of TFL or TFL′ there is a normal interpretation making all of the sentences of Σ true.

We first set out a normal interpretation I satisfying this theorem, then prove that it is one. If α is a singular term of TL or TL′, then $EC(\alpha)$ will be the set of all singular terms, λ, such that $(+\lambda+\alpha)\in\Sigma$. In effect, $EC(\alpha)$ is the set of all singular terms which are, by Σ, identical to α. Metatheorem 1 assures us that $EC(\alpha)$ is in fact an equivalence class. Further, let $|\alpha|$ be the result of applying a choice function to $EC(\alpha)$ which picks out one member of $EC(\alpha)$ to represent α and the other singular terms identical to α according to Σ. We can appeal here to the axiom of choice, but that is not necessary. In any particular case we can easily define an appropriate choice function. For example, in the case of Γ^* we choose the new singular term with lowest subscript.

We can now specify the normal interpretation I which makes all of the sentences in our given mdc ω-complete set of sentences Σ true. The domain is $\{|\alpha|: \alpha$ is a singular term of TL (or TL′)$\}$. The assignments are: (1) each propositional letter ρ is assigned the value true iff $(+\rho)\in\Sigma$; (2) each term letter η is assigned the set $\{|\lambda|: \lambda$ is a singular term and $(+\lambda+(+\eta))\in\Sigma\}$, with 'T' being assigned D, the whole domain; (3) each n-place relation symbol $+\xi^{n,123\cdots n}$ is assigned the set of all n-tuples $\langle|\lambda_1|,|\lambda_2|,\ldots,|\lambda_n|\rangle$ such that $(+\lambda_1+\xi^{n,123\cdots n}+\lambda_2+\ldots$

$+ \lambda_n) \in \Sigma$, where $\lambda_1, \lambda_2, \ldots, \lambda_n$ are singular terms. All other terms and relations are assigned extensions by the rules given in the definition of an interpretation.

I is clearly an interpretation of TL or TL′. We need to show that I is a normal interpretation. Since $(+ \alpha + \alpha)$, α a singular term, is an axiom, it is in Σ. Thus, $EC(\alpha)$ will be nonempty whenever α is a singular term, and $|\alpha|$ will denote one and only one element of D by Metatheorem 1. Hence, I is a normal interpretation. To show that I is a normal model of Σ, we show that, for all sentences ϕ, $\phi \in \Sigma$ iff ϕ is true under I. The proof proceeds by induction on the order of sentences and terms, which we must first define.

Df: A sentence χ is a *sentence of order 1* iff χ is $(\pm \zeta)$, ζ an elementary sentence, of *order n* iff χ is $(\pm \psi)$, ψ a sentence of order $n - 1$, and of *order $m + k + l$* iff χ is $(\pm (\pm \psi \pm \theta))$, ψ and θ sentences of order m and k respectively. A term α is a *term of order 1* if α is a singular term, of *order 2* if α is $(\pm \eta)$, η a general term letter or if α is $(-\eta)$, η a singular term letter, of *order n* if α is $(\pm \beta)$, β a term of order $n - 1$, of *order $m + k + l$* if α is $(\pm \langle \pm \beta \pm \gamma \rangle)$, β and γ terms of order m and k respectively, and *of order $m_1 + m_2 + \ldots + m_{n-1} + 1$* if α is $(\pm \xi^n \pm \beta_1 \pm \ldots \pm \beta_{n-1})$, $\beta_1, \ldots, \beta_{n-1}$ terms of order $m_1, m_2, \ldots, m_{n-1}$ respectively.

We now proceed to the details of the proof that $\phi \in \Sigma$ iff ϕ is true under I, which proceeds by induction on the order of ϕ. We begin with ϕ of order 1. Then ϕ is $(\pm \zeta)$, ζ an elementary sentence, either a proposition letter or $(\pm \alpha \pm \beta)$, α and β terms. Suppose ζ is a proposition letter, and, that ϕ is $(+ \zeta)$. Then $\phi \in \Sigma$ iff ϕ is true under I by construction. If ϕ is $(- \zeta)$ and $\phi \in \Sigma$, then $(+ \zeta) \notin \Sigma$. Then, by what was said for $(+ \zeta)$, $(+ \zeta)$ is false under I and $(- \zeta)$ is true under I. If $(- \zeta)$ is true under I, then $(+ \zeta)$ is false under I and $(+ \zeta) \notin \Sigma$. Hence, by Lemma 2, $(- \zeta) \in \Sigma$.

To deal with the case in which ϕ is $(\pm \alpha \pm \beta)$, we first prove the following lemma, which makes the proof very smooth.

Lemma: If ϕ is $(+ \lambda + \beta)$, where λ is a singular term, then $\phi \in \Sigma$ iff ϕ is true under I.

Proof: (By induction on the order of the term β) Suppose β has order 1 or 2, i.e., β is $(\pm \mu)$, where μ is a term letter. If β is $(+ \mu)$, the lemma holds by construction. If β is $(- \mu)$ and $\phi \in \Sigma$, then

$(+\lambda + (+\mu)) \notin \Sigma$. By construction it is false under I. Hence, $|\lambda| \notin [(+\mu)]$. By construction, $|\lambda| \in [(-\mu)]$ and ϕ is true under I. If β is $(-\mu)$ and ϕ is true under I, then $|\lambda| \in [(-\mu)]$. Hence, $|\lambda| \notin [(+\mu)]$ and, by construction, $(+\lambda + (+\mu)) \notin \Sigma$. Hence, by the duality of singular terms and Lemma 1, $\phi \in \Sigma$. We now assume the lemma is false and proceed by contradiction. If it is false, then, by the least number principle, there is some least number, call it k, such that the lemma fails for β of order k but holds for β of order less than k. By what has been proved so far we know that $k > 2$. Let ϕ be $(+\lambda + \beta)$, where β is of order n. There are three main cases: (1) β is $(\pm \gamma)$, (2) β is $(\pm \langle \pm \gamma \pm \nu \rangle)$, and (3) β is $(\pm(\pm \zeta^{n, i_1 i_2 \cdots i_n} \pm \gamma_1 \pm \gamma_2 \cdots \pm \gamma_{n-1}))$.

Case (1): Suppose β is $(+\gamma)$ and $\phi \in \Sigma$. Then by Neg $(+\lambda + \gamma) \in \Sigma$, which is true by the induction hypothesis. If β is $(+\gamma)$ and ϕ is true under I, then $(+\lambda + \gamma)$ is true under I. The latter is, by the induction hypothesis, in Σ, and, by Neg, $(+\lambda + (+\gamma)) \in \Sigma$. Suppose β is $(-\gamma)$ and $\phi \in \Sigma$. Then, by Neg and the duality of singular terms, $(+\lambda + \gamma) \notin \Sigma$. By the induction hypothesis it is false, which makes ϕ true. Suppose ϕ is true. Then, $(+\lambda + \gamma)$ is false under I, and, by the induction hypothesis, is not in Σ. Hence, $(-(+\lambda + \gamma))$ and $(+\lambda + (-\gamma))$, or ϕ, are in Σ.

Case (2): β is $(\pm \langle \pm \gamma \pm \nu \rangle)$. By driving in negations, we can reduce the cases to be considered to two: β is $\langle +\gamma + \nu \rangle$, and β is $\langle -\gamma + \nu \rangle$. Suppose β is $\langle +\gamma + \nu \rangle$ and $\phi \in \Sigma$. Then, by Lemma 2 and T(4), so are $(+\lambda + \gamma)$ and $(+\lambda + \nu)$. By the induction hypothesis both are true under I (since γ and ν are of order less than k). Hence, $|\lambda| \in [\gamma] \cap [\nu]$ and ϕ is true under I. Suppose β is $\langle +\gamma + \nu \rangle$ and ϕ is true under I. Then $|\lambda| \in ([\gamma] \cap [\nu])$ and $(+\lambda + \gamma)$ and $(+\lambda + \nu)$ are true. By the induction hypothesis both are in Σ. By the duality of singular terms and Theorem 12, $(+\lambda + \langle +\gamma + \nu \rangle)$, or ϕ, is also in Σ.

Suppose β is $\langle -\gamma + \nu \rangle$ and $\phi \in \Sigma$. Therefore, by T(5), $(-(+(+\lambda + \gamma)) + (+(+\lambda + \nu))) \in \Sigma$. By Lemma 2, either $(+\lambda + \nu) \in \Sigma$ or $(-(+\lambda + \gamma)) \in \Sigma$. If $(+\lambda + \nu) \in \Sigma$, then, by the induction hypothesis (ν being of order less than k), it is true under I. Hence, $|\lambda| \in [\nu]$ and $|\lambda| \in [\bar{\gamma}] \cup [\nu]$ or ϕ is true under I. If $(-(+\lambda + \gamma)) \in \Sigma$, then, by the duality of singular terms, $(+\lambda + (-\gamma)) \in \Sigma$. Since $(-\gamma)$ has order less than k, the latter is true under I. Hence, $|\lambda| \in [(-\gamma)]$ or $[\bar{\gamma}]$. Thus, $|\lambda| \in [\bar{\gamma}] \cup [\nu]$ and ϕ

is true under I. Suppose ϕ, $(+\lambda + \langle -\gamma + \nu \rangle)$, is true under I. Hence, either $(+\lambda + \nu)$ or $(+\lambda + (-\gamma))$ is true under I. If $(+\lambda + \nu)$ is true under I, then it is Σ. By Theorem 14, so is ϕ. If $(+\lambda + (-\gamma))$ is true under I, then it is in Σ, and by Theorem 15, so is its immediate consequence, ϕ.

Case (3): β is $(\pm (\pm \xi^{n, i_1 i_2 \cdots i_n} \pm \gamma_1 \pm \ldots \pm \gamma_{n-1}))$. We will not treat the case in which the initial '$\pm$' is a '$-$', since terms preceded by '$-$' merely get the complement of those preceded by '$+$' and the reasoning concerning them is straightforward. This makes it possible to skip consideration of relational terms with '$-$' directly before ξ. By Neg and the semantics, those terms are equivalent to terms with '$+$' before ξ and preceded by '$-$'. Thus, we need consider only the case in which the first two '$\pm$'s are '$+$'s.

Suppose $\phi = (+\lambda + (+\xi^{n, i_1 i_2 \cdots i_n} \pm \gamma_1 \pm \ldots \pm \gamma_{n-1}))$ is in Σ. First, we assume that all of the γ_i are singular terms. Then by the use of T(1) and T(7) together with Lemma 2 the sentence resulting from ϕ by changing all '$-$' signs on the terms behind ξ to '$+$' and rearranging the terms so that the index on ξ is '1 2 3 ... n' is in Σ. By construction that sentence is true under I, and by the truth-preserving nature of T(1) and T(7), so is ϕ (since ϕ can be derived from it). Second, suppose that not all of the γ_i are singular terms. Call the one with the least subscript γ_j; all the terms with smaller index are singular terms. Suppose now that γ_j has algebraic sign '$+$'. Then, by T(1), the result of changing any '$-$'s on terms with lower subscripts to '$+$'s is in Σ. By T(7), the result of interchanging γ_j and λ with suitable change in the index of ξ is in Σ. By Lemma 3, there is a singular term σ such that both $(+\sigma + \gamma_j)$ and $(+\sigma + (+\xi^{n, i_j i_1 \cdots 1 \cdots i_n} + \gamma_1 + \ldots + \lambda \pm \ldots \pm \gamma_{n-1}))$ are in Σ. Both have predicate terms of order less than k and hence, by the induction hypothesis, are true under I. Hence, so is $(+\gamma_j + (+\xi^{n, i_j i_1 \cdots 1 \cdots i_n} + \gamma_1 + \ldots + \lambda \pm \ldots \gamma_{n-1}))$. By the soundness of T(1) and T(7) and the fact that all the steps above are reversible, ϕ is true under I. Finally, suppose that γ_j is preceded by '$-$'. By T(1) the result of changing any '$+$'s on terms with lower subscripts than j to '$-$'s is in Σ. By a similar change on the sign of λ, we can use T(7) to ensure that the result of interchanging λ and γ_j with suitable changes in the index of ξ is also in Σ. Notice that these transformations are reversible. The result of the above transformations will be called ϕ'; it is $(-\gamma_j + (+\xi^{n,i_j i_1 \ldots 1 \ldots i_n} - \gamma_1 - \ldots - \lambda \pm \ldots \pm \gamma_{n-1}))$. By Lemma 3 we know that for every singular term σ, if $(+\sigma + \gamma_j)$ is in Σ, then so too is $(+\sigma + (+\xi^{n,i_j i_1 \ldots 1 \ldots i_n} - \gamma_1 - \ldots - \lambda \pm \ldots \pm \gamma_{n-1}))$. Both of these sentences have predicate terms of order less than k, and hence, if true are in Σ and vice-versa. For σ such that $|\sigma| \in [\gamma_j]$ both will be true and hence in Σ. Therefore, ϕ' is true under I. By the soundness of T(7) and T(1) and the reversibility of the transformations, so is ϕ.

Suppose that ϕ is true under I. We need to show that ϕ is in Σ. Again, first suppose that all of the γ_i are singular terms. By the fact that ϕ is true under I, we know that the sentence ϕ', resulting from ϕ by giving all terms '+' signs and rearranging them so that the index on ξ is '123 . . . n', is also true under I. By construction, ϕ' is in Σ. Since ϕ is derivable from ϕ' by T(1) and T(7), ϕ is in Σ. Second, suppose that not all of the γ_i are singular terms and let γ_j be the non-singular term with least subscript in ϕ. Suppose now that γ_j has algebraic sign '+'. Let ϕ' be the result here of changing any '−' signs on γ_i with subscript less than j to '+'s, interchanging λ and γ_j, and suitably modifying the index on ξ. Since all these changes are truth-preserving, ϕ' is true under I. Let $|\sigma|$ be the element in $[\gamma_j]$ making ϕ' true. Then by definition $(+\sigma + \gamma_j)$ and $(+\sigma + (+\xi^{n,i_j i_1 \ldots 1 \ldots i_n} + \gamma_1 + \ldots + \lambda \pm \ldots \pm \gamma_{n-1}))$ are both true under I. Since the predicate terms of both are of order less than k, both are in Σ by the induction hypothesis. By one use each of T(1) and DDO, ϕ' is in Σ (by lemma 2). Finally, suppose that γ_j has a '−' sign. Let ϕ^* be the result of changing any '+' signs on γ_i with subscript less than j to '−'s, interchanging λ and γ_j, and suitably modifying the index on ξ. Since all of these are truth-preserving (and reversible) ϕ^* is also true under I. Thus, $[\gamma_j] \subseteq [(+\xi^{n,i_j i_1 \ldots 1 \ldots i_n} - \gamma_1 - \ldots - \lambda \pm \ldots \pm \gamma_{n-1})]$. Hence, for all singular terms σ, if $(+\sigma + \gamma_j)$ is true under I, so is $(+\sigma + (+\xi^{n,i_j i_1 \ldots 1 \ldots i_n} - \gamma_1 - \ldots - \lambda \pm \ldots \pm \gamma_{n-1}))$. Since both sentences have predicate terms of order less than k, both are in Σ iff they are true under I. Therefore, for every singular term, σ, if the first sentence is in Σ, then the second is. And, by Lemma 3, $\phi^* \in \Sigma$. Since ϕ is derivable from ϕ^* by the reverse of the above steps, $\phi \in \Sigma$. Therefore, our lemma is established.

We can now prove that if ϕ is $(+(\pm\alpha \pm \beta))$, then $\phi \in \Sigma$ iff ϕ is true under I. There are two cases: ϕ is $(+\alpha+\beta)$ and ϕ is $(-\alpha+\beta)$. Suppose first that ϕ is $(+\alpha+\beta)$. If $\phi \in \Sigma$, then by Lemma 3 there is a singular term σ such that $(+\sigma+\alpha)$ and $(+\sigma+\beta)$ are in Σ. By our lemma both are true under I. Hence, $|\sigma| \in ([\alpha] \cap [\beta])$ and it is non-empty. Therefore, ϕ is true under I. If ϕ is true under I, then $[\alpha] \cap [\beta]$ is non-empty. Let σ be an element of the intersection. Then $(+\sigma+\alpha)$ and $(+\sigma+\beta)$ are true under I, and, by our lemma, in Σ. Therefore, by one use of T(1) and DDO, ϕ, which is derivable from the two sentences, is in Σ. Suppose now that ϕ is $(-\alpha+\beta)$. If $\phi \in \Sigma$, then, by Lemma 3, for every singular term σ if $(+\sigma+\alpha) \in \Sigma$, then $(+\sigma+\beta) \in \Sigma$. By our lemma these two sentences are in Σ iff they are true under I. Therefore, $[\alpha] \subseteq [\beta]$ and ϕ is true under I. If ϕ is true under I, then $[\alpha] \subseteq [\beta]$. Hence, for any singular term σ if $(+\sigma+\alpha)$ is true under I, so is $(+\sigma+\beta)$. By our lemma these sentences are in Σ iff they are true under I. Hence, for any singular term σ, if $(+\sigma+\alpha) \in \Sigma$, then $(+\sigma+\beta) \in \Sigma$. By Lemma 3, $\phi \in \Sigma$.

We have now established Metatheorem 3 for sentences of order 1. We assume the metatheorem to be false and proceed by contradiction. If the metatheorem is false, then, by the least number principle, there is some least order of sentence such that the metatheorem fails. Call that least order m. Then the metatheorem holds for any sentence of order less than m but fails for order m. We know by the above that $m > 1$. Suppose then that ϕ is of order m and that it is not true that $\phi \in \Sigma$ iff ϕ is true under I. There are three possibilities: (1) ϕ is $(\pm \psi)$, (2) ϕ is $(+\psi+\chi)$, and (3) ϕ is $(-\psi+\chi)$.

Case (1): ϕ is $(\pm \psi)$. The case in which ϕ is $(+\psi)$ is obvious. ϕ and ψ are true or false together and in or out of Σ together. Suppose then that ϕ is $(-\psi)$. If $\phi \in \Sigma$, then ψ is not. By the induction hypothesis, ψ is false. Hence, ϕ is true under I. If ϕ is true under I, then ψ is false. And, by the induction hypothesis, $(-\psi) \in \Sigma$. Therefore, ϕ cannot be $(\pm \psi)$.

Case (2): ϕ is $(+\psi+\chi)$. If $\phi \in \Sigma$, then, by Lemma 2, so are ψ and χ. By the induction hypothesis, both are true under I. Hence, ϕ is true under I. If ϕ is true under I, then ψ and χ are true under I. Hence, they are in Σ, and, by Lemma 2, so is ϕ. Hence, ϕ cannot be $(+\psi+\chi)$.

Case (3): ϕ is $(-\psi+\chi)$. If $\phi \in \Sigma$, then, by Lemma 2, either

$\chi \in \Sigma$ or $\psi \notin \Sigma$. If $\chi \in \Sigma$, then, by the induction hypothesis, χ is true under I, and so is ϕ. If $\psi \notin \Sigma$, then $(-\psi) \in \Sigma$. Hence, by case (1), ψ is false under I and ϕ is true under I. If ϕ is true under I, then either χ is true under I or ψ is false under I. If χ is true under I, then $\chi \in \Sigma$. By Lemma 2, $\phi \in \Sigma$. If ψ is false under I, then $\psi \notin \Sigma$. By Lemma 2, $\phi \in \Sigma$. Hence, ϕ cannot be $(-\psi + \chi)$, and we have proved that Metatheorem 3 holds.

Metatheorem 4: Every d-consistent set of sentences, Σ, of TFL has a normal model.

Proof: Extend Σ to a mdc and ω-complete set of sentences by Lemma 6. By Metatheorem 3 that extended set has a normal model. Therefore, Σ has a normal model.

Metatheorem 5: TFL is complete. If ϕ is logically valid, then it is derivable from Λ in TFL.

Proof: Suppose that ϕ is logically valid and yet not derivable from Λ in TFL. Then $(-\phi)$ is d-consistent. Hence, by Metatheorem 4, it has a normal model. Hence, it is not true that ϕ is true in every normal model.

ADDENDUM

One central aim of the treatment of traditional formal logic presented here is to make the translation of most simple English sentences into notation for logical reckoning easy and direct. To this end the subject–predicate surface structure of such sentences is retained in the symbolic representations of these sentences. This results in easier translation at the expense of somewhat more complex rules of inference. The most innovative feature of the present treatment is the ability to handle simple sentences involving relations by a term approach, i.e., within a subject–predicate structure. Were this feature removed we would have only a simple and elegant Boolean algebra of propositions and classes. With it a sentence like 'Every relative of a senator was given a pass by Carter' can be represented by '$(-(+R^{2,12}+S)+(+G^{3,321}+P+c))$', where 'x gave y to z' is taken to be $G^{3,123}$, the basic form of the relation.

The natural first question to ask about the expressive capacity of TL is 'What sentences of English can be translated into a suitably interpreted TL?' An approximate answer can be given by comparing the expressive capacity of TL to that of quantification theory. Let MPL be the language of a standard first-order system with identity. We will deny MPL the machinery for treating demonstratives and definite descriptions since it is clear that they cannot be handled by TL as it stands.

The sentences of MPL that can be represented in TL are:

(a) any sentence of MPL not involving quantifiers,

(b) any non-vacuously quantified sentence of MPL that by relativization and other transformations can be put into either of the forms $(QxCx)$ $(C'x)$ or $(Q_1x_1C_1x_1)$ $(Q_2x_2C_2x_2) \ldots (Q_nx_nC_nx_n)$ $(R^nx_1 \ldots x_n)$, where Cx, $C'x$, and C_ix_i are conditions on x and x_i respectively, and R^n is an n-place relation letter followed by n distinct variables, and

(c) any truth functional compound of the above.

Where there is no condition present, we automatically supply 'Tx'. Thus, a sentence like '$\forall'xFx$' is treated as if it were '$\forall x(Tx \to Fx)$'. We mean by a condition on x a sentence form of MPL with one free variable, x, such that were it closed it could itself be represented in TL.

Sentences of MPL in which the quantifiers have minimum scope can not be handled by TL if any matrix involves (a) repetitions of a variable, (b) more than one relation, or (c) relations with different numbers of places. The latter, (c), is mentioned separately because TL can be extended to handle matrices containing more than one relation when those relations involve the same number of places and the same variables. The necessary modifications are discussed below. Thus, if an English sentence can be expressed by an interpreted sentence of MPL meeting the above conditions, it can be represented by a sentence of TL. This is not a very informative answer to our question but it will do as a first approximation.

The limitations on TL so far mentioned are the result of eschewing an explicit apparatus of bound variables. The term approach necessarily relies on implicit devices to convey information about how the various predicates and relations are linked by variables and bound by quantifiers. Because of this, only a portion of the sentences of MPL can be treated by TL.

Looking now to English sentences, the sentences that present the above problematic features when rendered into MPL are those that contain ineliminable occurrences of pronouns, especially those we will call cross-referencing pronouns. Central examples of these are the reflexive and possessive pronouns. TL, as it stands, cannot treat 'All men love themselves' or 'All parents love their children'. This suggests that the answer to our question is that TL can represent those sentences of English which do not involve pronouns. We assume that numerical terms involve pronouns since the analysis of a sentence containing them (e.g. 'There is only one president') involves pronouns ('There is a president and anything that is a president is identical with him').

Extensions of TL are motivated by two considerations: (a) translating most English sentences, and (b) equalling the expressive power of MPL. Both considerations require that we extend TL in such a way to treat pronouns within the term approach. The first extension of TL along this line treats demonstratives, and by virtue of that, definite descriptions and some cross-referencing pronouns.

According to Sommers (see especially [5]) the paradigm of reference is the indefinite reference carried by phrases of the form 'some α', when embedded in an appropriate context. For example, if someone says 'Some men are at the door', on Sommers's view the phrase 'some men' refers indefinitely to all or some of the men at the door, if any. This reference is then picked up by terms like 'he', 'she', 'it', and 'they' as well as by proper names and definite descriptions. The formal treatment of this doctrine requires that we introduce into TL an infinite list of subscripts for the present terms. We will let i, j, k, i′, j′, k′, . . . bear singular import and l,m,n,l′,m′,n′, . . . bear plural import. In effect, these indices are associated with particular occasions of utterance. On some occasion a person utters 'Some α_i is β' in such a way that indefinite reference occurs. The index i picks up the reference of 'some α' on that occasion. It can henceforth function as a singular term, detached from 'some α' and standing on its own (e.g., as in '$(+i+\gamma)$', he (or it) is γ).

Definite descriptions become treatable once this apparatus is present. Consider the definite description, 'the α'. On

Sommers's view first we get an introduction, $\ulcorner(+\alpha_i+T)\urcorner$(the existence claim), then a restriction, $\ulcorner(-\alpha+i)\urcorner$ (the uniqueness claim), and in any subsequent occurrence 'i' refers to the α and does the job of 'the α'.

A limited amount of cross-referencing can also be represented. Consider 'Some man loves himself', represented as '($\exists$x)(Mx & Lxx)' in MPL. In TL with demonstratives we would treat it as follows: $(+M_i+T)$ and $(+i+(L^{2,12}+i))$, (some man (he) exists and he loves himself). In effect, we are able to treat cross-referencing in cases in which the pronoun can be treated as having a reference. This will not capture the use of pronouns in 'Every man loves himself' or in 'Every man gives himself credit', since they involve universal quantification and no specific reference. A different approach is required to treat such cross-reference.

Our attempts to extend TL have thus far taken place under a requirement that the result be straightforwardly translatable into English. In effect, this requires something like a 1–1 correspondence between English phrases and pieces of TL. To accommodate within this restriction the cross-referencing pronouns that do not have particular reference (those with universal import or functionally dependent on such) it appears that we must allow an analogue of variables in TL. That is, we must extend TL to allow for variable terms. This modification is, to be sure, a significant departure from the present term approach since variable terms cannot be given the semantics the terms of TL now enjoy. In a rigorous treatment of a language including such terms, some recourse to the notion of satisfaction would be necessary. The details of the needed modifications are not yet worked out, but a sentence like 'Every man loves himself' would be treated something like '$(-(+x+M)+(+x+(+L^{2,12}+x)))$' (as 'if x is a man then x loves himself'). A distinct set of variable terms would be required to treat certain existentially quantified variables lying in the scope of a universal quantifier. This approach shares with MPL the correspondence to such English sentences as 'If a and b sign a contract in which a promises . . . and b pays . . . then . . . .' This modification to TL, which appears capable of allowing the expression of all sentences of MPL, retains the apparatus of TFL although it diverges from a strict term approach on which every term has a determinate extension in all of its occurrences. However, as mentioned, the details of the modifications to the semantics of TL and to the rules of TFL are not yet worked out.

If we relax the 1–1 translatability requirement, we can retain the strict term approach. It has been known since the work of Schönfinkel in 1924 that variables are theoretically eliminable. In a more recent paper, [2], Quine develops a variable free language equivalent to MPL which is algebraic in nature. The devices used by Quine to achieve this result can be transplanted to TL. We need devices for (a) compounding relations, (b) for adding vacuous positions to relations, (c) for identifying positions within relations, and (d) for subtracting positions from relations. To accomplish (a), we allow the analogue of compound terms for relations. That is, '$(-T+(+ \langle -R^{2,12} + R^{2,21} \rangle -T))$' would represent '$\forall x \forall y (Rxy \rightarrow Ryx)$'. Notice that there is no English correlate for the relational term. We add various operators on relations and terms for (b) and (c), one which adds a final but vacuous position and one, r_{ij}, which identifies the ith and j^{th} positions of a relation. With these devices we can, as it were, line up the various relations and terms within a matrix whose quantifiers are all prenex. By adding positions all relations within the matrix are made into n-place relations for n equal to the largest naturally occurring relation. The details of the operators, their semantics, and the rules of inference necessary are partially worked out, but they are not important here. What is important is that this sort of thing can be done. It shows that the term approach is theoretically adequate.

REFERENCES

[1] Mates, Benson, *Elementary Logic*, 2nd edn, (New York: Oxford University Press, 1969).
[2] Quine, W. V. O., 'Algebraic Logic and Predicate Functors', in *The Ways of Paradox and Other Essays*, rev. edn, (New York: Random House, 1976).
[3] Sommers, Fred, 'Do We Need Identity', *Journal of Philosophy* 66 (1969), 499–504.
[4] ——, 'The Calculus of Terms', *Mind* 79 (1970), 1–40.

[5] ——, 'The Grammar of Thought', *Journal of Social and Biological Structures* 1 (1978), 39–51.

[6] Schönfinkel, Moses, 'On the Building Blocks of Mathematical Logic', transl. and repr. in *From Frege to Gödel*, (Cambridge, Massachusetts: Harvard University Press, 1967), 355–366.

Appendix G

Michael Lockwood

The Logical Syntax of TFL

Three related matters are dealt with in this Appendix. First we present a rigorous formulation of TFL (traditional formal logic) which differs somewhat from Sommers' own, being more economical, more comprehensive and also, in certain respects, in closer accord with Sommers' own notational practice. Second, we show how, without the use of pronouns or any other embellishments, Sommers' notation may be rendered equal to the task of expressing anything formulable in modern first-order predicate logic (MPL). Finally, we present an algorithm for translating formulae of MPL into this extended system, so that in favourable cases the result will be a well-formed formula of TFL.

We begin by giving a formal description of TFL, where by TFL we mean the pronoun-free combinatory core of Sommers' system. A word on terminology: *term*, here, will be used in a broader sense than in the body of this book, so as to include relations and propositions. We follow Quine in speaking of the *degree* of a term, degree being to terms what place is to predicates. Thus, 'is a man' is a one-place predicate; accordingly, 'man' is a term of degree one. Similarly, 'loves', which for MPL is a two-place predicate, corresponds to a term of degree two: 'lover of'. And just as logicians sometimes think of propositions as zero-place predicates, so we shall regard them as terms of degree zero. This point of view is reflected in our use of the same style of letters and bracketing for propositions, singular and general terms and relations. Any ambiguity as to degree that might otherwise result is resolved, at the level of term letters, by the use of numerical superscripts, whilst the degree of a compound term is given as a function of the degree of its components.

The vocabulary of TFL we take to consist of

(i) for each natural number n, an infinite stock of term letters of degree n, A^n, B^n, . . ., S^n, A_1^n, B_1^n . . ., S_1^n, . . .;
(ii) an infinite stock of singular term letters, of degree one, a, b, . . ., h, a_1, b_1, . . ., h_1, . . .;
(iii) a term letter T, of degree one, with the intuitive meaning 'thing';
(iv) superscripts 1, 2, . . .;
(v) signs of quality and quantity, $+$, $-$, and of wild quantity, $*$;
(vi) brackets, $\langle$ $\rangle$, and parentheses, ( ).

(Note: the propositional letters are simply the term letters of degree zero, A^0, B^0 etc.) We also make use of certain meta-linguistic symbols. U^n signifies an arbitrary term letter; X and Y, with or without subscripts or superscripts, signify arbitrary terms. $\pm$ and $\textcircled{\pm}$ mean, respectively, 'either $+$ or $-$' and 'either $+$, $-$ or $*$'. With this, we are in a position to give a strikingly concise statement of the formation rules for TFL:

(1) A term letter of degree n is a term of degree n.
(2) If U^n is a relation letter, i.e. a term letter of degree n > 1, and i_1, . . ., i_n is a sequence of n distinct numerals such that $1 \leqslant i_j \leqslant n$, then $U^{i_1 \cdots i_n}$ is a term of degree n.
(3) If X^n and Y^n are terms of degree n, so are $\langle \pm X^n \pm Y^n \rangle$.
(4) If X_1^1, . . ., X_n^1 are n terms of degree one and Y^m is a term of degree m, where $0 \leqslant n \leqslant m$, then $(\textcircled{\pm} X_n^1 \textcircled{\pm} X_{n-1}^1 \cdots \textcircled{\pm} X_1^1 \pm Y^m)$, in which $\textcircled{\pm}$ is $*$ only where it is followed by a singular term letter, are terms of degree m − n.
(5) An expression is well-formed just in case, for some natural number n, it follows from (1)–(4) that it is a term of degree n; an expression is a well-formed *formula*, or *proposition*, just in case it follows from (1)–(4) that it is a term of degree zero.

Observe that, by (1)–(5), a term of positive quality is not ill-formed for want of an initial $+$, though one is free to insert one if one wishes. This seems preferable to Sommers' policy of making an initial $+$ or $-$ a condition of well-formedness, and then in practice almost invariably suppressing the former.

These rules have been chosen expressly for their economy: we are given, in (3) and (4), just two modes of compounding terms, one binary and homogenous, the other heterogenous and multigrade. Note the portmanteau character of (4). (4) can obviously be used to generate what Sommers calls relational terms. But not only that. Whereas Sommers (in Chapter 9) and McIntosh (in Appendix F) invoke separate rules to generate $(\pm X)$ from X, and $(\underline{\oplus} X^1 \pm Y^1)$ from X^1 and Y^1, these now emerge simply as special cases of (4), where n = 0, and where m = n = 1, respectively. In their manner of generating relational terms, these rules actually work a little differently from those presented by Sommers and by McIntosh. First, (4) always places a relation at the end of a sequence of one-degree terms with which it is compounded. In this respect, the syntax we are proposing for TFL resembles that of a language such as Latin, in which a verb characteristically occurs at the end of the clause or sentence in which it figures. It would seem desirable, however, that our manner of transcribing sentences, in practice, should broadly coincide with Sommers' own, and thus with English word order. This is easily contrived. We define the *E-transform* of a term, T, to be the result of applying to it the following sequence of transformations:

(T1) Wherever there occurs, in T, a term of the form ($\underline{\oplus}$ X^1_n $\underline{\oplus}$ X^1_{n-1} ... $\underline{\oplus}$ $X^1_1 \pm Y^m$), shift $\pm Y^m$ to the left of the initial min (m, n − 1) elements of the sequence $\underline{\oplus}$ $X^1_1, ...,$ $\underline{\oplus}$ X^1_n; where 0 < n < m, replace $+ Y^m$ by $\underline{Y^m}$.

(T2) Delete the superscripts on propositional letters.

(T3) Strip the outer parentheses from any term of the form $(\pm X)$.

(T4) Delete outer enclosing brackets or parentheses, if any.

In the sequel, we shall generally, for the purpose of informal discussion, represent terms standing alone by their E-transforms. Think, if you like, of (1)–(5) as defining a set of base strings from which (T1)–(T4) then generate surface structures, in the manner of a transformational grammar. In part, we are simply formalizing, here, what Sommers does anyway; he himself makes implicit use of abbreviatory conventions corresponding to (T3) and (T4). The transformations (T1)–(T4), applied in strict succession, can be seen to be *formally acceptable*, in the technical sense that the original term, T, is uniquely recoverable from its E-transform, so defined. By contrast, the operation, allowed by Sommers, of replacing $(+X)$ by X violates this condition, since information is lost upon iteration; thus we have no way, in general, of knowing whether a given expression, X, derives from $(+X)$ or $(+(+X))$ or any other of an infinity of (admittedly equivalent) expressions. (This is not intended as a criticism; it is merely an observation.)

A more substantial difference is this. Sommers and McIntosh only admit relational terms of degree one, each compounded of a relation of degree n and $n-1$ terms of degree one. (4), however, allows one to combine a term of degree n with any number of terms of degree one, not exceeding n. And where the result is a term of degree greater than one, (3) and (4) allow one to treat it as a relation for the purposes of further compounding. When Sommers expresses a formula in subject–predicate normal form, he is, in effect, exploiting just the generalized mode of composition that (4) is intended to sanction. For the SNF of a formula is built up by a nested set of operations of combining a term of degree n with a single term of degree one, something that Sommers' own formation rules allow only in the special case where n = 1 or n = 2. So the SNF of a formula is, by our rules but not by Sommers', to be counted as, in its own right, a well-formed formula of TFL. That, while convenient, represents, of course, no increase in expressive power. But the very same feature of our rules that enables them to accommodate formulae in subject-predicate normal form does, in fact, make it possible to provide symbolic transcriptions of certain English sentences that would defy direct translation into Sommers' own version of TFL.

Take the following two sentences:

(a) Some sailor gives every chorus girl a rose,

and (b) Some sailor gives a rose to every chorus girl.

If (a), rather than (b), is seen as displaying the relation 'gives' in its primary syntactic role, then the first of these sentences may be transcribed as

(a') $+ S^1 + G^3 - C^1 + R^1$.

But how then, *without departing from the word order of the original*, is one to represent (b)? One might suppose that it could be transcribed as $+S^1 + G^{132} + R^1 - C^1$. This is incorrect, however, for it implies, as (b) does not, that every chorus girl receives the same rose. It would, therefore, be an appropriate way to represent 'Some sailor gives a certain rose to every chorus girl' (surreptitiously taking it back, perhaps, in order to pass it on to the next recipient). No, the correct transcription of (b) is

(b′) $+S^1 + (G^3 + R^1) - C^1$;

'gives a rose to' is now seen for what it is: a relation of degree two compounded out of the relation 'gives', of degree three, and the term 'rose', of degree one. This immediately explains why 'a rose', in (b), in spite of preceding 'every chorus girl', nevertheless lies within the scope of the latter term. And it preserves the equivalence between (a) and (b). Observe that (a′) and (b′) have the same SNF, namely $(+S^1 + (-C^1 + (+R^1 + G^3)))$. Pairs such as (a) and (b), in which the second sentence is arrived at by transposing direct and indirect objects and prefacing the latter with a preposition, are ubiquitous in English. Compare 'Some cook baked every soldier a cake' and 'Some cook baked a cake for every soldier'. Our analysis elegantly accounts for the fact that (in the absence of contrary indicators, such as 'certain') the indirect object of a verb, regardless of its position in the sentence, has a scope intermediate between that of the subject and the direct object.

In sentences such as (b), just because they may be rewritten along the lines of (a), the mode of composition we have been discussing adds nothing new. But now consider the sentence

(c) Every sailor admires and gives a rose to some chorus girl.

Sommers would be unable to transcribe this without falling back on cross-referential pronominalization, as follows:

(d′) $-S^1 + \langle + (A^2 + C_i^1) + (G^3 * i + R^1) \rangle$,

a formalization which translates back into English as

(d) Every sailor admires some chorus girl and gives her a rose.

Our rules, however, permit us to transcribe (c) directly into TFL as

(c') $-S^1 + \langle A^2 + (G^3 + R^1) \rangle + C^1$;

'admires and gives a rose to' is now represented as a relation of degree two, homogenously compounded out of the relation 'admires' and the relation of degree two that results from heterogenously combining the relation 'gives', of degree three, with the term 'rose', of degree one. It is gratifying to discover that a modification of the formation rules prompted solely by considerations of elegance and simplicity should thus turn out to increase the expressive resources of TFL—all the more so, seeing that its resemblance to ordinary English is thereby enhanced.

We turn our attention, now, from syntax to semantics. As in the standard semantics for MPL, we start with a *domain of discourse*, D, which may be any non-empty set. A TFL *assignment*, ϕ, is a function which

  (i) maps T onto D,
  (ii) maps every singular term letter onto some some unit subset of D,
  (iii) maps every remaining term letter of degree n onto some set of n-tuples of elements of D.

(By convention, no distinction is made between elements of D and the corresponding one-tuples.)

Now propositional letters are simply term letters of degree zero. Accordingly, they are mapped, under ϕ, onto either $\{\langle \rangle\}$, the set whose only member is the unique zero-tuple $\langle \rangle$ (otherwise referred to as the *empty sequence*), or onto the null set, $\emptyset$. These two sets may therefore be identified, respectively, with the truth-values T and $\perp$.

The modes of combination introduced in clauses (3) and (4) of our formation rules may be explained semantically in terms of just three concepts from set theory: we need the *Boolean complement*, *Boolean intersection* and the *image*. Let α^n and β^n be sets of n-tuples, that is sequences of length n. Then the Boolean complement of $\alpha^n, -\alpha^n$, is the set of sequences of length n that are not contained in α^n—or more precisely, the set-theoretic complement of α^n relative to some universe of n-tuples, in the present case D^n. The Boolean intersection of α^n and β^n, $\alpha^n \cap \beta^n$, is simply the set-theoretic intersection of α^n and β^n, but unlike the latter is undefined for sets of sequences of different lengths or sets of sequences of the same length but different for each set. (We shall later explore the consequences of employing an operator for which the latter restriction is dropped.) Finally, the n:1 image, α^n "β^1, is the set of sequences $\langle x_1, \ldots, x_{n-1} \rangle$ such that $\langle x_1, \ldots, x_{n-1}, y \rangle$ is in α^n for some object y in β^1. Thus, if α^2 is the relation *is the father of* and β^1 is the set of great men, then α^2 "β^1 is the set of fathers of great men. (The example is borrowed from *Principia Mathematica*,[1] where Whitehead and Russell make extensive use of this notation.) Notice that α^n "β^1 is always a set of $(n-1)$-tuples. Consequently, α^1 "β^1 is a set of zero-tuples or truth-values, the null set or $\perp$, if $\alpha^1 \cap \beta^1$ is empty, $\{ \langle \ \rangle \}$ or T, otherwise.

The set-theoretic notion corresponding to the sequence of superscripts introduced in (2) is that of a *permutation operator*. Bernays has a set of operators p_{ij} which generate from a set of sequences α^n the set of sequences $p_{ij}\alpha^n$ obtainable from those in α^n by switching their ith and jth elements. Adapting this notation, we can let $p_{i_1} \ldots i_n \alpha^n$ be the set of sequences obtainable from those in α^n by so rearranging their elements that the i_1th element is put in first place, the i_2th element in second place, ... and the i_nth element in last place. Then $p_{312}\alpha^3$, for example, will be what Bernays would represent as $p_{12} p_{13} \alpha^3$, $p_{13} p_{23} \alpha^3$ or $p_{23} p_{12} \alpha^3$.

The mode of combination introduced in clause (4) of the formation rules, since it is multigrade in character, demands in its own right a semantic characterization that is recursive in form. For n terms of degree one, (4) yields $(\bigoplus X_n^1 \bigoplus X_{n-1}^1 \ldots \pm X_1^1 \pm Y^m)$; when $n = 0$, this reduces simply to $(\pm Y^m)$. If we abbreviate the general formula, holding as it does for arbitrary n, as (Y^{m-n}), then the corresponding formula for $n+1$ becomes $(\bigoplus X_{n+1}^1 Y^{m-n})$. It suffices, therefore, that the semantics (i) yield a *basis* for the recursion, in the shape of an interpretation, under a given assignment, of the forms $(\pm Y^m)$ and (ii) contain recursion clauses yielding an interpretation of

[1] A. N. Whitehead and B. Russell, *Principia Mathematica*, vol. i, 1st ed. (Cambridge, 1910), p. 37.

the forms $(\pm X^1_{n+1}\, Y^{m-n})$ as a function of the interpretations assigned to $(\,Y^{m-n})$ and X^1_{n+1}; any arbitrary instance of the general form will then have been catered for. The entire semantics has, of course, a recursive structure; but more specifically, (5) and (6), below, may be thought of as constituting a recursion base with respect to the recursion clauses (11), (12), and (13).

As a minor addition to the stock of metalinguistic symbols so far introduced, let s be an arbitrary singular term letter; other such symbols are to retain their previous meanings. We can now extend ϕ to a TFL *valuation*, v_ϕ, mapping every term of degree n into D^n, by way of the following conditions:

(1) $v_\phi\ulcorner U^n\urcorner = \phi\ulcorner U^n\urcorner$;

(2) $v_\phi\ulcorner s\urcorner = \phi\ulcorner s\urcorner$;

(3) $v_\phi\ulcorner T\urcorner = \phi\ulcorner T\urcorner = D$,

(4) $v_\phi\ulcorner U^{i_1\cdots i_n}\urcorner = p_{i_1\ldots i_n}\phi\ulcorner U^n\urcorner = \{\langle x_{i_1},\ldots,x_{i_n}\rangle:$
$\langle x_i,\ldots,x_n\rangle \in \phi\ulcorner U^n\urcorner\}$;

(5) $v_\phi + \ulcorner X\urcorner = v_\phi\ulcorner X\urcorner$;

(6) $v_\phi\ulcorner -X^n\urcorner = -v_\phi\ulcorner X^n\urcorner = \{\langle x_1,\ldots,x_n\rangle : \langle x_1,\ldots,x_n\rangle$
$\in D^n \& \langle x_1,\ldots,x_n\rangle \notin v_\phi\ulcorner X^n\urcorner\}$;

(7) $v_\phi\langle +X^n + Y^n\rangle\urcorner = v_\phi\ulcorner X^n\urcorner \cap v_\phi\ulcorner Y^n\urcorner = \{\langle x_1,\ldots,x_n\rangle:$
$\langle x_1,\ldots,x_n\rangle \in v_\phi\ulcorner X^n\urcorner \& \langle x_1,\ldots,x_n\rangle \in v_\phi\ulcorner Y^n\urcorner\}$;

(8) $v_\phi\ulcorner \langle +X^n - Y^n\rangle\urcorner = v_\phi\ulcorner X^n\urcorner \cap -v_\phi\ulcorner Y^n\urcorner$;

(9) $v_\phi\ulcorner\langle -X^n + Y^n\rangle\urcorner = -(v_\phi\ulcorner X^n\urcorner \cap v_\phi\ulcorner Y^n\urcorner)$;

(10) $v_\phi\ulcorner\langle -X^n - Y^n\rangle\urcorner = -(v_\phi\ulcorner X^n\urcorner \cap v_\phi\ulcorner Y^n\urcorner)$;

(11) $v_\phi\ulcorner (+X^1_{n+1}\, Y^{m-n})\urcorner = v_\phi\ulcorner Y^{m-n}\urcorner \text{``}v_\phi\ulcorner X^1_{n+1}\urcorner$
$= \{\langle x_1,\ldots,x_{(m-n)-1}\rangle : \exists x_{m-n}(x_{m-n} \in v_\phi$
$\ulcorner X^1_{n+1}\urcorner \& \langle x_1,\ldots,x_{m-n}\rangle \in v_\phi\ulcorner Y^{m-n}\urcorner)\}$;

(12) $v_\phi\ulcorner (-X^1_{n+1}\, Y^{m-n})\urcorner = -(-v_\phi\ulcorner Y^{m-n}\urcorner\text{``}v_\phi\ulcorner X^1_{n+1}\urcorner)$;

(13) $v_\phi\ulcorner (*X^1_{n+1}\, Y^{m-n})\urcorner = (v_\phi\ulcorner Y^{m-n}\urcorner\text{``}v_\phi\ulcorner X^1_{n+1}\urcorner)$
$= -v_\phi\ulcorner Y^{m-n}\urcorner\text{``}v_\phi\ulcorner X^1_{n+1}\urcorner)$, since X^1_{n+1} is here required to be a singular term letter.

We proceed to define an entailment relation for TFL. Let X^n be a term of degree n and Γ^n a set of terms of degree n. Then Γ^n will be said *semantically to entail* X^n, formally $\Gamma^n \models_{TFL} X^n$, just in case, for every assignment ϕ, with respect to every (nonempty) domain D, if $v_\phi\ulcorner Y^n\urcorner = D^n$, for every $Y^n \in \Gamma^n$, then $v_\phi\ulcorner X^n\urcorner = D^n$. This definition has the unusual feature of applying to any terms of homogenous degree, not just well-formed formulae or propositions. It thus has the effect of conferring legitimacy on familiar ways of speaking that might otherwise be thought impossible to accept at face value. We would quite naturally say, for example, that 'either rich or handsome' and 'not rich' jointly entail 'handsome'. In spite of the fact that neither 'rich' nor 'handsome' is a proposition, this may now be regarded as a perfectly genuine instance of the entailment pattern $\langle -(-X)-(-Y)\rangle, \ (-X) \models_{TFL} Y$. That is rather satisfactory. Our main reason, however, for adopting this generalized definition of entailment is proof-theoretic: it seems likely that a proof procedure for TFL could profitably operate with a similarly extended concept of a valid sequent or theorem. (This suggestion, as applied to algebraic logic in general, derives from Nolin[2] and is endorsed by Quine.[3]) But these are matters that cannot be pursued here. Suffice it to say that one gets the desired definition of entailment for propositions, simply by setting n = 0. Then D^n becomes $\{\langle \ \rangle\}$, which is to say T.

Consider, now, the following algorithm for translating an arbitrary well-formed formula of TFL into a logically equivalent formula of MPL =, the first-order predicate calculus with identity. (In what follows, X and Y stand, not merely for terms, but also for expressions into which terms are transformed by successive steps of the algorithm.)

(1) Convert the formula to subject-predicate normal form, i.e. rewrite $(\oplus X_n^1 \pm X_{n-1}^1 \ldots \oplus X_1^1 \oplus Y^m)$ throughout as $(\oplus X_n^1 + (\oplus X_{n-1}^1 \ldots + (\oplus X_1^1 \oplus Y^m) \ldots))$.
(2) Rewrite $\langle +X+Y\rangle$ as $(X \ \& \ Y)$ and $\langle -X+Y\rangle$ as $(X \rightarrow Y)$.
(3) Rewrite $\langle +X-Y\rangle$ as $(X \ \& -Y)$ and $\langle -X-Y\rangle$ as $(X \rightarrow -Y)$.
(4) Rewrite $(-X)$ as $-X$.
(5) Rewrite $(+X+Y)$ as $\exists(X \ \& \ Y), (-X+Y)$ as $\forall(X \rightarrow Y)$ and $(*s+X)$ as $*(s+X)$.

[2] L. Nolin, 'Sur l'Algèbre des Prédicats', in *Le Raisonnement en Mathematiques et en Sciences Experimentales, Colloquui Internationaux du Centre National de la Recherche Scientifique*, 70 (1958), pp. 33–37.

[3] W. V. O. Quine, 'Algebraic Logic and Predicate Functors', in *The Ways of Paradox*, revised and enlarged edition (Cambridge, Mass., 1976), p. 306.

(6) Rewrite $(+X-Y)$ as $\exists(X\ \&\ -Y)$, $(-X-Y)$ as $\forall(X\to-Y)$ and $(*s-X)$ as $*(s+-X)$.

(7) Rewrite $\forall(T\to X)$ as $\forall X$ and $\exists(T\ \&\ X)$ as $\exists X$.

(8) Replace any remaining occurrences of $-T$ by $(F^1\ \&\ -F^1)$ and then any remaining occurrences of T by $(F^1\ \vee\ -F^1)$.

(9) Let $*$ now be construed as a quantifier symbol, along with $\forall$ and $\exists$. Attach to each quantifier symbol a variable letter, subject to the constraint that no quantifier may stand within the scope of another with the same variable. (Expressions of the form $*v$ will henceforth be referred to as *wild* quantifiers; $*v(X(v)+Y(v))$ may be regarded as definitionally equivalent to $(\exists v(X(v)\ \&\ Y(v))\ \&\ \forall(X(v)\to Y(v)))$.)

(10) Attach to each term letter of degree one the variable associated with the rightmost quantifier within the scope of which it lies.

(11) Attach to each relation letter in its basic form, U^n, the variable string associated with the n rightmost quantifiers within the scope of which it lies, taken in their order of occurrence.

(12) Consider, for each relational term $U^{i_1\cdots i_n}$, the sequence of variables, S, corresponding to the n rightmost quantifiers within the scope of which it lies, taken in their order of occurrence. Attach to $U^{i_1\cdots i_n}$ the variable string S', obtained by putting the first element of S in i_1th place, the second element of S in i_2th place, . . . and the final element of S in i_nth place. Replace $U^{i_1\cdots i_n}$ with U^n.

(13) Rewrite $*v(sv+X(v))$ as $X(s)$.

(14) Rewrite any remaining occurrences of sv as $v=s$.

(15) Rewrite s_1s_2 as $s_1=s_2$.

The result is a well-formed formula of MPL$=$.

To illustrate the operation of the algorithm, we take the sentence

(e) No contemporary biologist accepts every idea put forward by Darwin.

This may be transcribed as

(e') $-(+\langle +C^1+B^1\rangle+A^{12}-\langle +I^1+(P^{21}*d)\rangle)$, which is the E-transform of the formula

$$(-(+\langle C^1 + B^1 \rangle - \langle +I^1 + (*d + P^{21}) \rangle + A^{12})).$$

From this we derive, successively

$$(-(+\langle +C^1 + B^1 \rangle + (-\langle +I^1 + (*d + P^{21}) \rangle + A^{12})))$$ by (1) SNF

$$(-(+(C^1 \& B^1) + (-(I^1 \& (*d + P^{21})) + A^{12})))$$ by (2)

$$-(+(C^1 \& B^1) + (-(I^1 \& (*d + P^{21})) + A^{12}))$$ by (4)

$$-\exists((C^1 \& B^1) \& \forall((I^1 \& *(d + P^{21})) \to A^{12}))$$ by (5)

$$-\exists x((C^1 \& B^1) \& \forall y((I^1 \& *z(d + P^{21}) \to A^{12}))$$ by (9)

$$-\exists x((C^1 x \& B^1 x) \& \forall y((I^1 y \& *z(dz + P^{21})) \to A^{12}))$$ by (10)

$$-\exists x((C^1 x \& B^1 x) \& \forall y((I^1 y \& *z(dz + P^2 zy)) \to A^2 xy))$$ by (12)

$$-\exists x((C^1 x \& B^1 x) \& \forall y((I^1 y \& P^2 dy)) \to A^2 xy))$$ by (13)

The formulae of MPL= that issue from this algorithm have a rather specific form, which we now proceed to characterize. Let us say that a formula of MPL= is *pure* if every predicate letter that stands within the scope of one or more quantifiers has as one of its arguments the variable associated with the rightmost such quantifier. What we have just defined is a normal form; there are a variety of mechanical procedures whereby any arbitrary formula of MPL= may be purified. (The terminology, by the way, is Quine's.) The above algorithm transforms formulae of TFL into pure formulae of MPL= with the following key features:

  (i) The identity sign, =, only occurs flanked on one or both sides by individual constants.

 (ii) The sequence of variables associated with each predicate letter, whether or not interrupted by one or more individual constants, is either a terminal subsequence of the variable sequence associated with the quantifiers within the scope of which it lies, taken in their order of occurrence, or some permutation of such a subsequence.

(iii) For every quantifier, Qv, there is some number n ⩾ 1, such that every truth-functional component of the subformula governed by Qv either has v as its only free variable, or contains n free variables, including v (where 'free' means not bound by quantifiers situated to the right of Qv).

(i)–(iii) fall short of constituting an exhaustive characterization of the formulae that are generated by the algorithm. To complete the description, two things must be added. First, the only connectives that figure in these formulae are $-$, & and $\rightarrow$. Second, if a quantifier, Qv, has as its scope a truth-functional compound, $X(v)$, some components of which have v as their sole free variable, while others contain, in addition, free variables other than v, then, according as Q is $\forall$ or $\exists$, $X(v)$ will be a conditional or a conjunction, where the antecedent or first conjunct contains all and only those components of $X(v)$ that have v alone free. These last two conditions are included only for the sake of completeness; for any formula of MPL$=$ that satisfies (i)–(iii) can be cast in a form that has these further characteristics as well. (This is not altogether obvious, in the case of the final condition, but is easily demonstrated.[4]) That being so, we can say the following: it is a necessary and sufficient condition for a formula of MPL$=$ to be translatable into TFL that it can be converted to a pure form that satisfies (i)–(iii) above.

[4] Suppose we have a formula, S, that satisfies (i)–(iii), and that $QvX(v)$ is a subformula of S such that some but not all truth-functional components of $X(v)$ contain free variables other than v. Let $Y_1(v), \ldots, Y_n(v)$ be those truth-functional components of $X(v)$ that have v as their sole free variable. $X(v)$ may then be represented as $X(Y_1(v), \ldots, Y_n(v))$. Further, let T and F be the constant true and false propositions, respectively. If Q is $\forall$, we may then rewrite $QvX(Y_1(v), \ldots, Y_n(v))$ as

$$(\forall v((Y_1(v)\& \ldots \& Y_{n-1}(v)\& Y_n(v))\rightarrow X(T, \ldots, T, T))\&$$
$$\forall v((Y_1(v)\& \ldots \& Y_{n-1}(v)\& - Y_n(v))\rightarrow X(T, \ldots, T, F))\& \ldots \&$$
$$\forall v((- Y_1(v)\& \ldots \& - Y_{n-1}(v)\& - Y_n(v))\rightarrow X(F, \ldots, F, F))).$$

If Q is $\exists$, we rewrite it as

$$(\exists v((Y_1(v)\& \ldots \& Y_{n-1}(v)\& Y_n(v))\& X(T, \ldots, T, T))v$$
$$\exists v((Y_1(v)\& \ldots \& Y_{n-1}(v)\& - Y_n(v))\& X(T, \ldots, T, F))v \ldots v$$
$$\exists v((- Y_1(v)\& \ldots \& - Y_{n-1}(v)\& - Y_n(v))\& X(F, \ldots, F, F))).$$

T and F may then be eliminated from the resultant formula by simplifying in accordance with the usual truth-table definitions of the connectives. As a result, $QvX(v)$ becomes a conjunction of universally quantified conditionals or a disjunction of existentially quantified conjunctions, according as Q is $\forall$ or $\exists$, such that all and only components with v as their sole free variable are to be found in the antecedents or first conjuncts. If this is done for every suitable subformula in S, the result will be a formula that satisfies the second of the two conditions cited in the text. (The connectives $\leftrightarrow$ and v may then be eliminated, in the usual way, in favour of $\rightarrow$ and $-$, so that the first of these conditions is satisfied also.)

It is instructive to consider separately the system TFL⁻, obtained by discarding clause (2) of the formation rules and clause (4) of the valuation function. This is TFL stripped of the superscript sequences that allow one to form, from a relation of degree n, its $n! - 1$ converses. For a formula of MPL= to be translatable into TFL⁻, it must be expressible in a pure form that, in addition to satisfying (i) and (iii) above, satisfies a condition more stringent than (ii), namely:

(ii′) (a) The sequence of variables associated with every predicate letter, leaving aside individual constants, is an *unpermuted* terminal subsequence of the variable sequence associated with the quantifiers within the scope of which it lies, taken in their order of occurrence. (b) No individual constant immediately precedes a string of the form $s_1 \ldots s_n v$, where $s_1 \ldots s_n$ is a (possibly empty) sequence of individual constants and v is a variable, if $s_1 \ldots s_n v$ is, elsewhere within the scope of the quantifier that binds v, immediately preceded by a variable or by a different constant.

Formulae that satisfy (a) are said to be *uniformly quantified*, in the sense that the order of the variables associated with each predicate letter matches that of the quantifiers that bind them. (b) is simply the condition under which such uniformity may be maintained when, by way of reversing step (13) of the above algorithm, individual constants are reconstrued as predicates and relinquish their original positions in favour of variables bound by wild quantifiers; it is only where condition (b) is met that one can slot these wild quantifiers into the formula in a way that preserves sequence.

It is easy to see that, in the case of formulae of MPL=, lacking individual constants, which are both pure and uniformly quantified, the individual variables are strictly superfluous. Given a sequence of quantifiers and a predicate letter that lies within the scope of these quantifiers, all one need know, in order to understand the construction, is which quantifiers govern which argument places. The sole function of the variables is to effect this coordination; beyond that it is a matter of indifference which variable letters occur where. This being the case, one could, if one wished, adopt the convention that, where a formula is both pure and uniformly quantified, its variables may be suppressed. For one would know, in the absence of variables, that the ith argument place of any n-place predicate letter, P^n, was governed by the ith quantifier in the sequence comprising the n rightmost quantifiers that include P^n in their scope. That is one way of explaining why TFL^- is able to dispense with the use of variables, or any surrogates for the latter.

Departures from uniformity may take any of three forms. Let P^n be an n-place predicate letter and S the sequence of variables associated with the n rightmost quantifiers that include P^n within their scope. (Again, we assume, for the sake of simplicity, that there are no individual constants.) Then the argument string attached to P^n may be a *permutation* of S, or it may contain repetitions of one or more variables in S, what Quine calls *identifications*, or it may, skip some elements of S altogether, what we shall call *omissions*. It is here, as Quine observes, that 'the bound variable enters essentially', serving 'to keep track of permutations and identifications of arguments of polyadic predicates'.[5] But the permutation job, at any rate, can be discharged as well by Sommers' superscript sequences as by bound variables. If we were to import this device into $MPL =$, we should be able to discard the variables from all pure formulae (free of individual constants) that satisfied (ii) above. Confronted with the predicate $P^{i_1 \cdots i_n}$, bereft of variables, one would be able to interpret it as the predicate P^n, with its i_jth argument place, for all j such that $1 \leqslant j \leqslant n$, governed by the jth quantifier in the sequence comprising the rightmost n quantifiers that include $P^{i_1 \cdots i_n}$ within their scope.

That leaves identifications and omissions. Now the requirement that a formula of $MPL =$, if it is to be translatable into TFL, must be expressible in a pure form that satisfies (ii) above just is the requirement that it be possible to express it in a pure form that is free of identifications and omissions. It is impossible to translate into TFL formulae of $MPL =$ that contain ineliminable departures from uniformity of either of these two kinds. For example,

(f) $\exists x F^2 x x$

[5] W. V. O. Quine, 'The Variable', in *The Ways of Paradox*, op. cit., p. 282.

is not translatable into TFL, since the identification of the two argument places is ineliminable. Nor is there any obvious way of translating into TFL the formula

(g) $\forall x \forall y \forall z((R^2xy \ \& \ R^2yz) \to R^2xz)$

which says that R^2 is transitive. In its pure form

$\forall x \forall y(R^2xy \to \forall z(R^2yz \to R^2xz))$

the final occurrence of R^2 is associated with an argument string in which y is skipped; and it seems more than probable that *any* pure rendering of the original formula would embody a similar omission.

The final limitation on the expressive capacity of TFL has quite a different source. Consider the formula

(h) $\forall x(F^1x \to \exists y(G^1y \ \& \ \exists z(H^1z \ \& \ (R^2yz \ \& \ S^3xyz))))$.

This satisfies (i) and (ii′) above, but not (iii), the reason being that R^2yz, which has two free variables, is here conjoined with S^3xyz, which has three. It is impossible to translate into TFL a formula of MPL= every pure representation of which incorporates one or more truth-functional compounds in which, for distinct m, n > 1, an expression with m free variables is combined with one with n. That is the force of (iii). (h) is thus not translatable into TFL, unless (as seems unlikely) it can be recast in a pure form in which no such heterogeneous combination occurs. The point is that, in TFL, as in natural languages, conjunction, disjunction and conditionalization are homogeneous operations.

Natural language, of course, has its own means of overcoming these limitations: it resorts to cross-referential pronominalization. And this is the device that Sommers himself uses to bridge the gap between the full first-order power that we find in MPL= and what can be expressed employing only the combinatorial resources of TFL. Using pronouns, (f), (g) and (h) can be transcribed, respectively, as

(f′) $+T_i + F^2 *i,$
(g′) $-T + \langle -(R^2 + (R^2 + T_i)) + (R^2 *i) \rangle,$
and (h′) $-F^1 + S^{123} + G_i^1 + \langle +H^1 + (R^{21} *i) \rangle.$

But a remarkable fact now emerges. Formally speaking, there is no need to introduce pronouns. The notation of TFL, without pronouns, is *as it stands* adequate for the expression of anything that can be said in MPL (first-order predicate logic without identity). All we need do is relax the formation rules slightly, so that more expressions count as well-formed, and then modify the interpretation, as embodied in the valuation function.

We begin by generalizing the binary mode of composition introduced in clause (3) of the formation rules, so that it extends to terms of unlike degree; (3) is accordingly replaced by

(3′) If X^m and X^n are terms of degree m and n, respectively, then $\langle \pm X^m \pm Y^n \rangle$ are terms of degree max(m, n).

To interpret $\langle \pm X^m \pm Y^n \rangle$ we shall need to generalize the homogeneous Boolean intersection, $\cap$, to a *heterogeneous intersection*, $\bullet$, so defined that $\alpha^m \bullet \beta^n$ (where α^m and β^n are sets of sequences of length m and n, respectively) is the set of all sequences in α^m that end with sequences in β^n, or conversely, according as $m \geqslant n$ or $m \leqslant n$.[6] Clause (7) of the valuation function then becomes

(7′) $v_\phi {}^\ulcorner \langle + X^m + Y^n \rangle {}^\urcorner = v_\phi {}^\ulcorner X^m {}^\urcorner \bullet v_\phi {}^\ulcorner Y^n {}^\urcorner$
$= \{ \langle x_1, \ldots, x_{\max(m,n)} \rangle :$
$(\langle x_1, \ldots, x_m \rangle \in v_\phi {}^\ulcorner X^m {}^\urcorner \ \& \ \langle x_{m-n}, \ldots, x_m \rangle \in v_\phi {}^\ulcorner Y^n {}^\urcorner) \lor$
$(\langle x_1, \ldots, x_n \rangle \in v_\phi {}^\ulcorner Y^n {}^\urcorner \ \& \ \langle x_{n-m}, \ldots, x_n \rangle \in v_\phi {}^\ulcorner X^m {}^\urcorner) \}$

and clauses (8)–(10) give way to (8′)–(10′), where the latter differ from the former merely by the substitution of $\bullet$ for $\cap$.

With this, we are free to translate (h), above, as

(h″) $(- F^1 + G^1 + H^1 + \langle + R^2 + S^3 \rangle)$

and thence, by (T1)–(T4), into its E-transform

$- F^1 + \langle + R^2 + S^3 \rangle + G^1 + H^1.$

(h″) is now a well-formed, interpretable formula, not of TFL, but of an extension of it.

TFL may be further enriched, again without introducing any

---

[6] Cf. W. V. O. Quine, 'Algebraic Logic and Predicate Functors', op. cit., p. 297. (Note that Quine's functor is distinct from ours, inasmuch as a sequence from one set is required to match an *initial* segment of a sequence in the other, rather than a terminal segment, if it is to belong to Quine's heterogenous intersection.)

fresh notation. Consider the following prescription for eliminating the variables from an arbitrary formula of MPL that
does not contain any individual constants:

(i) Convert the formula to a pure form F.
(ii) Consider, for each n-place predicate letter P^n, in F, the
terminal subsequence S, of the sequence of variables that
include P^n within their scope, taken in their order of
occurrence, that has as its first element the variable
associated with the leftmost quantifier that binds some
variable in the variable string associated with P^n. Rewrite
P^n as $P^{i_1 \cdots i_n}$, where each i_j gives the position that the jth
variable in the string associated with P^n occupies within S.
(iii) Delete all individual variables.

This works because the superscripts introduced in (ii), unlike
Sommers', are capable of encoding absolutely any pattern of
coordination, as between quantifiers and argument places, that
is consistent with F's being pure, including those that involve
identifications or omissions. $P^{i_1 \cdots i_n}$ is now to be read as the
predicate P^n, where the jth argument place, for all j such that $1
\leqslant j \leqslant n$, is governed by the i_jth quantifier symbol in the
sequence comprising the $\max(i_1, \ldots, i_n)$ rightmost quantifier
symbols within the scope of which $P^{i_1 \cdots i_n}$ lies.
It may be illuminating to compare this method of eliminating
variables from MPL with Quine's. The connectives and
quantifier symbols $\forall$ and $\exists$ are all now interpretable as *predicate
functors*, in Quine's sense. In terms of the system presented in
his 'Variables Explained Away',[7] $\exists$ corresponds to Quine's
derelativization functor, Der, which has the effect, in the
underlying semantics, of *cropping* the rightmost element of
each of a set of sequences, thereby reducing by one the degree of
the term to which it is applied. $-$ corresponds to Neg, which is
interpreted, semantically, in terms of Boolean complemen-
tation. & has no direct counterpart, in this particular system of
Quine's, but may be interpreted by the heterogeneous intersection just introduced. $\forall$ then corresponds to Neg Der Neg, and

[7] W. V. O. Quine, 'Variables Explained Away', in *Proceedings of the American
Philosophical Society*, 104 (1960), pp. 343–47, reprinted in *Selected Logic Papers* (New
York, 1966), pp. 227–35.

the remaining connectives may be defined, in the standard way, in terms of & and $-$.

That leaves the superscript sequences. What do they amount to semantically? Well, each distinct sequence $i_1 \ldots i_n$ is really a predicate functor in its own right, and may be interpreted by a corresponding *redistribution operator*, $r_{i_1 \ldots i_n}$. If α^n is a set of sequences of length n, then $r_{i_1 \ldots i_n} \alpha^n$ is the set of sequences of length max $(i_1, \ldots, i_n)$ which, for some sequence σ, in α^n, have the first element of σ in i_1th place, the second element of σ in i_2th place, ... and the nth element of σ in i_nth place. In the special case where $1 \leqslant i_j \leqslant n$ for all i_j, and $i_j \neq i_k$ for all $j \neq k$, $r_{i_1 \ldots i_n} \alpha^n$ has the effect of permuting the elements of the sequences in α^n. Thus, $r_{231} \alpha^3 = p_{312} \alpha^3$ and, symmetrically, $r_{312} \alpha^3 = p_{231} \alpha^3$. Here, r is related to p in a very simple way. It is a question of whether one takes the elements of the unpermuted sequence, in their order of occurrence, and then gives, for each in turn, its position in the permuted sequence, or whether one takes the elements of the permuted sequence, in their order of occurrence, and gives, for each in turn, its position in the unpermuted sequence. r does the first, p the second. But of course it is arbitrary which of these two sequences we regard as the permuted one; hence the symmetry.

Previously, we have used the superscripts in a manner corresponding to p, both because this is the way Sommers (following a suggestion of Bennett's) uses them, and because it is slightly more perspicuous. Now, however, we switch to the alternative convention, based on r, because r yields useful operations that are not permutations, in a way that no straightforward generalization of p could. Take our earlier example, $\exists x F^2 xx$. Under the procedure just sketched, this becomes $\exists F^{11}$. Here, the superscripts fulfil the function that, in Quine's system, is served by the *reflection* functor, Ref, which fuses the final and penultimate argument places of an n-place predicate, so as to convert, for example, the two-place predicate 'kicks' into the one-place predicate 'kicks self'. $\exists F^{11}$ is what, in the notation of 'Variables Explained Away', would be written Der Ref F^2. From identifications we turn to omissions. (g), above, goes over to the pure form $\forall x \forall y (R^2 xy \rightarrow \forall z (R^2 yz \rightarrow R^2 xz))$ and then becomes $\forall \forall (R^{12} \rightarrow \forall (R^{12} \rightarrow R^{13}))$. The superscripts in R^{13} fulfil the function which Quine, in his more recent writings, calls *padding*: they expand the relation R^2 into a relation of degree three that embraces every triple the first element of which stands to the third in the relation R^2. (Actually, Quine can only pad at one end of a sequence, so the superscripts here do directly what, on Quine's approach, can only be done by padding and then permuting.)

This, then, is the key idea that allows us to extend TFL to a system, TFL^+, the expressive power of which slightly exceeds that of MPL. (Slightly exceeds, rather than equals, inasmuch as equations involving singular terms can be handled in TFL^+ without recourse to an identity sign, which TFL^+ and MPL both lack.) The superscripts, under their new interpretation, call, once again, for certain modifications of the formation and valuation rules. Clause (2) of the formation rules is relaxed so as to yield

(2') If U^n is a relation letter, i.e. a term letter of degree $n > 1$, and $i_1, \ldots, i_n$ is a sequence of n numerals denoting positive integers, then $U^{i_1 \cdots i_n}$ is a term of degree $\max(i_1, \ldots, i_n)$;

and clause (4) of the valuation function becomes

(4') $v_\phi \ulcorner U^{i_1 \cdots i_n} \urcorner = r_{i_1 \ldots i_n} \phi \ulcorner U^n \urcorner = \{ \langle x_1, \ldots, x_{\max(i_1, \ldots, i_n)} \rangle : \langle x_{i_1}, \ldots, x_{i_n} \rangle \in \phi \ulcorner U^n \urcorner \}$.

Adding these to the changes made earlier, in order to accommodate constructions of the form $\langle \pm X^m \pm Y^n \rangle$ where $m \neq n$, we now have a system into which any formula of MPL is translatable.

Actually, the substitution of (2') for (2), in the formation rules, and (4') for (4), in the valuation function, suffices by itself to convert TFL into a system that can express anything that is expressible in MPL. Only in respect of relational terms is there a need for the kind of heterogenous compounding which clause (4') of the formation rules and clauses (7')–(10') of the valuation function are designed to accommodate; and there it can always be accomplished indirectly by way of homogeneous compounding, as is permitted by the original formation rules, and our new superscript sequences. Thus, instead of writing $\langle + R^2 + S^3 \rangle$, we could write $\langle + R^{23} + S^{123} \rangle$. (We leave, as an exercise for the reader, the task of formulating a general prescription for the construction of a homogenous surrogate for $\langle \pm X^m \pm Y^m \rangle$, where X^m and Y^n may be of arbitrary complexity.) Incidentally, the *relative product* of two relations R^2 and S^2, commonly written $R^2|S^2$, can now be expressed, without recourse to our new heterogenous mode of composition, as $(+ T + \langle + R^{13} + S^{32} \rangle)$. This is the relation of degree two that embraces all pairs, the first element of which stands in the relation R^2 to something that stands to the second element in the relation S^2. Thus, if R^2 is the relation 'mother of' and S^2 is the relation 'parent of', the relative product of R^2 and S^2 is the relation 'mother of a parent of', i.e. 'grandmother of'.

To gain the expressive power of the first-order predicate calculus with identity, MPL =, we supplement the vocabulary of TFL$^+$ with an identity letter, I. I, in its unsubscripted forms, is accordingly removed from the stock of general purpose term letters. For the purposes of clause (2') of the formation rules and clause (4') of the valuation function, I must now be included among the substituends for U^n, where n = 2; correspondingly, U must be understood as resulting from U^n by the deletion of the superscript *if any*. We introduce the further valuation rule

(14) $v_\phi \ulcorner \Gamma = \phi \ulcorner \Gamma = \{\langle x, x \rangle : x \in D\}$.

The resulting enriched system we call extended traditional formal logic with identity, TFL$\overset{+}{=}$·

It only remains to give an algorithm for translating formulae of MPL = into logically equivalent formulae of TFL$\overset{+}{=}$. An obvious desideratum is that the algorithm be fairly efficient at yielding translations into a weaker, rather than a stronger subsystem, TFL or better TFL$^-$, where this is possible. It is the attempt to meet this desideratum that makes for much of the complexity of the algorithm. Basically, it just involves a prescription for getting to a pure form that may then be mechanically transcribed. The method of purification is that of converting the formula to prenex normal form, converting the matrix to conjunctive or disjunctive normal form, according as the rightmost quantifier in the prefix is universal or existential, simplifying, and then distributing the quantifier through the resultant conjunction or disjunction, iterating the procedure until all quantifiers have been driven in as far as they will go.

As a practical matter, the simplest way of arriving at a conjunctive or disjunctive normal form is to proceed as though one were constructing a semantic tableau. For disjunctive normal forms the appropriate rules are:

$$
\begin{array}{cccc}
(X_1 \,\&\, \ldots \,\&\, X_n) & (X_1 \lor \ldots \lor X_n) & (X \to Y) & (X \leftrightarrow Y) \\
X_1 & \diagup|\diagdown & \diagup\diagdown & \diagup\diagdown \\
\vdots & X_1 \,\cdots\, X_n & -X \quad Y & X \quad -X \\
X_n & & & Y \quad -Y
\end{array}
$$

$$
\begin{array}{ccccc}
-(X \,\&\, Y) & -(X \lor Y) & -(X \to Y) & -(X \leftrightarrow Y) & --X \\
\diagup\diagdown & -X & X & \diagup\diagdown & X \\
-X \quad -Y & -Y & -Y & X \quad -X & \\
& & & -Y \quad Y &
\end{array}
$$

For conjunctive normal forms one employs their duals:

$$
\begin{array}{cccc}
(X_1 \,\&\, \ldots \,\&\, X_n) & (X_1 \lor \ldots \lor X_n) & (X \to Y) & (X \leftrightarrow Y) \\
\diagup|\diagdown & X_1 & -X & \diagup\diagdown \\
X_1 \,\cdots\, X_n & \vdots & Y & X \quad -X \\
& X_n & & -Y \quad Y
\end{array}
$$

$$
\begin{array}{ccccc}
-(X \,\&\, Y) & -(X \lor Y) & -(X \to Y) & -(X \leftrightarrow Y) & --X \\
-X & \diagup\diagdown & \diagup\diagdown & \diagup\diagdown & X \\
-Y & -X \quad -Y & X \quad -Y & X \quad -X & \\
& & & Y \quad -Y &
\end{array}
$$

The result of making all possible applications of these rules will, in either case, be a tree. In the first case, where one wants a disjunctive normal form, take each branch in turn and form a conjunction the conjuncts of which are the truth-functionally noncomposite formulae which occur on that branch, then disjoin the resultant conjunctions. In the second case, where one wants a conjunctive normal form, take each branch in turn and form a disjunction the disjuncts of which are the truth-functionally noncomposite formulae which occur on that branch, then conjoin the resultant disjunctions. (For present purposes, $-X$ counts as noncomposite if X is noncomposite and does not itself have the form of a negation.)

We now give a rigorous account of the method of translation, which we shall illustrate with an example. Let MPL= be a formulation of the first-order predicate calculus with identity, the vocabulary of which comprises (i) for each natural number n, an infinite stock of n-place predicate letters, A^n, B^n, ..., S^n (excluding I^n), A_1^n, B_1^n, ..., S_1^n, ...; (ii) a two-place predicate,

=, connoting identity; (iii) an infinite stock of individual variables, x, y, z, x_1, y_1, z_1, . . . ; (iv) an infinite stock of individual constants, a, b, . . . , h, a_1, b_1, . . . , h_1, . . . ; (v) connectives, $-$, &, v, $\rightarrow$ and $\rightarrow$; (vi) quantifier symbols, $\forall$ and $\exists$; (vii) left and right parentheses, (,). (The propositional letters are the zero-place predicate letters.) We use italicized upper case letters for formulae or parts of formulae (many of which will be chimeras, belong neither to MPL $=$ nor to TFL$_=^+$ proper); v and t, with or without subscripts, denote arbitrary individual variables and constants, respectively. Certain italicized words and phrases are defined at the end. In what follows, 'conjunction' and 'conjunct', 'disjunction' and 'disjunct' are to be understood in such a sense that there can be one-membered 'conjunctions' which are their own conjuncts and one-membered 'disjunctions' which are their own disjuncts. X is a limiting case, for n $=$ 1, both of the conjunctive form (X_1 & . . . & X_n) and of the disjunctive form (X_1 ∨ . . . ∨ X_n). With this we proceed to a statement of the algorithm. To translate an arbitrary well-formed formula, F, of MPL $=$ into an equivalent well-formed formula of extended traditional formal logic with identity, TFL$_=^+$, perform the following steps.

(1) Convert F to prenex normal form. Call the result G.
(2) Locate those atomic subformulae (henceforth *atoms*) of G, if any, in which the variables fail to constitute an unbroken consecutive substring of the variables corresponding to the string of quantifiers in the prefix. Giving absolute priority to minimizing the number of atoms in which the variables fail even to constitute a permuted substring of the string of variables associated with the prefix, reduce the number of atoms in which the variables are out of sequence to a minimum by permuting quantifiers in the prefix and/or left-right interchange of variables within equations. Note: universal quantifiers may be shifted only within blocks of adjacent universal quantifiers; likewise, existential quantifiers may be shifted only within blocks of adjacent existential quantifiers. Let $Qv_1 \ldots Qv_n M(v_1, \ldots, v_n)$ be the resultant formula, where $Qv_1, \ldots, Qv_n$ are quantifiers and $M(v_1, \ldots, v_n)$ is the matrix.
(3) Convert $M(v_1, \ldots, v_n)$ to conjunctive or disjunctive

normal form (CNF or DNF) according as Qv_n is universal or existential.

(4) Discard each of a pair of *mutually exclusive* subformulae that either constitute or are disjuncts of otherwise *identical* conjuncts of a CNF, unless this would cause the entire formula, upon deletion of vacuous quantifiers, to vanish. If it would, do not discard these subformulae, but note that the formula is inconsistent.

(5) Discard each of a pair of *jointly exhaustive* subformulae that either constitute or are conjuncts of otherwise identical disjuncts of a DNF, unless this would cause the entire formula, upon deletion of vacuous quantifiers, to vanish. If it would, do not discard these subformulae, but note that the formula is tautologous.

(6) If any conjunct, in a CNF, contains two disjuncts that are jointly exhaustive, discard it unless this would cause the entire formula, upon deletion of vacuous quantifiers, to vanish. If it would, note that the formula is tautologous and discard instead all disjuncts except for the jointly exhaustive pair.

(7) If any disjunct, in a DNF, contains two conjuncts that are mutually exclusive, discard it unless this would cause the entire formula, upon deletion of vacuous quantifiers, to vanish. If it would, note that the formula is inconsistent and discard instead all conjuncts except for the mutually exclusive pair.

(8) Discard all duplicate conjuncts of a CNF, or disjuncts of a DNF, and then all duplicate or *redundant* disjuncts or conjuncts within those disjunctions or conjunctions that remain.

(9) Where not all the component disjuncts of a conjunct or conjuncts of a disjunct of the resultant CNF or DNF contain v_n, group together those that do as a terminal segment of the corresponding disjunction or conjunction. Enclose each such segment in parentheses, if it has more than one component, and preface it with Qv_n.

(10) Call the result, excluding what remains of the prefix, N. Discard all quantifiers, in the truncated prefix $Qv_1 \ldots Qv_{n-1}$, that in consequence of steps (5)–(9) have become vacuous. Call the thinned quantifier string P, so that what remains is of the form PN.

(11) Iterate steps (3)–(10), successively substituting each new P and N for $Qv_1 \ldots Qv_n$ and $M(v_1, \ldots, v_n)$, respectively, and the rightmost quantifier in P for Qv_n, until every quantifier in the original prefix, $Qv_1 \ldots Qv_n$, has been dealt with. Apply steps (4)–(8). Call the result H.

(12) Locate those blocks of adjacent quantifiers in H, within the scope of which there are one or more atoms whose variables fail to constitute an unbroken consecutive substring of the variable string associated with the quantifiers that bind them, taken in their order of occurrence. Giving absolute priority to minimizing the number of atoms, within the scope of each such block, in which the variables fail even to constitute a permuted substring of the sequence of variables associated with the quantifiers within whose scope they lie, taken in their order of occurrence, reduce (as before) the number of atoms in which the variables are out of sequence to a minimum by permuting quantifiers in the block (subject to the constraints stated under (2) above) and/or left-right interchange, within equations, of variables one or both of which are bound by these quantifiers. Then, taking 'Qv_n', in (9), now to mean the rightmost quantifier in the block, and 'v_n' the corresponding variable, subject the conjunction or disjunction that constitutes the scope of the rightmost quantifier to any of steps (4)–(9) that are applicable. Repeat this procedure, as many times as is possible, for each successive new rightmost quantifier, discarding vacuous quantifiers after each application. Apply steps (4)–(8) to the resultant subformula. Do this for each such block in H.

(13) Iterate (12), as many times as is possible, substituting each successive new formula for H.

(14) Replace every instance of $Qv_1 \ldots Qv_n - X(v_1, \ldots, v_n)$ by $- Q'v_1 \ldots Q'v_nX(v_1, \ldots, v_n)$, where Q' is $\exists$ if Q is $\forall$ and $\forall$ if Q is $\exists$. Call the resulting formula J.

(15) Consider, for each universal and existential quantifier Qv_k in J, the (possibly one-membered) conjunction or disjunction of subformulae that lie within its scope, and let $Qv_1, \ldots, Qv_{k-1}$ be the quantifiers, listed in their order of occurrence, within whose scope Qv_k itself lies. Determine, for each conjunct (if Qv_k is existential) or disjunct (if Qv_k

is universal), which, of all the variables it contains that figure in the sequence $v_1, \ldots, v_{k-1}, v_k$, occurs earliest in that sequence. If it be v_i, assign that conjunct or disjunct (henceforth *component*) the *rank* $(k-i)+1$. If there is only a single component, or if all are of the same rank n, for some $n > 1$, add the extra conjunct, Tv_k, if Qv_k is existential, or disjunct, $-Tv_k$, if Qv_k is universal. Arrange the components of the conjunction or disjunction governed by Qv_k in ascending order of rank, with Tv_k or $-Tv_k$, if it occurs, taking overall precedence, and with unnegated components taking precedence over negated ones, or conversely, according as Qv_k is existential or universal. Unless all components are of rank one, enclose in parentheses each subsegment of the resulting conjunction or disjunction, with more than one component, that comprises all components of the same rank. Reorder all remaining disjunctions so that negated disjuncts take precedence over unnegated ones, and all remaining conjunctions so that unnegated conjuncts take precedence over negated ones.

(16) Rewrite each conjunction $(X_1 \& \ldots X_{n-1} \& X_n)$ as $(X_1 \& (\ldots \& (X_{n-1} \& X_n) \ldots))$ and each disjunction $(X \vee \ldots \vee X_{n-1} \vee X_n)$ as $(-X_1 \rightarrow (\ldots \rightarrow (-X_{n-1} \rightarrow X_n) \ldots))$. Delete all occurrences of $--$.

(17) Rewrite $-(X_1 \rightarrow (\ldots \rightarrow (X_{n-1} \rightarrow X_n) \ldots))$ as $(X_1 \& (\ldots \& (X_{n-1} \& -X_n) \ldots))$. Delete all occurrences of $--$. Call the resultant formula K.

(18) Locate those atoms of K in which there occur one or more individual constants. Let C be such an atom. If C is of the form $v = t$ or $t = v$, replace it with tv. Otherwise, let t_1 be the rightmost occurring individual constant within C and let v_1 be some variable distinct from those associated with the quantifiers that include C within their scope. Substitute v_1 for t_1 at this occurrence within C; call the result C'. If v_1 is the final argument of C', replace C' with $*v_1(t_1v_1 + C')$; if C' is of the form $t_2 = v_1$, where t_2 is an individual constant, replace $(t_1v_1 + C')$ by $(t_2v_1 + t_1v_1)$. If, on the other hand, v_1 immediately precedes a variable v_2, see whether v_2, elsewhere within the scope of the quantifier, Qv_2, that governs v_2, is immediately preceded

by a variable v_3, associated with a quantifier Qv_3, that includes Qv_2 in its scope. If it is, replace C', as before, with $*v_1(t_1v_1 + C')$; otherwise, take the subformula $Qv_2X(v_1, v_2)$, where $X(v_1, v_2)$ comprises everything within the scope of Qv_2, and replace it with $*v_1(t_1v_1 + Qv_2X(v_1, v_2))$. Iterate this procedure for the rightmost occurring individual constant in C', and so on until all occurrences of individual constants within C have been dealt with. Do this for each atom of K in which individual constants appear. (For the purposes of (20), below, $*$ is to be treated as a quantifier symbol, along with $\forall$ and $\exists$.)

(19) Replace every equation of the form $v_1 = v_2$ by the corresponding formula $I^2v_1v_2$, where I^2 is to count as a two-place predicate letter. Call the resulting formula L.

(20) Examine L to see whether or not the sequence of variables associated with every one of its atoms is an unpermuted terminal subsequence of the variable sequence associated with the quantifiers that include the atom within their scope, taken in their order of occurrence. If it is, replace I^2, at each occurrence, with I and proceed immediately to (21). Otherwise, consider, for each atom C, the terminal subsequence S, of the sequence of variables corresponding to the quantifiers that include C within their scope, which has as its first element the variable associated with the leftmost quantifier that binds some variable within C. (The above steps ensure that the final element of S will also figure in C.) Let P^n be the predicate letter of C. If $n > 1$, replace the superscript, n, by a sequence of n numerals, the ith element of which gives the position that the ith variable of C occupies within S. Replace I^{12} with I.

(21) Delete all individual variables.

(22) Replace $-\forall(X \to Y)$ by $\exists(X \& - Y)$, $-\exists(X \& Y)$ by $\forall(X \to - Y)$ and $-*(t + X)$ by $*(t + - X)$. Repeat until no longer applicable, deleting emergent occurrences of $- -$ after each application.

(23) Rewrite $-X$ as $(- X)$.

(24) Rewrite $\forall(X \to (- Y))$ as $(- X - Y)$, $\exists(X \& (- Y))$ as $(+ X - Y)$ and $*(t + (- X))$ as $(*t - X)$.

(25) Rewrite $\forall(X \to Y)$ as $(- X + Y)$, $\exists(X \& Y)$ as $(+ X + Y)$ and $*(t + X)$ as $(*t + X)$.

(26) Rewrite $(X \rightarrow (- Y))$ as $\langle - X - Y \rangle$ and $(X \& (- Y))$ as $\langle + X - Y \rangle$.

(27) Rewrite $(X \rightarrow Y)$ as $\langle - X + Y \rangle$ and $(X \& Y)$ as $\langle + X + Y \rangle$.

The result is a well-formed formula of TFL $\overset{+}{=}$, in subject–predicate normal form. To simplify the formula apply, wherever possible, the further step

(28) Rewrite $(\oplus X_n^1 + (\oplus X_{n-1}^1 \ldots + (\oplus X_1^1 \pm Y^m) \ldots))$ as $(\oplus X_n^1 \oplus X_{n-1}^1 \ldots \oplus X_1^1 \pm Y^m)$.

(T1)–(T4) may then, if one wishes, be invoked to produce the E-transform of the resulting formula. If the formula has been translated successfully into TFL, one may wish to replace superscript sequences by their equivalents, according to the convention adopted by Sommers. To this end, one can apply a further transformation, governed by the rule:

(T5) Given a term of the form $U^{i_1 \cdots i_n}$, where $1 \leqslant i_j \leqslant n$ for all i_j, and $i_j \neq i_k$ for all $j \neq k$, replace $i_1 \ldots i_n$ with the sequence obtained by putting 1 in i_1th place, 2 in i_2th place, ... and n in i_nth place.

Suppose, finally, the result of applying the algorithm is not a formula of TFL or TFL$^-$, as hoped. If the formula has been ruled tautologous or inconsistent, at some stage in the application of the algorithm, and one is concerned only with translation up to logical equivalence, then one may replace the formula, as the case may be, with some standard tautology, such as $(- T + T)$, or standard contradiction, such as $(+ T - T)$.

The point, of course, is that the translation algorithm doubles as a weak decision procedure for MPL $=$. At least, it does so when we specify which formulae are to be regarded as pairwise *identical, mutually exclusive* or *jointly exhaustive* and which *redundant*. This we now proceed to do.

We count two formulae as *identical*, if they differ, at most, only in the ordering of conjuncts within a conjunction or of disjuncts within a disjunction, or in the order of flanking variables or constants within an equation, or in the labelling of bound variables (bound, that is to say, by quantifiers within the subformula in question: such quantifiers will make their appearance only as steps (4)–(11) are iterated). In what follows, the X, Y etc. may be taken to refer to equivalence classes of identical formulae.

Partial definition of mutual exclusion and joint exhaustiveness
 (i) X and $-X$ are both mutually exclusive and jointly exhaustive.
 (ii) If $X(v)$ and $Y(v)$ are mutually exclusive, so are $\forall vX(v)$ and $\forall v\ Y(v)$, and $\forall vX(v)$ and $\exists v\ Y(v)$.
 (iii) If $X(v)$ and $Y(v)$ are jointly exhaustive, so are $\exists vX(v)$ and $\exists v\ Y(v)$, and $\forall vX(v)$ and $\exists v\ Y(v)$.

Partial definition of relative strength
 (i) X is as strong as X.
 (ii) $(X\ \&\ Y)$ is as strong as X.
 (iii) X is as strong as $(X\ \lor\ Y)$.
 (iv) $(X\ \&\ Y)$ is as strong as $(X\ \lor\ Y)$.
 (v) $\forall vX(v)$ is as strong as $X(t)$, where t is an individual constant.
 (vi) $X(t)$ is as strong as $\exists vX(v)$.
 (vii) $\forall vX(v)$ is as strong as $\exists vX(v)$.
 (viii) $QvX(v)$ is as strong as $Qv\ Y(v)$ if and only if $X(v)$ is as strong as $Y(v)$.

Definition of redundancy
 (i) In a CNF, a conjunct C_1 is redundant if and only if there is some other conjunct C_2 which, under some ordering and grouping of its disjuncts, or of conjuncts or disjuncts within embedded conjunctions or disjunctions, is, by the above definition, as strong as C_1.
 (ii) In a DNF, a disjunct D_1 is redundant if and only if, under some ordering and grouping of its conjuncts, or of conjuncts or disjuncts within embedded conjunctions, it is, by the above definition, as strong as some other disjunct D_2.

Our 'partial definitions' are obviously expandable without limit. They merely encapsulate, with an eye to the simplification of conjunctive and disjunctive normal forms, certain logical relations the holding of which can be ascertained by simple

Worked example

We take a formula that is already in prenex normal Form:

$$\exists x \forall y \exists z ((F^1 x \to G^2 xy) \lor (H^2 yz \lor (K^1 z \to J^2 ay)))$$

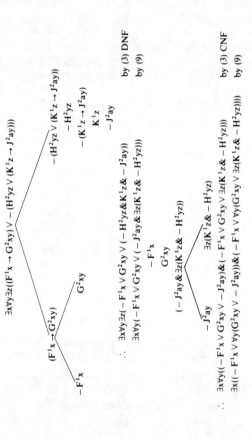

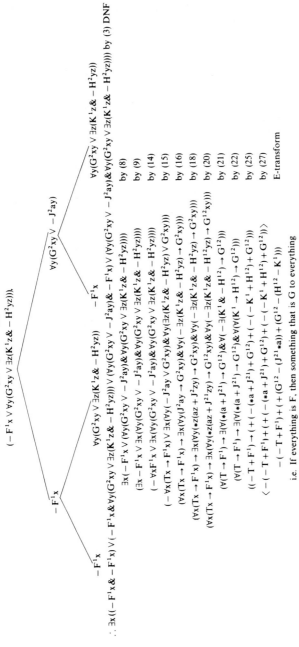

by (8)
by (9)
by (14)
by (15)
by (16)
by (18)
by (20)
by (21)
by (22)
by (25)
by (27)
E-transform

i.e. If everything is F, then something that is G to everything

J'd by a is G to everything that is H to every K.

inspection. Were we to expand them, we should thereby increase the number of formulae that our algorithm will translate into well-formed formulae of TFL or TFL⁻. Since the relation of logical equivalence, as between formulae of MPL =, is undecidable, so is the property of being translatable, up to logical equivalence, into TFL or TFL⁻. There is, therefore, no best algorithm for this purpose; any algorithm could be improved upon.

The complexity of the algorithm just presented is, in a sense, a measure of the semantic distance between quantification theory and natural language. Philosophically minded linguists, such as Chomsky (in his more recent writings), and philosophers with an interest in linguistics, such as Montague, have alike tended to suppose that an apparatus of quantifiers and bound variables must somehow lurk beneath the surface of our speech, whenever we employ such words as 'some', 'all', 'no', 'a', and 'the'. We repudiate this supposition. The natural logic of natural language, we believe, is what, to philosophers and grammarians alike, it always appeared to be before the advent of Frege, a logic of terms. It need hardly be said that the *de facto* philosophical dominance of quantification theory is no argument at all for preferring a semantic theory that ascribes to sentences of natural language a quantificational structure to one that does not. For this dominance is itself a sheer historical accident. Had the medieval logicians stumbled upon the possibility, explored in this book, of extending term logic to the polyadic case, quantification theory would most probably never have been invented.

Bibliography

Aristotle, *Analytica Priora*, in *Aristotelis Analytica*, Oxford University Press 1964; translated in *The Works of Aristotle translated into English*. Oxford University Press (*AE*), vol. 1, 1928.

——, *De Interpretatione*, in *Aristotelis Categoriae et Liber De Interpretatione*, Oxford University Press, 1949; translated in *Aristotle's Categories and De Interpretatione* by J. L. Ackrill, Oxford University Press, 1963; also translated in *AE* vol. 1, 1928.

——, *Ethica Nicomachea*, Oxford University Press, 1894; translated in *AE* vol. 9, 1925.

——, *Sophistici Elenchi*, in *Aristotelis Topica et Sophistici Elenchi*, Oxford University Press, 1958; translated in *AE* vol. 1, 1928.

——, *Topica*, references as for previous entry.

Angelelli, J., 'Friends and Opponents of the Substitutivity of Identicals', in M. Schirn, ed., *Studies on Frege II*, Frommann Holzboog, 43, 1976.

Anscombe, G. E. M. and Geach, P. T., *Three Philosophers*, Oxford, 1961.

Austin, J. L., *Philosophical Papers*, London, 1961.

——, *How To Do Things With Words*, Oxford, 1962.

Ayer, A. J., 'Negation', *Journal of Philosophy*, 49, 1952.

Bach, E., 'Nouns and Noun-Phrases', in E. Bach and R. Harms, eds., *Universals in Linguistic Theory*, New York, 1968.

Bacon, J., 'Ontological Commitment and Free Logic', *Monist*, 53, 1969.

Bar-Hillel, Y., *Aspects of Language*, Jerusalem, 1970.

Bennett, J., 'Note on Sommers', *Journal of Symbolic Logic*, 32, 1968.

——, 'Note on Sommers', *Journal of Symbolic Logic*, 36, 1971.

Black, M., 'Russell's Philosophy of Language', in P. A. Schilpp, ed., *The Philosophy of Bertrand Russell*, New York, 1944.

Bochenski, I. M., *Ancient Formal Logic*, North-Holland, 1957.

Brody, B., 'Sommers on Predicability', *Philosophical Studies*, 23, 1972.

Buridan, John, *Sophismata*, trans. T. K. Scott as *Sophisms on Meaning and Truth*, Appleton-Century-Crofts, 1966.

Boole, G., *Studies in Logic and Probability*, ed. R. Rhees, London, 1952.

Carnap, Rudolf, *Meaning and Necessity*, University of Chicago Press, 2nd edn, 1956.

Castaneda, H. N., 'Leibniz's Syllogistico-Propositional Calculus', *Notre Dame Journal of Formal Logic*, 17, 1976.

Chomsky, N., *Syntactic Structures*, The Hague, 1957.

——, *Aspects of the Theory of Syntax*, Cambridge, 1965.

——, *Studies on Semantics in Generative Grammar*, The Hague, 1972.

——, *The Logical Structure of Linguistic Theory*, New York and London, 1976.

——, *Reflections on Language*, London, 1976.

Cohen, L. J., *The Diversity of Meaning*, Methuen, 1962.

Davidson, D., 'Truth and Meaning', *Synthese*, XVII, 1967.

——, 'True to the Facts', *Journal of Philosophy*, LXVI, 1969.

——, 'The Logical Form of Action Sentences', in N. Rescher, ed., *The Logic of Decision and Action*, Pittsburgh, 1967.

Davidson, D. and Harman, G., eds., *Semantics of Natural Language*, Dordrecht-Holland, 1972.

Davidson, D. and Hintikka, J., eds., *Words and Objections*, Dordrecht-Holland, 1969.

Davidson, D. and Harman, G., eds., *The Logic of Grammar*, Encino, California, 1975.

DeMorgan, A., *Formal Logic*, London, 1926.

Donnellan, K., 'Reference and Definite Descriptions', in S. P. Schwartz, ed., *Naming, Necessity and Natural Kinds*, Ithaca, 1977.

Drange, T., *Type Crossongs*, The Hague, 1966.

Dummett, M., 'A Comment on "A Fregean Dogma" ', in I. Lakatos, ed., *Problems in the Philosophy of Mathematics*, Amsterdam, 1967.

——, *Frege: Philosophy of Language*, New York and London, 1973.

——, *Elements of Intuitionism*, Oxford, 1977.

——, *Truth and Other Enigmas*, Cambridge, Mass., 1978.

Englebretsen, G., 'Sommers' Theory and the Paradox of Confirmation', *Philosophy of Science*, 38, 1971.

——, 'A Note on Contrariety', *Notre Dame Journal of Formal Logic*, 15, 1974.

——, 'The Square of Opposition', *Notre Dame Journal of Formal Logic*, 17, 1976.

——, 'Notes on the New Syllogistic', *Logique et Analyse*, 85–86, 1979.

——, 'Singular Terms and the Syllogistic', *The New Scholasticism*, 54, 1980.

——, *Logical Negation*, Assen (forthcoming).

——, *Three Logicians: Aristotle, Leibniz and Sommers And the New Syllogistic*, Assen (forthcoming).

Evans, G., 'Pronouns, Quantifiers and Relative Clauses', *Canadian Journal of Philosophy*, Vol. VII, Number 3 1977.

Frege, G., *Frege: Philosophical Writings*, ed. M. Black and P. T. Geach, Ithaca, 1962.

——, 'Begriffsschrift', in J. Van Heijenoort, ed., *From Frege to Gödel*, Cambridge, Mass., 1967.

——, 'The Thought', in P. F. Strawson, ed., *Philosophical Logic*, Oxford, 1967.

Fillmore, C. J. and Langendeon, D. T., *Studies in Linguistic Semantics*, New York, 1971.

Fodor, J. A. and Katz, J. J., eds., *The Structure of Language*, Englewood Cliffs, N. J., 1964.

Fodor, J. D., *Semantics*, New York, 1977.

Friedman, W. H., 'Calculemus', *Notre Dame Journal of Formal Logic*, 19, 1978.

Gangadean, A. K., 'Formal Ontology and Movement Between Worlds', *Philosophy East and West*, 26, 1976.

Geach, P. T., *Reference and Generality*, Ithaca, N. Y., 1962.

——, *Logic Matters*, Oxford, 1972.

——, *Reason and Argument*, University of California Press, 1976.

——, 'Distribution and *Suppositio*', *Mind*, 85, 1976.

——, 'Back Reference', in Asa Kasher, ed., *Language in Focus: Essays in Memory of Yehoshua Bar-Hillel*, Dordrecht, 1976.

Grice, H. P., 'Meaning', *The Philosophical Review*, LXVI, 1957.

Grice H. P. and Strawson, P. F., 'In Defense of a Dogma', *The Philosophical Review*, LXV, 1956.

Goodman, N., 'On Likeness of Meaning', in L. Linsky, ed., *Semantics and the Philosophy of Language*, Urbana, Ill., 1952.

Harman, G., 'Deep Structure as Logical Form', *Synthese*, 21, 1970.

Howell, W. S., *Eighteenth Century British Logic and Rhetoric*, Princeton, 1971.

Jespersen, O., *Negation in English and Other Languages*, Copenhagen, 1917.

Joseph, H. W. B., *An Introduction to Logic*, Oxford, 2nd edn, 1916.

Kalmar, L., 'Not Fregean and not a Dogma', in I. Lakatos, ed., *Problems in the Philosophy of Mathematics*, Amsterdam, 1967.

Kaplan, D., 'What is Russell's Theory of Descriptions?', in Wolfgang Yourgrau and Allen D. Breck, eds., *Physics, Logic and History*, New York, 1970.

——, 'Quantifying In', in D. Davidson and J. Hintikka, eds., *Words and Objections*, Dordrecht-Holland, 1969.

Katz, J. J., *The Philosophy of Language*, New York, 1966.
——, *Semantic Theory*, New York, 1972.
Kasher, A., 'On Sommers' Concept of Natural Syntax', *Philosophical Studies*, 20, 1972.
Keenan, E. L., ed. *Formal Semantics of Natural Language*, London and New York, 1975.
Keil, F. C., *Semantics and Conceptual Development*, Cambridge, Mass., 1979.
Kirwan, C., *Logic and Argument*, London, 1978.
Klemke, E. D., *Essays on Frege*, Urbana, Ill., 1968.
Kneale, W. and Kneale, M., *The Development of Logic*, Oxford, 1962.
Kripke, S., 'Naming and Necessity', in D. Davidson and G. Harman, eds., *Semantics of Natural Language*, Dordrecht, 1972.
Lakoff, G., 'Linguistics and Natural Logic', in D. Davidson and G. Harman, eds., *Semantics of Natural Language*, Dordrecht, 1972.
Lakoff, R., 'Some Reasons Why There Can't be Any *Some-Any* Rule', *Language*, 45, 1969.
Lees, R. B., *The Grammar of English Nominalizations*, Bloomington, Indiana, 1960.
Leibniz, G. W., in G. H. R. Parkinson, ed., *Logical Papers*, Oxford, 1966.
Leibniz, G. W., *Philosophische Schriften*, C. I. Gerhardt, Berlin, 1895.
Lejewski, C., 'The Logical Form of Singular and General Statements', in I. Lakatos, ed., *Problems in the Philosophy of Mathematics*, Amsterdam, 1967.
Lewis, C. I., *A Survey of Symbolic Logic*, New York, 1960.
Linsky, L., ed., *Semantics and the Philosophy of Language*, Urbana, Ill., 1952.
——, *Referring*, London, 1967.
——, ed., *Reference and Modality*, London, 1971.
Lockwood, M., 'On Predicating Proper Names', *The Philosophical Review*, 84, 1975.
Lyons, J., *Introduction to Theoretical Linguistics*, London and New York, 1968.
——, ed., *New Horizons in Linguistics*, Harmondsworth, 1970.
——, *Semantics*, London and New York, 1977.
Martin, R. M., *Truth and Denotation*, Chicago, 1958.
Massey, G., *Understanding Symbolic Logic*, New York, 1970.
Massie, D., 'Sommers' Tree Theory: A Reply to De Sousa', *Journal of Philosophy*, 64, 1967.
Mates, B., *Elementary Logic*, Oxford, 2nd edn, 1972.
Mill, J. S., *A System of Logic, ratiocinative and inductive*, Longmans, 6th edn, 1865; first published 1843.

Montague, R., in R. Thomason, ed., *Formal Philosophy*, New Haven, 1974.

Noah, A., 'Singular Terms and Predication', Ph.D. thesis, Brandeis University, 1973.

——, 'Predicate-Functors and the Limits of Decidability in Logic', *Notre Dame Journal of Formal Logic*, 21, 1980.

Pap, A., 'Types and Meaninglessness', *Mind*, 69, 1960.

Peter of Spain (Petrus Hispanus, Pope John XX or XXI): *Summulae Logicales*, ed. I. M. Bochenski, Marietti 1947.

Prior, A. N., *The Doctrine of Propositions and Terms*, London, 1976.

Purtill, R., *Logic: Argument, Refutation and Proof*, New York, 1979.

Putnam, H., 'Is Logic Empirical', in R. S. Cohen and M. Wartofsky, eds., *Boston Studies in the Philosophy of Science*, Boston, 1969.

Quine, W. V. O., *Word and Object*, Cambridge, Mass., 1960.

——, *Philosophy of Logic*, Englewood Cliffs, N. J., 1970.

——, *The Ways of Paradox and Other Essays*, Second rev. edn, New York, 1976.

——, *Methods of Logic*, 3rd edn, New York, 1972.

——, *The Roots of Reference*, La Salle, Ill., 1974.

——, 'Variables Explained Away', in *Selected Logic Papers*, New York, 1966.

——, 'On the Limits of Decision', *Acts of the XIV International Congress of Philosophy*, Vol 3, Vienna, 1968.

Ramsey, F. P., *The Foundations of Mathematics*, ed. R. B. Braithwaite, London, 1931.

Richmond, S. A., 'A Possible Empirical Violation of Sommers' Rule for Enforcing Ambiguity', *Philosophical Studies*, 28, 1975.

Russell, B., *Logic and Knowledge, Essays 1901–1950*, ed. R. C. Marsh, London, 1956.

——, *Our Knowledge of the External World*, New York, 1960.

——, *An Inquiry Into Meaning and Truth*, London, 1940.

Ryle, G., *The Concept of Mind*, London, 1949.

——, 'Categories', in *Logic and Language*, Series 2, ed. A. Flew, Oxford, 1955.

Sayward, C., 'A Defense of Sommers', *Philosophical Studies*, 29, 1976.

Sayward, C. and Voss, S., 'The Structure of Type Theory', *Journal of Philosophy*, 77, 1980.

Schönfinkel, M., 'On the Building Blocks of Mathematical Logic', in J. Van Heijenoort, ed., *From Frege to Gödel* 1967.

Searle, J. R., *Speech Acts*, London and New York, 1969.

——, ed., *The Philosophy of Language*, London, 1971.

Slater, B. H., 'A Fragment of a New Propositional Logic', *International Logic Review*, 9, 1978.

——, 'Singular Subjects', *Dialogue*, 18, 1979.

Sommers, F., 'The Ordinary Language Tree', *Mind*, 68, 1959.

——, 'Meaning Relations and the Analytic', *Journal of Philosophy*, 60, 1963.

——, 'Types and Ontology', *Philosophical Review*, 72, 1963. Reprinted in P. F. Strawson, ed., *Philosophical Logic*, Oxford, 1967.

——, 'Truth-functional Counterfactuals,' *Analysis Supplement*, 24, 1964.

——, 'A Program for Coherence', *Philosophical Review*, 73, 1964.

——, 'Truth-value Gaps: A reply to Mr. Odegard', *Analysis*, 25, 1965.

——, 'Predicability', in M. Black, ed., *Philosophy in America*, Ithaca, 1965.

——, 'Why Is There Something and Not Nothing', *Analysis*, 26, 1966.

——, 'Reply', in I. Lakatos, ed., *Problems in the Philosophy of Mathematics*, Amsterdam, 1967.

——, 'What We Can Say About God', *Judaism*, 15, 1966.

——, 'On a Fregean Dogma', in I. Lakatos, ed., *Problems in the Philosophy of Mathematics*, Amsterdam, 1967.

——, 'Do We Need Identity?' *Journal of Philosophy*, 66, 1969.

——, 'On Concepts of Truth in Natural Languages', *The Review of Metaphysics*, 23, 1969.

——, 'The Calculus of Terms', *Mind*, 79, 1970.

——, 'Confirmation and the Natural Subject', *Philosophical Forum*, 2, 1970–71.

——, 'Structural Ontology', *Philosophia*, 1, 1971.

——, 'Distribution Matters', *Mind*, 84, 1975.

——, 'Logical Syntax in Natural Language', *Issues in the Philosophy of Language*, eds. A. Mackay and D. Merrill (New Haven, 1976).

——, 'On Predication and Logical Syntax', in A. Kasher, ed., *Language in Focus*, Dordrecht, 1976.

——, 'Frege or Leibniz?' Studien Zu Frege III Logik und Semantic fromman-holzboog 44 Stuttgart-Bad Cannstatt 1976.

——, 'The Grammar of Thought', *Journal of Social and Biological Structures*, 1, 1978.

'Strawson, P. F., 'On Referring', *Mind*, LIX, 1950.

——, *Introduction to Logical Theory*, London, 1952.

——, *Individuals*, London, 1959.

——, *Logico-Linguistic Papers*, London, 1971.

——, *Subject and Predicate in Logic and Grammar*, London, 1974.

——, ed. *Philosophical Logic*, Oxford, 1967.

Tarski, A., 'The Concept of Truth in Formalized Languages', in J. H. Woodger, ed., *Logic, Semantics, Metamathematics*, London, 1956.

——, 'The Semantic Conception of Truth and the Foundations of Semantics', *Philosophy and Phenomenological Research*, IV, 1943–44.

Wald, J., 'Geach on Atomicity and Singular Propositions', *Notre Dame Journal of Formal Logic*, 20 1979.

Whorf, B. L., *Language, Thought and Reality*, ed. J. B. Carroll, New York, 1956.

Wiggins, D., *Identity and Spatio-Temporal Continuity*, Oxford, 1967.

Wittgenstein, L., *Tractatus Logico-Philosophicus*, trans. D. Pears and B. McGuinness, London, 1961.

——, *Philosophical Investigations*, ed. G. E. M. Anscombe, G. H. Von Wright and R. Rhees, Oxford, 1953.

Zabeeh, F., Klemke, E. D. and Jacobson, A., eds., *Readings in Semantics*, Urbana, Ill., 1974.

Ziff, P., *Semantic Analysis*, Ithaca, 1960.

Index